# Pain: Its Nature and Management

# Pain: Its Nature and Management

Edited by

**Veronica Nicky Thomas** BSc, PhD, DipN, RGN, CPsychol, DipCouns

*Department of Nursing Studies*
*King's College London, UK*

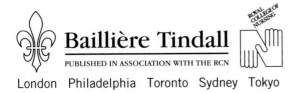

**Baillière Tindall**
PUBLISHED IN ASSOCIATION WITH THE RCN

London  Philadelphia  Toronto  Sydney  Tokyo

Baillière Tindall     24–28 Oval Road
London NW1 7DX, UK

The Curtis Center
Independence Square West
Philadelphia, PA 19106-3399, USA

Harcourt Brace & Company
55 Horner Avenue
Toronto, Ontario, M8Z 4X6, Canada

Harcourt Brace & Company, Australia
30–52 Smidmore Street
Marrickville
NSW 2204, Australia

Harcourt Brace & Company, Japan
Ichibancho Central Building
22-1 Ichibancho
Chiyoda-ku, Tokyo 102, Japan

© 1997 Baillière Tindall

This book is printed on acid-free paper

A catalogue record for this book is available from the British Library

ISBN 0-7020-2293-4

Typeset by Florencetype Ltd, Stoodleigh, Devon
Printed and bound in Great Britain by WBC Book Manufacturers, Bridgend,
Glamorgan

'To have great pain is to have certainty;
to hear that another person has pain is to have doubt'

Elaine Scarry, 1985

*The Body in Pain*

# Contents

# List of contributors

**Eloise Carr**
MSc BSc RGN PGCEA RNT
Senior Lecturer, Practice and Research
Institute of Health and Community
    Studies
Bournemouth University
Royal London House
Christchurch Road
Bournemouth BH1 3LT


**Chris Eccleston**
BSc PhD
Clinical Director
Pain Management Unit
Royal National Hospital for Rheumatic
    Diseases, and
Lecturer in Psychology
School of Social Sciences
University of Bath
Claverton Down
Bath BA2 7AY


**Dinah Gould**
BSc MPhil PhD RGN CertEd RNT
Senior Lecturer in Nursing Studies
Department of Nursing Studies
King's College London
Cornwall House
Waterloo Road
London SE1 8WA


**Margaret L Heath**
MB BS FRCA
Consultant Anaesthetist
Lewisham Hospital NHS Trust
High Street
Lewisham
London SE13 6LH

**Lindy King**
BN Dip AppSc (Nsg) RGN
Lecturer in Nursing Studies
Department of Nursing Studies
King's College London
Cornwall House
Waterloo Road
London SE1 8WA


**Noelle E Llewellyn**
SRN RSCN DPSN BA
Clinical Nurse Specialist – Pain Control
    Service
Great Ormond Street Hospital for
    Children NHS Trust
Department of Anaesthesia
Great Ormond Street
London WC1N 3JH


**Alison Richardson**
PhD MSc BN RGN PG DipEd RNT
Clinical Nurse Manager – Cancer
    Services
Bromley Hospitals NHS Trust
Farnborough Hospital
Farnborough Common
Orpington
Kent BR6 8NB


**Kate Seers**
BSc PhD RGN
Senior Research Fellow
Royal College of Nursing
    Institute
Radcliffe Infirmary
Woodstock Road
Oxford OX2 6HE

**Veronica (Nicky) J Thomas**
BSc PhD RGN DipN DipCouns
    CPsychol
Senior Research Fellow
Department of Nursing Studies
King's College London
Cornwall House
Waterloo Road
London SE1 8WA


**Janet M Walker**
PhD BSc RGN RM RHV CPsychol
Reader in Health Studies
King Alfred's College
Winchester
SO22 4NR

**Amanda C de C Williams**
BSc MSc PhD CPsychol
Senior Lecturer in Clinical Health
    Psychology
UMDS, University of London
INPUT Pain Management Unit
St Thomas' Hospital
London SE1 7EH

**Jenifer Wilson-Barnett**
PhD MSc BA SRN DipN RNT FRCN
    FKCL
Head of Department of Nursing
    Studies and Head of Nursing and
    Midwifery Division
King's College London
Cornwall House
Waterloo Road
London SE1 8WA

# Preface

This book is intended to encourage health care professionals to reflect the multidimensional nature of pain in their assessment, management and evaluation of patients' pain. The contributors to the book come from different disciplines – clinical nursing, nursing education, psychology, and sections of the medical profession currently involved in pain management. This variety is meant to reflect the fact that successful pain management requires the combined efforts of the multidisciplinary team and I hope that this will encourage recognition of each contribution to the delivery of care.

I have stressed the subjective nature of pain experience and the importance of involving the patient as an active participant in his/her care. Although I am essentially appealing to nurses in calling for reforms in care within this book, it is also of value to all health care professionals because the strategies can be translated to other disciplines. I have tried to present the information in a style that is user friendly but not too simplistic, since I wanted it to be of value to clinical practitioners, researchers and educationalists.

The coverage of pain conditions is selective, focusing on those which are known to be problematic and drawing heavily on research to inform strategic solutions. Inevitably the topics reflect our interests and biases, and the suggested solutions are by no means a panacea. The book is not a 'how-to-do-it' recipe book – rather the aim is promote a reflective, evidence-based approach to care that challenges routine non-critical methods. I invite the reflective health care practitioner to read this book with a healthy scepticism and constantly to have the following questions uppermost in his/her mind: What are the implications of these ideas for my practice? Will these ideas improve patient care within my practice?

This book is designed to help all those involved in pain management to question their practice, and hopefully to improve the standard of pain relief strategies within the hospital and the community.

V J Thomas

Veronica Nicky Thomas

# Important notice

Every effort has been made to check any drug dosages given in this book. However, as it is possible that dosage schedules have been revised, the reader is strongly urged to consult the drug companies' literature before administering any of the drugs listed.

# Introduction

During the last 30 years following the introduction and refinement of the Gate Control theory (Melzack and Wall, 1965), pain has been conceptualized as a multidimensional and highly subjective experience. Physiological, sensory, affective, cognitive, behavioural and sociocultural factors are combined to contribute to the overall subjectivity of the experience. In recent years there have been other numerous advances in our understanding of the mechanisms of pain and, with these advances, have come improvements in the control of acute and chronic pain. However, despite these advances, pain remains one of the most common symptoms in and outside of hospital.

Severe pain causes misery, which affects the quality of life; therefore its relief should be seen as an important objective which is relatively straight-forward. However, this activity is fraught with problems. Within hospital the provision of pain relief is seen essentially as the balancing of two distinct activities: the relief of pain and achieving the main objective. The main objective is concerned with carrying out procedures associated with treating specific diseases whilst the relief of pain is accorded a low priority.

## ■ PROFESSIONAL CURRICULUM ON PAIN

Professional bodies such as the International Association for the Study of Pain (IASP) have called for more commitment and vigilance from health care professionals to improve the current situation. They attribute the main difficulties to a lack of education among health professionals and a task force on professional education has developed a core curriculum for professional education on pain (IASP, 1991, 1995), which has been modified to reflect the nursing perspective (IASP, 1993). This professional curriculum emphasizes the need for an appreciation of the way in which physiological, pharmacological, psychological, cultural and social factors influence pain experience, and strongly recommends that professionals use this multidimensional framework in the assessment, intervention and evaluation of pain.

In this book the message we try to convey is that pain control can be seen as part of a general scheme of facilitating personal control in our patients, and that allowing patients to be involved in their care empowers them. The IASP professional pain curriculum is used to guide the contents in the following manner.

Chapter 1 presents a description of the basic anatomy and physiology of pain, pain pathways and the neurochemistry of pain. The physiological differences between acute and chronic pain are discussed and, within Chapter 13, the physiological disturbances that occur in cancer and give rise to pain are described. Pain modulation is also dealt with in Chapter 1 and we use the Gate Control theory as a primary vehicle for demonstrating the brain regions involved in modulation, nociceptive transmission, their interconnections and spinal projections. The Gate Control theory also allows us to acknowledge the elaborate interaction between physiology and psychological processes in contributing to the pain experience.

In Chapter 2, we follow on by describing the ways in which psychosocial and cultural variables account for individual differences in the experience of pain. However, this is prefaced by a strong reminder to health professionals that pain exists whenever the experiencing person says it does, and we urge them always to undertake individual assessment of patients' pain and to individualize pain relief according to their patient's needs. In this chapter it is suggested that knowledge of psychosocial and cultural influence is double-edged, and professionals should be careful not to use this information to label and stereotype their patients' main responses.

Cognitive psychology has in recent years contributed enormously to our understanding of ways in which information processing and styles of thinking influence pain perception and response. In Chapter 3, we acknowledge this contribution by presenting the psychology involved in pain and thinking. This chapter makes explicit the downward inhibitory mechanism identified in the Gate Control theory by focusing on the central role of thinking, which is presented in the context of normal psychology rather than the abnormal. The intention here as it is throughout the book, is to focus on the processes and variables that are more likely to lead to successful strategies and effective pain relief interventions. The chapter provides extensive coverage of cognitive processes involved in acute and chronic pain by drawing on recent research.

As stated above, the provision of effective pain relief is fraught with difficulties and remains largely inadequate, therefore Chapter 4 considers the ethical issues and dilemmas surrounding pain management. In this chapter we use the principles of autonomy, beneficence, non-maleficence, justice, accountability and responsibility to highlight the deficiencies and make suggestions for solutions. Variables are identified on both the patients' and the professionals' perspectives as potential barriers to ethical decision making, and we encourage professionals to enter into partnerships with their patients in order to achieve effective solutions.

Chapter 5 presents an overview of pain assessment tools. In this chapter there is an emphasis on assessment tools that seek to reflect the multidimensional nature of pain. There is a discussion of a range of pain scales used in managing pain in children as well as adults and some of the strategies that can be employed when assessing pain in patients from different cultures.

The rest of the book is concerned with current pharmacological and psychological pain management strategies, and some types of clinical pain that are known to give rise to problematic issues in their management. In applying psychosocial theory and research to pain management, this book endeavours to enhance the education of health care professionals in caring for patients with pain.

## ■ EVIDENCE-BASED PRACTICE IN PAIN MANAGEMENT

This book draws very heavily on research evidence from the fields of physiology, psychology and nursing. We make no apologies for this because we are seeking to help nurses and other health care professionals bridge the gap between theory and practice. This is considered to be very important because, although much has been written about pain mechanisms, little has been applied to clinical practice and, in the current 'climate' of clinical effectiveness, any book on pain experience has a responsibility to ensure that health care professionals have access to up-to-date research with which to inform patient care. According to Sackett et al. (1996), 'the practice of evidence-based health care means integrating individual clinical expertise with the best external, clinical evidence from systematic research'. However, even good research evidence may be unsuitable for particular patient groups and pain conditions.

Chapter 7 reveals research findings which highlight the importance of psychological interventions such as cognitive behaviour therapy for the management of chronic non-malignant pain. In applying this model to manage pain in sickle cell disease, we attempt to provide examples of how to transfer models across pain conditions. The community-based focus of the interventions described in Chapters 11, 13 and 14 highlight the importance of transferring exemplars of good practice across settings in order to respond to the expressed Department of Health policy initiative to move care away from the hospital and into the community.

The final chapter (Chapter 15) presents findings which suggest that simply learning about pain is not sufficient to guarantee improvement in pain management. Rather it seems that nurses who use a reflective appproach that includes a synthesis of theoretical and experiential knowledge are more able to make accurate clinical decisions resulting in the provision of effective pain relief. Therefore, recognition of the changing ability of nurses and other health care professionals to make clinical judgements in relation to their level of knowledge, skills and expertise appears to be vital for effective teaching in both clinical and educational settings.

## ■ REFERENCES

**International Association for the Study of Pain** (1991) Core curriculum for professional education in pain. IASP, Seattle.

**International Association for the Study of Pain** (1993) Newsletter, September–October. Technical corner: pain curriculum for basic nurse education. Edited by C.B. Berde, pp. 4–6.

**International Association for the Study of Pain** (1995) Core curriculum for professional education in pain, 2nd edn. IASP, Seattle.

**Melzack, R. & Wall, P.D.** (1965) Pain mechanisms: a new theory. *Science* **150**, 971–979.

**Sackett, D.L., Rosenberg, W.M., Gray, J.A., Haynes, R.B. & Richardson, W.S.** (1996) Evidence-based medicine: what it is and what it isn't (Editorial) *British Medical Journal* **312**, 71–72.

# Pain mechanisms: The neurophysiology and neuropsychology of pain perception

The purpose of this chapter is to discuss different types of pain, to describe the physiological mechanisms which result in its manifestation and to provide an account of the main theories of pain.

## ■ NEUROANATOMY

An understanding of the anatomy and physiology of the nervous system is central to understanding the physiology of pain. The nervous system receives sensory input from the external and internal environment of the body, processes the data it receives and initiates an appropriate response, e.g. moving muscles in the fingers so that a hot object is dropped (Brooker, 1993). The two major components of the nervous system are the central nervous system (CNS) and the peripheral nervous system (PNS).

*The central nervous system* consists of the brain and spinal cord. Its function is to receive and process information.

*The peripheral nervous system* consists of 12 pairs of cranial nerves arising from the brain and 31 pairs of nerves arising from the spinal cord. It can be divided into two functional parts: the sensory division and the motor division. The sensory division consists of afferent nerves which carry sensory data, including the awareness of pain, from receptors in the skin, muscles, joints and internal organs to the CNS. The motor division consists of efferent nerves which carry nervous impulses from the CNS to the rest of the body. Voluntary efferent nerves serve the musculoskeletal system which can be moved consciously. The autonomic nervous system supplies the glands, blood vessels, the gastrointestinal and respiratory systems, and other internal organs, which are not under voluntary control.

### ▪ Neurones

Nervous tissue consists of excitable cells called neurones. Neurones are complex, highly differentiated cells, which are very sensitive to changes within the environment. Each neurone consists of three fundamental structural units: an axon, the soma or cell body, and a number of highly branching dendrites (Fig. 1.1). Information is received by the dendrites. The cell body is responsible for organizing this information and the axon transmits it to other parts of the nervous system.

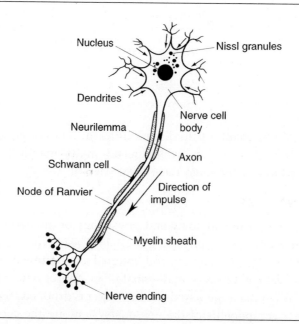

*Figure 1.1. The structure of a typical neurone.*

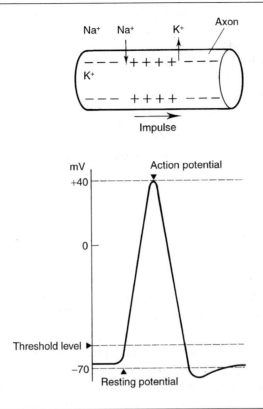

*Figure 1.2. Transmission of a nervous pulse.*

## ■ The nervous impulse

The nervous impulse (action potential) is a change in electrical charge across a cell membrane, occurring when a neurone transmits information or a muscle contracts (Dolphin, 1983). The nervous impulse is generated at the juncture of the axon and cell body, a point known as the axon hillock. As it travels along the neurone, sodium ions move into the axon while potassium ions move from within the axon out into the surrounding extracellular space (Catton, 1970). The portion of the neurone which has just been stimulated then repolarizes and enters a refractory (inactive) period as the ions return to their original location (Fig. 1.2).

The speed at which the nervous impulse travels is determined by two factors: the diameter of the axon and the presence of myelin. Larger nerves which have a greater diameter, transmit impulses more swiftly than smaller nerves. The presence of myelin also increases the speed of transmission. Myelin is a white, fatty substance covering the axons of the larger neurones. Its function is to provide insulation, preventing leakage of the electrical charge generated by the action potential: it is analogous to the plastic covering around an electrical wire. The action potential travels more rapidly along myelinated neurones, at a speed of up to 130 metres per second, leaping from one node of Ranvier to the next (see Fig. 1.1), a phenomenon called saltatory conduction.

### ■ Synapses and neurotransmitters

A synapse is a gap or junction between two neurones, or between a neurone and a muscle or a gland (Fig. 1.3). A typical synapse between two neurones consists of:

- A pre-synaptic neurone with a terminal knob containing vesicles filled with a chemical neurotransmitter substance.
- A post-synaptic neurone with a membrane containing sites for the specific neurotransmitter produced by the pre-synaptic neurone.
- A narrow cleft between the two neurones.

When the nervous impulse reaches the terminal knob of the axon of the pre-synaptic neurone, a neurotransmitter is released from the vesicles and diffuses across the gap, then attaches to the receptor sites on the membrane of the post-synaptic neurone. Neurotransmitters either have an excitatory effect or an inhibitory effect. If the neurotransmitter is excitatory, the action potential is transmitted to the next neurone, allowing the passage of the nervous impulse. If its effect is inhibitory, no action potential is generated and the nervous impulse does not travel further (Bisby, 1976). A number of neurotransmitters have been discovered. Chemically, they fall into three groups:

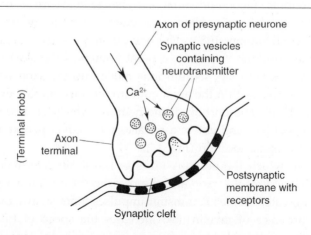

Axon of presynaptic neurone

Synaptic vesicles containing neurotransmitter

$Ca^{2+}$

(Terminal knob)

Axon terminal

Postsynaptic membrane with receptors

Synaptic cleft

*Figure 1.3. A synapse.*

- Monoamines
- Amino acids
- Neuropeptides

Some neurotransmitters have other functions in addition to their role in transmission of the nervous impulse and are known to be important in the physiology of pain.

Once the action potential has been passed between adjacent neurones across a synapse, further action of the neurotransmitter is blocked by the release of an enzyme. Any individual neurone interacts with many others so that it is continually receiving large numbers of stimuli, some excitatory, others inhibitory, all at the same time. The system is therefore highly complex.

## ■ PSYCHOLOGICAL THEORIES OF PAIN

Theories of pain have undergone evolutionary changes and, as a direct result of experimental and psychological evidence, it now seems that any plausible theory must take the following two things into account.

1. There is a specific anatomical pain pathway, and
2. This pathway does not operate in a simple push-button manner.

There have been four main theories put forward over the centuries to explain the experience of pain. These are Affect theory, Specificity theory, Pattern theory and the Gate Control theory.

### ■ Affect theory

The Affect theory dates back to Aristotelian times and considers pain to be an affect, distinct from the five senses. Pain in this analysis has an emotional quality rather like sadness, and colours all sensory events (Marshall, 1894). This theory is clearly inadequate in its explanation of pain experience. However, it introduces an important yet hitherto neglected element: the affective quality. Some researchers have tended to view the emotional aspect of pain as secondary to the sensory element (Hardy et al., 1952; Beecher, 1959), whilst other perspectives characterize the affective qualities as the most distinguished component of the experience (Melzack and Wall, 1965; Melzack and Casey, 1968).

### ■ Specificity theory

Specificity theory was first espoused by von Frey (1985), who suggested that pain experience is caused by a painful stimulus exciting specific nerve endings, from which information is carried via a specific pathway to the pain centre in the brain. The facts regarding physiological specialization make an important contribution in sensory physiology. However, the psychological assumption of this theory is undermined because the physiological and psychological evidence fail to support its conception of a simple one-to-one relationship between the extent of pain and the intensity of the stimulus.

### ▪ Pattern theory

The Pattern theory, which was proposed by Weddel (1962), states that there is no separate system for perceiving pain, rather that pain is due to intense peripheral stimulation of non-specific receptors. This in turn produces a pattern of nerve impulses, which is interpreted centrally as pain. Strong and mild stimuli produce different patterns; consequently, being hit hard is interpreted as painful whilst being touched is not. There are many difficulties with this theory but the most obvious stems from its requirement that there must be an intense stimulus to trigger pain. Thus it cannot account for allodynia, the fact that innocuous stimuli such as a gentle touch can trigger episodes of neuralgia.

### ▪ The Gate Control theory

The Gate Control theory (Melzack and Wall, 1965) is currently the most important pain theory. This theory has greatly enriched our understanding of pain mechanisms and takes account of both the physiological and psychological dimensions of pain. It also represents an attempt to integrate a number of aspects of the previous theories described above. The Gate Control theory

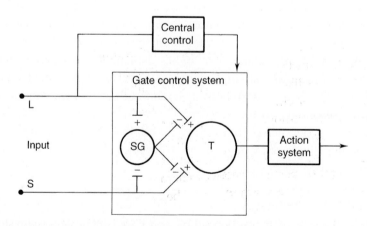

**Figure 1.4.** Diagram of the Gate Control concept (adapted from Melzack and Wall, 1965).

proposes that the complex, subjective experience of pain results from a pattern of neural activity within the brain (Melzack and Wall, 1965). The activity is initiated when nerve impulses conveying painful information arrive from the periphery via the ascending pathways of the spinal cord. Melzack and Wall propose that there is a neural mechanism in the dorsal horn of the spinal cord, which acts as a gating mechanism through which peripheral information passes. The gating mechanism consists of two types of neurones: cells in the substantia gelatinosa (SG cell) and transmission cell or T cell. Transmission of information about pain is achieved by activation of the T cell, whilst the SG cell inhibits activity (see Fig. 1.4). These cells are influenced both by myelinated and unmyelinated fibres. Small unmyelinated fibres facilitate pain, whilst the larger myelinated fibres inhibit pain. The T cell is influenced by the descending impulses from the brain, in other words, the state of mind. Therefore if the person is relaxed, descending impulses from the dorsolateral funiculus activate the SG cell and inhibit T cell activity. On the other hand, when the person is very anxious, impulses travel from the limbic system and activate the T cell, thereby increasing the perception of pain.

In simple terms, injury results in the stimulation of receptors. The amount of stimulation passing through the gate and hence the amount of stimulation which may give rise to pain is dependent upon the relative amounts of activity in A beta, large-diameter and small-diameter A delta and C fibres, and also upon descending influences from the brain. When the amount of information passing through the gate reaches a critical level, it activates the neural areas responsible for pain experience and response.

The descending control influences may be exerted through the following systems.

### Reticular projections

The brainstem reticular formation exerts a powerful inhibitory control over information projected by the spinal gate. This reticular inhibitory projection is also influenced by somatic input as well as input from the visual and auditory systems.

### Cortical projections

Fibres from the cortex, particularly the frontal cortex (which subserves cognitive processes such as past experience), project to the reticular formation, and influence the gate control system. Cognitive processes can also influence the spinal gate mechanism by means of large fast-conducting, corticospinal (pyramidal) fibres and directly modulate pain experience (see Chapter 3 for a detailed discussion of the important role of thinking in the perception and experience of pain). Some central activities, such as anxiety or excitement, may open or close the gate from all inputs and any part of the body, while others involve selective localized action. Melzack and Wall (1965) propose that there is a central mechanism called a central control trigger, which activates the particular selective brain processes, such as memories, past experiences and response strategies. These can then be used to influence information, which is still being transmitted via more slowly conducting pathways. These psychological processes have an extremely important role in pain perception and research has shown that psychological factors such as helplessness (Seligman and Maier, 1967; Thornton and Jacobs, 1971), anxiety (Johnston, 1980; Thomas et al., 1990), neuroticism (Taenzer et al., 1986; Thomas et al., 1990, 1995) and culture (Thomas and Rose, 1991) can intensify the pain experienced. Conversely inter-ventions that reduce anxiety (Hayward, 1975; Johnson et al., 1978; Ridgeway and Mathews, 1982; Johnson, 1983), helplessness and enhance personal control (Miller and Mangan, 1983; Thomas et al., 1995) can reduce the degree of pain experience and enhance coping.

Pain can be regarded as having three psychological components, the sensory–discriminative, the motivational–affective and the cognitive–evaluative.

### Sensory–discriminative component

This allows the injury to be identified in time and space, and its exact extent determined. In addition to transmission of nociceptive stimuli, this component requires large fibre transmission of touch, and other non-nociceptive stimuli to enable the source, site and severity of the pain to be identified. This component is subserved by the rapidly conducting projection systems of the spinothalamic tract (Willis, 1984; Dostrosvsky, 1993). The ventrobasal complex area of the thalamus (Chandler, 1992; Bushnell et al., 1993) and the lateral thalamus (Dostrosvsky, 1993) are also involved in the sensory–discriminative aspects of pain.

### Motivational–affective component

This component produces somatic and autonomic activity, which results in various protective processes, such as movement away from the source of injury, immobilization of damaged tissue or preparation for flight. The neural areas of reticular formation and the limbic system are involved in the motivational–affective features of pain (Melzack and Casey, 1968; Bowsher, 1976). In addition, the medial thalamus, in particular, the centre median and the parafascicular nuclei, have important roles in mediating the motivational–affective aspects of pain (Willis, 1985; Dostrosvsky, 1993).

### Cognitive–evaluative component

This is a complex component in which response to the painful stimulus is influenced by cultural values, anxiety, attention and many other factors. These activities, which are subserved partly by cortical processes, may affect the sensory–discriminative or the motivational–affective dimension. Thus, excitement in war appears to block both these dimensions of pain, while suggestion and placebo may modulate the motivational–affective component and leave the sensory–discriminative relatively undisturbed (Melzack and Dennis, 1978).

Thus the Gate Control theory provides the conceptual framework for the integration of three distinct psychological dimensions of pain experience. These are the sensory–discriminative, the motivational–affective and the cognitive–evaluative dimensions, respectively.

The first is associated with rapidly conducting spinal systems projecting to the thalamus, the second with the reticular systems and limbic structures, and the third with neocortical processes. Approaches to pain control can therefore be seen as not only directed towards the sensory component, but also towards the motivational and cognitive elements. One of the most obvious predictions of the Gate Control theory was that stimulation of large-diameter fibres would inhibit pain. The practical implication of this is that increasing large-diameter fibre input to the spinal cord with vibration, acupuncture and electric stimulation could inhibit upward transmission of pain impulses. The theory states that pain can on the one hand be controlled by blocking the transmission of impulses through S fibres, which facilitates transmission (opening the gate), or by blocking the activation of the action system by output of the T cells. On the other hand, pain can be controlled by facilitating the inhibiting mechanism (closing the gate). Indeed the theory has been responsible for the introduction of transcutaneous electrical nerve stimulation (TENS) as a method of pain relief. TENS provides a continuous low-intensity electrical current, which stimulates large fibres and causes inhibition of nociceptive cells (closing the gate) (Wall and Sweet, 1967). Simultaneously, TENS is thought to stimulate the production of endorphin, an endogenous opioid. It is now most commonly used for the management of chronic pain, and increasingly with acute postoperative pain (Tyler et al., 1982) and pain during childbirth (Augustinsson et al., 1977).

Although the Gate Control theory has undergone considerable revision and extension since it was first proposed in 1965 (Nathan, 1976; Melzack and Dennis, 1978; Wall, 1978; Melzack and Wall, 1988; Melzack, 1990), the function, location of the dorsal horn and the descending control remain conceptually the same. The activity of the endogenous opioid system, which alters synaptic transmissions, can also be conceptualized as a type of chemical gating mechanism (Bridgeman, 1988) and is accounted for within the framework of the Gate Control theory (Melzack and Wall, 1988). This chemical 'gate' is also thought to be extensive throughout the nervous system and very effective in reducing pain (Yaksh and Rudy, 1978; Terenius, 1984).

# ■ TYPES OF PAIN

Clinically pain can be classified as acute or chronic pain.

## ■ Acute pain

There are two major manifestations of acute pain – superficial and deeper.

*Superficial acute pain* is usually described as sharp or prickling. Despite its name, it may be severe enough to cause the victim to exclaim aloud, although it is generally of short duration (seconds). The term superficial refers to the location of the pain on the surface of the body rather than the degree of pain experienced. It is possible for the individual to locate the source of this type of pain sensation accurately on the skin or mucous membranes. Sustaining a sharp cut or sipping unexpectedly hot liquid will result in superficial acute pain.

*Deeper acute pain* usually presents as a burning or aching sensation. It originates from the deeper layers of the skin, membranes, muscles, joints or serous membranes, but in most cases the victim is unable to determine its origin precisely, although it tends to be more persistent than superficial acute pain. Deeper acute pain is indicative of tissue destruction.

It is possible to experience both superficial acute and deep acute pain rapidly in succession as responses to the same injury. Burns and scalds, for example, initially result in acute pain, which may be excruciating. This is superseded by a burning or gnawing sensation, which will persist for hours or days, depending on the extent of the damage and the amount of skin and underlying tissue lost.

## ■ Chronic pain

Chronic pain originates from the internal organs. It is usually described as a dull ache or a sensation of pressure, which may be similar to, or indistinguishable from, deep acute pain. It is often very severe, for example, the pain associated with bony metastases in the cancer patient.

# ■ THE PHYSIOLOGY OF PAIN

The physiology of pain can be divided into three steps:

1. Detection by receptors called nociceptors.
2. Transmission of a nervous impulse up the spinal cord to the brain.
3. Perception of pain.

Detection appears to be influenced by the nature of the damage causing the pain to be experienced, so detection of each of the types of pain will be discussed separately.

## ∎ The detection of pain

### Superficial acute pain

Superficial acute pain is generated when the skin or mucous membranes are damaged. The skin is sensitive to touch, temperature, pressure and pain. Each different stimulus is detected by specific receptors called nociceptors (Campbell, 1995). These are the free ends (dendrites) of sensory (afferent) neurones. There are two types of nociceptors:

- Mechano-nociceptors, which detect heavy pressure and pinching.
- Polymodal nociceptors, which respond to a wide range of painful stimuli, e.g. extremes of temperature and noxious chemicals.

Damaged skin and mucous membranes generate pain through inflammation. Damaged tissue releases several chemicals, including prostaglandins, histamine, serotonin and bradykinin, which increase the sensitivity of the nociceptors (Lakhani et al., 1993). The severity of superficial acute pain is influenced by the distribution of nociceptors and by the frequency with which nervous impulses are generated by them. Nociceptors are present in large numbers on the face, especially the lips and tongue, and on the hands, particularly the fingers, so pain is experienced more often from these regions. Nociceptors are scattered in smaller numbers over the trunk, including the back, where pain is less likely to be detected and is more difficult for the individual to localize. The intensity of the harmful stimulus influences the frequency of the pain stimulus. Thus severe heat or cold will be perceived as more painful than mild heat or cold.

### Deeper acute pain

Deeper acute pain is usually classified according to its cause:

- Ischaemia. This occurs when the metabolic demands of the tissues are greater than their blood supply, resulting in the production of lactic acid, which produces cramping pain. Patients usually describe ischaemic pain as sharp, continuous, grinding or heavy, e.g. myocardial infarction.
- Spasm occurs in hollow organs, e.g. the bile duct, colon, small bowel or ureter, giving rise to colicky pain, which is usually severe. Renal colic and cholecystitis are classic examples.
- Irritation of serous membranes, e.g. the pleurae, peritoneum or meninges, results in severe pain, which is worse when the patient moves. A patient with pleuritis will thus avoid taking deep inspirations or coughing. 'Guarding'

is the medical term used to describe the patient's reaction to the inflamed membranes. The neck stiffness typical of meningitis occurs because adjacent muscle groups contract to protect the inflamed membranes. Palpation of the abdomen of a patient with peritonitis will result in guarding as the abdominal muscles contract to protect the inflamed area. Rebound pain is experienced when pressure on an inflamed membrane is suddenly released during a medical examination. Both guarding and rebound pain are important diagnostic signs.

## ■ THE TRANSMISSION OF PAIN

### ▮ Superficial acute pain

A delta axons are associated with the transmission of the sharp, localized sensation typical of superficial acute pain. They are myelinated and transmit pain impulses rapidly (Jackson, 1995). The axons of nociceptive neurones serving the same area of skin converge to form spinal nerves, which enter the spinal cord via the dorsal horn (Fig. 1.5). The cell bodies of these neurones lie in the dorsal root ganglia. Nervous impulses travel along the axons of these nociceptor neurones into the dorsal horn and it is here that the gate control mechanism is thought to operate (see Fig. 1.5). The impulse then travels from the dorsal horn to the anterior horn of the spinal cord, then ascends to the brain via the spinothalamic tracts.

### ▮ Deeper acute pain

As with superficial acute pain, the impulse is carried from the site of origin along sensory neurones to the dorsal horn of the spinal cord. Pain from an

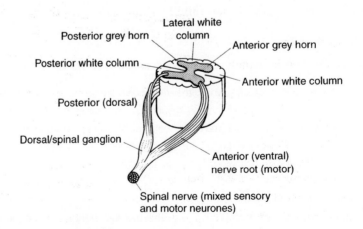

*Figure 1.5. The dorsal horn.*

internal organ or membrane may be experienced at some other location, a phenomenon known as referred pain. There are two explanations for this:

- The site where the pain originated may share the same common ascending nervous pathways as the site where the pain is perceived to occur.
- The site where the pain originated may share the same embryological origins as the site where the pain is perceived to occur. During development some tissues migrate to the position they eventually occupy, but retain their early sensory connections.

Myocardial infarction and angina are typical examples of referred pain. In both cases the pain radiates along the left arm, because tissue damage in the myocardium culminates in pain impulses which enter the spinal cord in the region of the upper thorax (spinal nerve roots T1–T4). These also receive impulses from the left side of the chest and arm. Thus the brain, which ultimately receives all nervous impulses in connection with pain, interprets the left arm as the source. Similarly, pain from the bladder may be perceived in the skin over the suprapubic region, while pain originating in the lung and diaphragm may be experienced around the root of the neck.

## ▪ Chronic pain

With this dull, poorly localized pain, nervous impulses travel slowly along unmyelinated C axons at a speed of 0.4–1 metres per second from the origin of the pain to the brain via the dorsal horn (Jackson, 1995).

## ▪ THE PERCEPTION OF PAIN

All neurones transmitting pain eventually synapse in the thalamus of the brain. Nervous pathways run from the thalamus to the sensory cortex. Here knowledge, memory of previous pain experience and cultural influences exert their effects on the perception of pain. Axons in the spinothalamic tracts also synapse with the medulla, hypothalamus and the limbic system before reaching the thalamus.

This pathway is important in determining the individual's emotional reaction to the pain. The medulla probably helps to initiate the response of the autonomic nervous system to painful stimuli, for example, the initiation of nervous impulses resulting in muscular contraction so that movement occurs away from the source of pain.

## ▪ The endogenous opiates

The endogenous opiates are neuropeptides that have analgesic properties, first isolated during research with morphine (Hughes et al., 1975). It became apparent that the pharmacological effect of morphine was produced when it became attached to receptors on the membrane of the neurone. As morphine is not present under normal circumstances, the pre-existence of receptors to which it could become attached implied that the body must already produce some naturally occurring chemical with a similar structure.

This eventually led to the discovery of the natural opiates – enkephalins and endorphins. The endogenous opiates modify pain transmission rather than alter pain perception or tolerance, and inhibit prostaglandin synthesis during the inflammatory response.

*Endorphins* are present in the anterior pituitary gland, which is the site of manufacture (Goldstein, 1978). Their function is to inhibit pain by blocking the release of Substance P (see below), but they may also play a role in temperature control, memory and learning, and have links with depressive conditions and schizophrenia.

*Enkephalins* are manufactured by neurones in the posterior pituitary gland (Hong et al., 1977), but are distributed throughout the thalamus, the hypo-thalamus, the limbic system and areas of the spinal cord which transmit pain impulses (Friederickson and Geary, 1982). They suppress pain by inhibiting the action of Substance P. In the medulla they intercept pain impulses travelling through the cortex, while in the spinal cord they exert an effect by activating inhibitory synapses.

Enkephalins appear to be most active when pain is present. At other times they are present in low quantities, indicating that their main function is probably the regulation of pain transmission rather than pain perception or tolerance. Levels of enkephalins in the blood rise during exercise, labour, delivery and when morphine is taken. However, levels decline if morphine is taken by the same individual for a long time. This helps to explain why patients in pain who receive morphine over a long period of time gradu-ally increase their tolerance and require a larger dose.

It has been suggested that the analgesic effect of acupuncture may be produced by stimulating the production of the natural opiates. It is also thought that they may play a role in the placebo effect: possibly the expec-tation that pain relief may be available could trigger the release of natural opiates.

*Substance P* is a neuropeptide which has been isolated from sensory neurones, the spinal cord and from all parts of the brain known to play a role in pain perception. Its function appears to be the transmission of pain from detectors into the central nervous system.

## ■ THE EFFECTS OF PAIN

### ı Acute pain

Acute pain evokes the stress response mediated through the action of the sympathetic nervous system and hormonal changes:

- Adrenalin is released from the adrenal medulla. This hormone complements the action of the sympathetic nervous system by acting directly on the blood vessels in the skin to cause vasoconstriction, so the patient appears pale. Blood is redirected to the brain, skeletal muscles and kidneys. The heart beats faster, cardiac output increases and blood pressure rises. Adrenalin has a direct effect on the nervous system, increasing arousal and consciousness, and heightening the emotional reaction to events. Vasodilation occurs and the respiratory rate is heightened.

- Antidiuretic hormone (ADH) is released by the posterior pituitary gland, causing water to be reabsorbed by the renal tubules and retained in the body's extracellular fluid compartment.

- Aldosterone released from the adrenal cortex increases the reabsorption of sodium and chloride ions by the renal tubules.

The patient in pain thus looks pale and frightened, has a rapid pulse and respiratory rate, feels anxious and is restless.

## ■ Chronic pain

The patient in chronic pain is less likely to exhibit the manifestations of the acute stress response, but will still be anxious. Other psychological reactions may include depression or resignation, if the pain has not been well controlled. The longer term manifestations of stress are likely to be apparent. These include the increased release of the glucocorticoid hormone cortisol from the adrenal cortex. Cortisol alters the metabolism of carbohydrates, fats and proteins, increasing the amount of carbohydrate available to the body, but depresses the immune response and slows wound healing.

## ■ THE PURPOSE OF PAIN

Acute pain has a protective function, warning the individual of damage and provoking movement away from the harmful stimulus, e.g. dropping a hot object and recoiling after stepping on something sharp. This is clearly illustrated in the case studies presented by Melzack and Wall in their book *The Challenge of Pain* (1982), which describes how the lives and safety of people are severely compromised if they cannot appreciate pain and do not recognize harmful stimuli which need to be avoided. However, the benefit of chronic pain is obscure. The pain resulting from osteoarthritis or from bony metastases is experienced once damage is underway and, in any case, the stimulus cannot be avoided in the same way as an environmental stimulus.

## ■ SUMMARY

In this chapter we have tried to explain the complexity of pain perception as simply as is possible, suggesting that pain perception occurs through an 'action system'. Nociception is limited to A delta and C fibres sending off impulses in these small fibres in the spinal cord. The central endings of afferent fibres terminate in the dorsal horn of the spinal cord, especially in the region of the substansia gelatinosa. Large-diameter afferent fibres ascending in the posterior column give off collaterals which enter the substansia gelatinosa medially and have important inhibitory functions. We have outlined the differences in physiology between acute and chronic, and superficial and deep pain.

Other information in addition to nociception is transmitted by the rapidly and slowly conducting spinothalamic systems, and is responsible for the discriminatory, motivational and emotional aspects of pain. The sensory discriminative dimension is influenced by the rapidly conducting spinal systems and the motivational drive is influenced by activities in the reticular and limbic structures, which are influenced primarily by the slow conducting spinal systems. Neocortical processes, which subserve information concerning past experiences, exert control over both discriminatory and motivational systems. Alogenic substances, such as bradykinin, serotonin, and prostaglandins that occur naturally in the environment of nociceptors, intensify pain by sensitizing nociceptive nerve endings. Inhibition of pain in the spinal cord is also achieved by large diameter fibres.

Melzack and Wall (1965) postulated that simultaneous activity in the adjacent large fibres could modulate small-fibre transmission by activating inhibitory cells in the substansia gelatinosa of the spinal cord. This mechanism is described as a gate. Central control systems in the brain further modulate pain by means of corticofugal fibres that carry information from the brain to the spinal cord to inhibit pain transmission (Melzack and Dennis, 1978). The descending raphe-spinal tract is another inhibitory mechanism and the fibres of this tract are serotoninergic, have an inhibitory effect on dorsal horn activity, and can be activated by opiates and electrical stimulation. Opiates act on specific and localized 'opiate receptors' situated in the central nervous system. These are normally acted upon by naturally occurring polypeptides, endorphins and enkephalins which exhibit analgesic properties similar to those of morphine.

# ■ REFERENCES

**Augustinsson, L.E., Bohlin, P., Bundsen, P., Carlsson, C.A., Forssman, L., Sjoberg, P. & Tyreman, N.O.** (1977) Pain relief during transcutaneous electrical nerve stimulation. *Pain* **4**, 59–65.

**Beecher, H.K.** (1959) *Measurement of Subjective Responses: Quantitative Effects of Drugs.* Oxford University Press, New York.

**Bisby, M.A.** (1976) Axonal transport. *General Pharmacology* **7**, 387–393.

**Bowsher, D.** (1976) Role of the reticular formation in response to noxious stimulation. *Pain* **2**, 361–378.

**Bridgeman, B.** (1988) *The Biology of Behaviour and Mind.* Wiley, New York.

**Brooker, C.** (1993) *Human Structure and Function.* Mosby, London.

**Bushnell, M.C., Duncan, G.H. & Tremblay, N.** (1993) Thalamic VPM nucleus in the behaving monkey: multimodal and discriminative properties of thermosensitive neurons. *Journal of Neurophysiology* **69**, 739–752.

**Campbell, J.** (1995) Making sense of pain management. *Nursing Times* **91**(27), 34–35.

**Catton, W.T.** (1970) Mechanoreceptor function. *Physiological Review* **50**, 35–56.

**Chandler, M.J., Hobbs, S.F., Fu, Q.G., Kenshalo, D.R., Jr, Blair, R.W. & Foreman, R.D.** (1992) Responses of neurons in the ventroposterolateral nucleus of primate thalamus to urinary bladder distension. *Brain Research* **571**, 26–34.

**Dolphin, N.W.** (1983) Neuroanatomy and neurophysiology of pain: nursing implications. *International Journal of Nursing Studies* **20**, 255–263.

**Dostrosvsky, J.O.** (1993) Ascending pathways, thalmus, cortex. In: *International Association for the Study of Pain Refresher Course Syllabus.* IASP Publications, Seattle, pp. 7–11.

**Frederickson, R. & Geary, L.E.** (1982) Endogenous opioid peptides, review of physiological, pharmacological and clinical aspects. *Programmes in Neurobiology* **19**, 19–69.

**Frey, M. von** (1895) Beiträge zur Sinnesphysiologie der Haut. *Ber. D. Kgl. Sachs. Ges.d. Wiss, Math-Phys.* Kl **47**, 166–184.

**Goldstein, A.** (1978) Endorphins. *Science* **18**, 14–19.

**Hardy, J., Wolff, H. & Goodell, H.** (1952) *Pain Sensations and Reactions.* Williams and Wilkie, Baltimore.

**Hayward, J.** (1975) *Information: A Prescription against Pain.* The Study of Nursing Care Project Report Series 2, no. 5. Royal College of Nursing, London.

**Hong, J., Yang, H. & Fratta, W.** (1977) Determination of methionine enkephalin in discrete regions of rat brain. *Brain Research* **134**, 383–386.

**Hughes, J., Smith, T.W., Kosterlitz, H.W. & Fothergill, L.A.** (1975) Identi-fication of two related peptides from the brain with potent agonist activity. *Nature* **258**, 577–579.

**Jackson, A.** (1995) Acute pain: its physiology and the pharmacology of analgesia. *Nursing Times* **91** (16), 27–28.

**Johnson, J.E.** (1983) Preparing patients to cope with stress. In: Wilson-Barnett, J. (ed.) *Patient Teaching.* Recent Advances in Nursing Series, Vol. 6. Churchill Livingstone, Edinburgh, pp. 231–237.

**Johnson, J.E., Rice, V.H., Fuller, S.S. & Endress, M.P.** (1978) Sensory information, instruction in coping strategy and recovery from surgery. *Research in Nursing and Health* **1**, 4–7.

**Johnston, M.** (1980) Anxiety in surgical patients. *Psychological Medicine* **10**, 145–152.

**Lakhani, S.R., Dilly, S.A. & Finlayson, C.J.** (1993) *Basic Pathology.* Edward Arnold, London.

**Marshall, H.R.** (1894) *Pain, Pleasure, and Aesthetics.* Macmillan, London.

**Melzack, R.** (1990) The tragedy of needless pain. *Scientific American* **262**, 27–33.

**Melzack, R. & Casey, K.L.** (1968) Sensory, motivational and central control determinants of pain. In: Kenshalo, D.L. (ed.) *The Skin Senses.* Charles C. Thomas, Springfield, IL, pp. 423–439.

**Melzack, R. & Dennis, S.G.** (1978). Neurophysiological foundations of pain. In: Sternbach, R.A. (ed.) *The Psychology of Pain.* Raven Press, New York, pp. 1–25.

**Melzack, R. & Wall, P.D.** (1965) Pain mechanisms: a new theory. *Science* **150**, 971–979.

**Melzack, R. & Wall, P.D.** (1988) *The Challenge of Pain.* Penguin, Harmondsworth.

**Miller, S.M. & Mangan, C.E.** (1983) The interacting effects of information and coping style in adapting to gynaecologic stress: should the doctor tell all? *Journal of Personality and Social Psychology* **45**, 223–236.

**Nathan, P.W.** (1976) The Gate Control theory of pain: a critical review. *Brain* **99**, 123–158.

**Ridgeway, V. and Matthews, A**. (1982) Psychological preparation for surgery: a comparison of methods. *British Journal of Clinical Psychology* **21**, 271–280.

**Seligman, M.E.P. & Maier, S.F.** (1967) Failure to escape traumatic shock. *Journal of Experimental Psychology* **74**, 1–9.

**Taenzer, P.A., Melzack, R. & Jeans, M.E.** (1986) Influence of psychological factors on postoperative pain, mood and analgesic requirements. *Pain* **24**, 331–342.

**Terenius, L.** (1984) Endogenous opioids and other central peptides. In: Wall, P.D. & Melzack, R. (eds) *Textbook of Pain.* Churchill Livingstone, Edinburgh, pp. 133–141.

**Thomas, V.J. & Rose, F.D.** (1991) Ethnic differences in the experience of pain. *Social Science and Medicine* **32**, 1063–1066.

**Thomas, V.J., Heath, M.L. & Rose, F.D.** (1990) Effect of psychological variables and pain relief system on postoperative pain experience. *British Journal of Anaesthesia* **64**, 388–389.

**Thomas, V.J., Heath, M., Rose, D. & Flory, P.** (1995) Psychological characteristics and the effectiveness of patient-controlled analgesia. *British Journal of Anaesthesia* **74**, 271–276.

**Thornton, J.W. & Jacobs, P.D.** (1971) Learned helplessness in human subjects. *Journal of Experimental Psychology* **87**, 367–372.

**Tyler, O., Caldwell, C. & Ghia, J.N.** (1982) Transcutaneous electrical nerve stimulation: an alternative approach to the management of postoperative pain. *Anaesthesia and Analgesia* **61**, 449–456.

**Wall, P.D.** (1978) The Gate Control theory of pain mechanisms: A re-examination and re-statement. *Brain* **101**, 1–18.

**Wall, P.D. & Sweet, W.H.** (1967) Temporary abolition of pain. *Science* **155**, 108–109.

**Weddel, G.M.** (1962) 'Activity pattern' hypothesis for sensation of pain. In: Grenell, G.R. (ed.) *Neural Physiopathology. Some Relationship of Normal to Altered Nervous System Activity.* Harper & Row, New York, pp. 134–177.

**Willis, W.D.** (1984) The origin and destination of pathways involved in pain transmission. In: Melzack, R. & Wall, P.D. (eds) *Textbook of Pain.* Churchill Livingstone, Edinburgh, pp. 88–100.

**Willis, W.D., Jr** (1985) Pain system: The neural basis of nociceptive transmission in the mammalian nervous system. In: Gildenberg, P.L. (ed.) *Pain and Headache.* Karger, Basel, p. 346.

**Yaksh, T.L. & Rudy, T.A.** (1978) Narcotic analgesics: CNS sites and mechanisms of action as revealed by intracerebral techniques. *Pain* **4**, 299–359.

# Psychological and social factors influencing pain: Individual differences in the experience of pain

Melzack and Wall (1989) argue that pain perception cannot be described simply in terms of stimulus intensity. In Chapter 1, we see that the complex interplay between physiological and psychological variables is central to our understanding of pain perception. In this chapter some of the psychological and social factors that contribute to this highly individual experience will be explored. These include the role of gender, age, culture and personality, the personal interpretation of pain, and other social factors. An extensive review of these factors are detailed in *Patient Controlled Analgesia: Confidence in Postoperative Pain Control* (Heath and Thomas, 1993) and some of the material for this chapter is quoted from this source with kind permission from Oxford University Press.

The contributors to the present book are largely in agreement with the philosophy that pain is a subjective phenomenon and therefore strongly endorse McCaffery's definition of pain: 'Pain is whatever the experiencing person says it is and exists whenever he says it does' (McCaffery, 1972). If we accept this nursing definition, then it follows that we should be encouraging nurses to undertake individual assessments of all their patients. So what is the rationale for including this chapter?

The author believes that an awareness of the role of psychosocial factors in the experience and expression of pain is very useful to health care professionals because it provides them with potential insights and explanations for understanding the patient's reaction and behaviour, and may also help them to avoid possible biases in their practice.

## ■ GENDER DIFFERENCES IN THE EXPERIENCE OF PAIN

The influence of an individual's gender on the experience of pain is contradictory. On the one hand, Glynn et al. (1976) found that, among chronic pain patients, pain scores were higher for females than for males. However, among postoperative patients, Khun et al. (1990) found no such difference, but Miller and Shuter (1984) found that females did experience significantly more pain than males. Similarly, Nayman (1979) found that females recorded higher pain scores than males, although this difference did not achieve statistical significance.

This appears to be a complex area of inquiry because, in assessing whether there were any sex differences in the amount of analgesic consumed (an indirect measure of pain), Bond (1981) found that 52 male cancer patients received less analgesia compared to females. However, among postoperative patients, neither Nayman (1979) nor Streltzer and Wade (1981) could find any significant differences in the amounts of pain medication given to male and female patients. Yet, Taenzer et al. (1986) found that females required significantly more analgesics than males in the postoperative context. It therefore appears that the gender of a patient can influence pain experience and the analgesic requirements, but there is no consistent pattern.

## ■ AGE DIFFERENCES IN THE EXPERIENCE OF PAIN

The literature addressing the influence of age on pain experience is also not straightforward. Kaiko (1980) attempted to determine the age-related variation in analgesia and pain experience among 946 surgical patients whose age groups ranged from 18 to 89 years old. The results showed that ageing was associated with enhanced analgesia, with 50% of the oldest groups experiencing an average duration of 5 hours pain relief compared to 3 hours for 50% of the youngest group. Kaiko argued that these results indicate that it is the duration of analgesia rather than the peak pain relief that is responsible for the age-related differences. He concluded that the decline in function of organs in drug elimination may also be expected to modify analgesic response. However, Homer and Stanski (1983), using electroencephalograhic (EEG) recordings to quantify the brain's sensitivity to centrally active drugs, found no significant changes in the brain's sensitivity to thiopental owing to age, even though the dose required to reach a surgical level of anaesthesia decreased with age. From this evidence it appears that the precise mechanism responsible for age-related differences is not clear.

Several other studies indicate that the elderly can obtain pain relief for longer periods with smaller doses of opioid analgesics (Belville et al., 1971; Berkowitz et al., 1975; Mather, 1983; Taenzer et al., 1986; Burns et al., 1989; Koh and Thomas, 1994) and younger patients express greater dissatisfaction with pain relief (Donovan, 1983; Koh and Thomas, 1994). The picture is further complicated by the differences in the amount of pain reported by different age groups. On the one hand, Miller and Shuter (1984) found that patients over 40 years reported more pain than those of a younger age group, whilst Khun et al. (1990) found no relation between the amount of reported pain and age.

These inconsistent findings support Williams' assertion (in Chapter 7) that psychological coping strategies are more useful in explaining the differences in pain experience and behaviour than variables such as age and gender.

## ■ ETHNIC DIFFERENCES IN THE EXPERIENCE OF PAIN

It is apparent from empirical studies and observations that pain experience cannot be fully explained without reference to cultural and ethnic differences. Culture seems to influence the expressiveness rather than the sensory experience itself (Melzack and Wall, 1989). Cultural norms determining when and where to express pain are learnt at an early age (Peck, 1986; Thomas and Rose, 1991). People from Latin origins are typically more expressive and are inclined to dramatize pain expression with excessive vocalization and posturing (Zborowski, 1952, 1969; Lipton and Marbach, 1984). The stoic Scandinavian on the other hand, has been shown to be more likely to become withdrawn and inexpressive (Chapman, 1984).

Black people have been found to report more pain than white people (Woodrow et al., 1972) but more recent research (Thomas and Rose 1991) shows that black people of Caribbean origin are better able to tolerate pain than white people of Anglo-Saxon origin, who in turn are better able to tolerate pain than South Asian people which does seem to contradict this view.

In a study designed to assess the variations in pain relief between black and white cancer patients, Kaiko et al. (1983) found that black patients reported significantly better relief on lower doses of morphine than white patients. Similar findings have been achieved by Miller and Shuter (1984).

Whilst these studies point to differences between groups the next two studies highlight similarities.

A study of episiotomy pain was carried out among 'Old American', Southern US black, Irish, Italian and Jewish subjects (Flannery et al., 1981). The latter three groups were all of immigrant parents. No differences were found on any of the measures, including several self-assessment measures of pain and behavioural measures such as the number of complaints to nurses and requests for medication.

Lipton and Marbach (1984) found a similar pattern when they administered a questionnaire about pain experience of facial pain to black, Jewish, Irish, Italian and Puerto Rican patients. The questionnaire included descriptions, attitudes and emotional expressiveness related to pain and illness behaviour. Assignment to one of the latter three groups required at least one grandparent to have been born in the appropriate foreign country. Overall, responses were relatively similar, with differences found in sections dealing with emotionality in response to pain and interference with daily lives. The pain experiences reported by black, Italian and Jewish patients were found to be the most similar. The Irish and Puerto Rican patients were relatively distinct from the other groups and from each other. Lipton and Marbach concluded that the relationship between pain experience and ethnicity may be more subtle than customarily thought, and that it may only be possible to describe certain responses as more or less characteristic of one group relative to another.

Overall, the number of comparative studies on pain expression and the response to pain are small in number and limited to relatively few ethnic groups. Ethnic groups of non-European origin (except for 'blacks') are virtually ignored. Most of the research on ethnicity has been carried out in North America with individuals who speak English and who are exposed to a variety of influences that would encourage both homogeneity across groups and variability within groups; therefore, no firm conclusions can be drawn. However, a recent review of the literature (Garro, 1990) states that the findings point to the importance of experiential factors of lifestyle and cultural upbringing in influencing judgements about pain intensity, but the role of genetic factors is not supported.

## ∎ The ethnic background of staff

The ethnic or cultural background of the nurses has been found to interact with that of the patients, and influence pain experience and analgesic consumption. In Chapter 10, Carr discusses this factor as a potential barrier to good pain management.

Research indicates that, in addition to holding common beliefs that certain operations, injuries and illnesses are more painful, nurses also have a stereotypical belief that patients from various ethnic or religious backgrounds differ markedly in the degree to which they suffer (Davitz and Davitz, 1981, 1985). For example, in a cross-cultural study of nurses' perceptions of pain and suffering, Davitz and Davitz found that nurses believed that Jewish and Hispanic patients suffered greatest physical and emotional pain, while Oriental, Asian and Anglo-Saxon patients suffered the least. Black nurses inferred a greater degree of psychological distress than white nurses regardless of patients' race, whilst nurses of northern European backgrounds inferred the least physical suffering (see Davitz and Davitz 1981, 1985, for a fuller discussion).

In the United Kingdom, stoicism is viewed as a positive characteristic which is to be admired. Both Bond (1981) and Seers (1987) found that nurses rewarded patients' stoicism by praise ('you are really courageous') and the administration of analgesics. On the other hand, complaints of pain, especially those considered by staff to be 'exaggerated', were penalized by the withholding of analgesic medication and verbal reproach (Bond, 1981). Garro (1990) suggests that these responses by staff are influenced by their expectations about what they consider to be appropriate pain behaviour.

In addition to making inferences about the suffering caused by pain, staff may consciously or unconsciously use the patients' ethnic background to make decisions about treatment. Streltzer and Wade (1981) conducted a study to assess the doses of analgesics given after surgery in relation to cultural background. They found that Caucasians and Hawaiians received significantly more analgesia than Chinese, Japanese or Philippino patients. These results should be interpreted with some caution, since the authors themselves believe that they may have arisen as a by-product of the nurse–patient interaction and the many other factors that influence this relationship.

According to Hartog and Hartog (1983), a caring individualized approach must be used to guide culturally based decisions in the management of pain, since cultural generalizations of a negative kind are prejudicial. In hospitals where there is a wide diversity of ethnic backgrounds among patient and staff populations, these cultural differences may significantly contribute to pain experience and should be the subject of more investigation.

## ■ PERSONALITY VARIABLES IN THE EXPERIENCE OF PAIN

The influence of personality on pain experience has been the subject of much research and it appears that personality can influence the sensory as well as the expressive aspects of pain.

### ■ Extraversion

Extraversion reflects the patient's sociability and has been associated with increased reports of pain in chronic pain patients (Bond, 1973), but this relationship has not been supported within the acute surgical pain populations (Dalrymple and Parbrook, 1976; Boyle and Parbrook, 1977; Thomas et al., 1995). Within an acute surgical setting, it seems that extraversion was a significant predictor of the amount of analgesic medication used among 40 patients recovering from cholecystectomy operations (Taenzer et al., 1986).

## ∎ Neuroticism

Neuroticism refers to the emotional stability and correlates highly with measures of trait anxiety (Eysenck, 1969; Loo, 1979). The studies to be reviewed used Eysenck's personality inventory (EPI) or the questionnaire (EPQ) to measure neuroticism. In a study of 190 patients undergoing abdominal surgery, Boyle and Parbrook (1977) found that pre-operative neuroticism correlated positively and significantly with pain experience in both men and women. This positive relationship between pain experience and neuroticism has been observed more recently (Thomas et al., 1990, 1995).

Since the amount of analgesic medication requested is an indirect measure of pain, it is therefore not at all surprising to find that other studies have found a positive relationship between this measure and neuroticism (Gourlay et al., 1982; Lim et al., 1983; Taenzer et al., 1986; Thomas et al., 1990, 1995).

## ∎ Anxiety and pain

The association between anxiety and pain is well known. Anxiety has been distinguished as: (1) a transitory emotional state – 'state anxiety' that varies in intensity and fluctuates over time, and is associated with threatening anticipatory circumstances; and (2) 'trait anxiety', a stable personality disposition, which is said to predict state anxiety, i.e. it predisposes people to react in a highly anxious manner in stressful situations (Spielberger, 1972). It is well known that people awaiting surgery become extremely anxious and Spielberger et al. (1973) have shown that anxiety trait remained stable in surgical patients before and after surgery, but those patients with high trait anxiety scores reacted in a highly anxious manner just before surgery.

Numerous studies have shown that both state and trait anxiety are positively correlated with the degree of pain experienced in acute and chronic pain settings (Auerbach, 1973; Spielberger et al., 1973; Martinez-Urrutia, 1975; Chapman and Cox, 1977; Johnston, 1980; Lim et al., 1983; Scott et al., 1983; Taenzer et al., 1986; Seers, 1987; Thomas, 1991; Thomas et al., 1995).

Overall it does appear that anxiety as an emotional state and a personality characteristic has an important role to play in the perception of pain. This consistent finding has led many researchers to attempt to reduce pain and distress by directly addressing state anxiety in the pre- and postoperative situations. The reader is referred to Chapter 7 and Heath and Thomas (1993) for a more detailed discussion.

**▪ Depression and pain**

Depression, like anxiety, is also considered to be a dysphoric mood or emotion, which may occur after a stressful episode and is a common feature of chronic pain (Romano and Turner, 1985; Tyrer et al., 1989; James, 1992). When people experience the prolonged stress of chronic pain and feel that nothing they do helps, they may stop striving to achieve goals and come to believe that they have no control over events in their lives. In other words they learn a sense of helplessness. There tends to be withdrawal and lethargy with accompanying feelings of worthlessness, and also sometimes of guilt and anxiety.

Romano and Turner (1985) reviewed the American literature and found varying prevalence of depression in pain patients as well as pain in those who were clinically depressed. Similarly Pilowski (1988) examined the pain-depression literature and found a variable prevalence ranging from 0% (Maruta et al., 1976) to 50% (Schaffer et al., 1980). In a study of British chronic pain patients, Tyrer et al. (1989) more recently found that 21% of patients had a depressive disorder.

Seligman (1975) and Beck (1976) first identified this learned helplessness (inability to effect change in spite of repeated efforts) to be the main component of depression.

**▪ Helplessness**

The psychological state of uncontrollability or helplessness is therefore a key feature of anxiety, depression and pain. There is an abundance of human and animal studies which supports the link between perceived control, anxiety and painful or aversive events (Lazarus, 1966; Mandler and Watson, 1966; Mandler, 1972; Henry and Stephens, 1977; Katz and Wykes, 1985). Psychological techniques aimed at enhancing personal control and reducing the sense of helplessness are a basic feature of the psychological treatments described in Chapter 7.

**▪ MAJOR LIFE EVENTS AND THE EXPERIENCE OF PAIN**

According to Roy (1992), significant personal losses resulting in feelings of guilt, which in turn are compounded by feelings of helplessness, are common features in many chronic pain patients. The following literature, which has examined the relationship between life events and the development of chronic pain, has been equivocal. For example, DeBenedittis et al. (1990) investigated a group of patients with chronic primary headache and found that they had a significantly greater incidence of life events than non-chronic pain controls. The chronic pain patients reported that these life events preceded the onset of their headache. Similarly, Smith et al. (1985) found a relationship between negative life events and the development of depression in patients with chronic back pain.

Other researchers such as Pilowski and Bassett (1982) and Jensen (1988), however, failed to find any relationship between life events and the onset of pain, or its treatment outcome. In trying to reconcile these disparate findings, Roy (1992) states that clinical experience does support the role of negative events in exacerbating chronic pain. In addition, minor trauma does have the capacity to trigger off a chain of events which lead to chronic pain.

## ■ THE PAIN-PRONE PERSONALITY

In 1959, the American psychiatrist Engel suggested that there are certain individuals for whom the presence of pain was necessary for the relief of emotional turmoil. In a paper entitled 'Psychogenic pain and the pain-prone patient', Engel suggested the clinical proposition that there is a relationship between childhood abuse and pain. Usually in their childhood these individuals experienced a great deal of emotional and physical abuse with the result that, when they become adults, they are unable to express anger.

According to Engel, 'for the most part, these patients are repeatedly chronically suffering from one or another painful disability, sometimes with and sometimes without any recognizable peripheral change'. These individuals he believed lead a 'life of pain' to expiate guilt. These patients fall into two categories: those indicative of abuse, and those where there is no direct evidence of abuse.

Engel provided the following five scenarios of childhood abuse and neglect:

1. Parents who are physically or verbally abusive to each other and/or their children.
2. One brutal parent and one submissive parent, the former sometimes an alcoholic father.
3. A parent who punishes frequently, but suffers remorse and overcompensates with a rare display of affection so that the child becomes accustomed to the sequence of pain and suffering to gain love.
4. A parent who is cold and distant who responds with affection when a child is ill or suffering pain to the point that the child invites injury to elicit such a positive response from the parent.
5. The child who deflects the aggression of a parent away from the other parent on to himself, usually with much guilt.

The child would be confronted with directly abusive situations in all five conditions.

Engel also put forward the following two non-abuse-related conditions, which could promote pain-proneness:

(a) Parental pain or pain in a significant figure close to the child for whom the child feels responsible and perhaps even guilt.

**(b)** A situation which led to the abandonment of feelings of aggression or pain by some sudden event where the abandonment was usually associated with guilt.

Basically the child has no means of understanding the reasons for the regular infliction of pain and abuse by an authority figure other than to associate it with his/her own badness. As a result pain is adopted as a means to atone for one's badness and thus expiate the guilt associated with being bad.

Even though this paper was published more than 30 years ago, Engel's idea continues to draw much attention. According to Roy (1992), there are many such patients in pain clinics today. Support for this has come from Green (1978) who looked at abused children receiving therapy and found evidence that they constantly invited punishment by behaving badly. Green suggested that these children engaged in subtle forms of pain-dependent behaviour, provocative and limit-testing activity, which easily resulted in punishment from parents. In another study Hunter et al. (1985) found an association between sexual abuse and abdominal pain in adolescent children.

The association between childhood abuse and adult pain has been investigated in the adult with chronic pain. For example, Violon (1980) found evidence of lack of affection, open rejection and physical abuse in chronic intractable pain patients. Similarly, in a study of patients with chronic pelvic pain, Gross et al. (1980) found that significant numbers had a history of incest or other forms of sexual abuse.

Violon (1990) conceptualized negative childhood experiences to culminate in the child using pain as a way of communication or, as Engel proposed, as a way of expiating guilt leading to proneness to pain. The other alternative intrapsychic mechanism proposed by Violon is one in which the negative experiences lead to neuroticism, which in turn lead to proneness to depression, leading to proneness to pain.

## ■ THE ROLE OF MEANING IN THE EXPERIENCE OF PAIN

People attach meaning to their pain and evidence suggests that such meaning may influence the ways individuals tolerate pain. The meanings associated with pain and suffering may dramatically affect the intensity and quality of the individual experience of pain. Pavlov's (1927) conditioning experiments were responsible for highlighting the relationship between personal meaning and pain experience. In these studies, Pavlov demonstrated that the dogs' negative reactions to electric shocks could be changed if the shocks consistently preceded food. Another early example of the powerful effect of meaning was described by Henry Beecher in 1956. He made a comparison between seriously wounded soldiers during World War II and civilians in an American hospital during peace time. He observed that, in spite of their extensive wounds, the soldiers reported significantly less pain than the civilians and required less analgesic medication. Beecher suggested that the soldiers' relief at finding themselves alive and being removed from the line of fire was significant. For the soldiers, their wounds marked the end of disaster, but for the civilians surgery heralded the start of personal disaster and disruption in their lives.

Rituals and rites of passage ceremonies also convey symbolic messages which can override pain. For example, 'hook swinging' is an example of a ritual which is powerful enough to obliterate pain. This ancient Indian ceremony is supposed to convey the desire of gods to bless the crops and a villager is chosen to represent 'god'. Steel hooks are driven into his back, which are attached by strong ropes to the top of a special cart. The cart is then driven from village to village and, at the climax of the ceremony in each village, the 'god' swings free, suspended only by the steel hooks in his back. His face conveys entrancement – but no indication of pain (Kosambi, 1967).

In addition to shaping the individual response or lack of it, such religious and cultural practices also provide examples on which to model pain behaviour. According to Illich (1976), pain behaviour responses, such as the saint, the warrior or the victim, are models that have been shaped by cultural meanings. In a study involving 148 hospital in-patients, Copp (1974) assessed personal meanings of pain. The results showed that more than half viewed pain as a challenge, something to fight and conquer, to promote self-searching and increasing understanding of others, and a quarter considered pain to be a weakness or punishment. These sociocultural meanings influence attitudes towards pain and the resultant behaviour. Fordham and Dunn (1994) have argued that the search for and attribution of meaning to pain is not only necessary for response, but provides a way of coping with pain.

Like pain, cancer has special meanings for people. It is commonly perceived to be uncontrollable and unpredictable, linked closely to extreme pain, suffering and death. Cassell (1982) provides an example of a patient who reported that when she believed the pain in her leg was due to sciatica, she was able to control it with small doses of codeine. However, when she discovered that the real cause was due to the spread of malignant disease, much greater amounts of medication were required for relief. In another study of cancer pain, patients who believed their pain indicated disease progression scored higher on several psychological measures assessing anxiety and depression (Ahles et al., 1983). Further, a study by Daut et al. (1982) found impairment of normal activities and life enjoyment to be greatest in patients who believed their pain to be caused by cancer, intermediate for those attributing pain to cancer treatment and lowest for those who did not believe cancer was causing their pain.

## ■ CONCLUSION

This chapter has discussed some of the factors that account for individual differences in the response to pain. Individuals with the same pathology may react in quite different ways depending on cultural values, personality, a sense of control, childhood experiences, the relationship to his/her family, the personal meanings of pain and the models from which pain behaviour was learnt. An awareness of the psychological factors in the experience and expression of pain is very useful to health care professionals because it provides them with potential insights and explanations for understanding patients' expressions and behaviour, and also helps to avoid possible biases in their own practices. However, a little knowledge can be dangerous because, as Sofaer (1992) has argued, there is a great danger of stereotyping people. This can be avoided by being mindful of the subjectivity of the experience, which is highlighted by McCaffrey's definition of pain. Every individual is unique and, therefore, nurses and other health care professionals should always engage in individual assessment of patients' pain and in individualizing pain relief.

## ■ REFERENCES

**Ahles, T.A., Blanchard, E. & Ruckdeschel, J.** (1983) The multidimensional nature of cancer-related pain. *Pain* **1**, 277–288.

**Auerbach, S.M.** (1973) Trait state anxiety and adjustment to surgery. *Journal of Consulting and Clinical Psychology* **40** (2), 264–271.

**Beck, A.T.** (1976) *Cognitive Therapy and the Emotional Disorders*. International Universities Press, New York.

**Beecher, H.K.** (1956) Relationship of significance of wound to pain experienced. *JAMA* **161**, 1609–1613.

**Belville, J.W., Forrest, W.H., Jr, Miller, E. et al.** (1971) Influence of age on pain relief from analgesics. *JAMA* **217**, 1835–1841.

**Berkowitz, B.A., Ngai, S.H., Yang, J.C. et al.** (1975) The disposition of morphine in surgical patients. *Clinical Pharmacology and Therapeutics* **17**, 629–635.

**Bond, M.R.** (1973) Personality studies in patients with pain secondary to organic disease. *Journal of Psychosomatic Research* **17**, 257–263.

**Bond, M.R.** (1981) Personality and pain. In: Lupton, S. (ed.) *Persistent Pain: Modern Methods of Treatment*, Vol. 2. Academic Press, London, pp. 1–25.

**Boyle, P. & Parbrook, G.D.** (1977) The interrelation of personality and postoperative factors. *British Journal of Anaesthesia* **49**, 259–263.

**Burns, J.W., Hodsman, N.B.A., McLintock, T.T., Gillies, G.W., Kenny, G.N. & McArdle, C.S.** (1989) The influence of patient characteristics on the requirements for postoperative analgesia. *Anaesthesia* **44**, 2–6.

**Cassell, E.** (1982) The nature of suffering and the goals of medicine. *New England Journal of Medicine* **306**, 639–645.

**Chapman, C.R.** (1984) New directions in the understanding and management of pain. *Journal of Social Science and Medicine* **19**(12), 1261–1277.

**Chapman, C.R. & Cox, G.B.** (1977) Anxiety, pain and depression surrounding elective surgery: a multivariate comparison of abdominal surgery patients with kidney donors and recipients. *Journal of Psychosomatic Research* **21**, 7–15.

**Copp, L.A.** (1974) The spectrum of suffering. *American Journal of Nursing* **74**(3), 491–495.

**Dalrymple, D.G. & Parbrook, G.D.** (1976) Personality assessment and postoperative analgesia. *British Journal of Anaesthesia* **48**, 593.

**Daut, R.L. & Cleeland, C.S.** (1982) The prevalence and severity of pain in cancer. *Cancer* **50**, 1913–1918.

**Davitz, J.R. and Davitz, L.L.** (1981) *Inferences of Patients Pain and Psychological Distress: Studies of Nursing Behaviours.* New York, Springer.

**Davitz, J.R. & Davitz, L.J.** (1985) Culture and nurses' inferences of suffering. In: Copp, L.A. (ed.) *Perspective on Pain.* Recent Advances in Nursing Series, Vol. 11. Churchill Livingstone, Edinburgh, pp. 17–28.

**DeBenedittis, G., Lovenzetti, A. & Pieri** (1990) The role of life events in the onset of primary headaches. *Pain* **40**, 65–75.

**Donovan, B.D.** (1983) Patients attitude to postoperative pain relief. *Anaesthesia and Intensive Care* **11**(2), 125–129.

**Engel, G.** (1959) Psychogenic pain and the pain prone disorder. *American Journal of Psychiatry* **26**, 899–918.

**Eysenck, H.** (1967) *The Biological Basis of Personality.* Thomas, Springfield, IL.

**Fordham, M. & Dunn, V.** (1994) *Alongside the Person in Pain: Holistic Care and Nursing Practice.* Bailliere Tindall, London.

**Flannery, R.B., Sos, J. & McGovern, P.** (1981) Ethnicity as a factor in the expression of pain. *Psychosomatics* **22**, 39–50.

**Garro, L.** (1990) Culture, pain and cancer. *Journal of Palliative Care* **6**(3), 34–44.

**Glynn, C.J., Lloyd, J.W. & Folkard, S.** (1976) The diurnal variations in perception of pain. *Proceedings of the Royal Society Journal* **28**, 501.

**Gourlay, G.K., Wilson, P.R. & Glynn, C.J.** (1982) Pharmacodynamics and pharmacokinetics of methadone during the perioperative period. *Anaesthesiology* **57**, 458.

**Green, G.** (1978) Psychopathology of abused children. *Journal of American Academy of Child Psychiatry* **17**, 92–103.

**Gross, R., Doerr, H. Caldirola, G. & Ripley, H.** (1980) Borderline syndrome and incest in chronic pain patients. *International Journal of Psychiatric Medicine* **10**, 79–96.

**Hartog, J. & Hartog, E.A.** (1983) Cultural aspects of health and illness behaviour in hospitals. Cross cultural medicine. *The Western Journal of Medicine* **139**, 910–916.

**Heath, M.L. & Thomas, V.J.** (1993) *Patient Controlled Analgesia: Confidence in Postoperative Pain Control.* Oxford University Press, Oxford.

**Henry, J.P. & Stephens, P.M.** (1977) *Stress, Health and the Social Environment: A Biologic Approach.* Springer, New York.

**Homer, T.D. & Stanski, D.R.** (1983) The effect of increasing age on thiopental dose requirement. *Anaesthesiology* **59**, A530.

**Hunter, R. Kilstrom, M. & Loda, F.** (1985) Sexually abused children: identifying masked presentations in a medical setting. *Child Abuse and Neglect* **9**, 17–25.

**Illich, I.** (1976) *Limits to Medicine. Medical Nemesis: The Exploration of Health.* Penguin, Harmondsworth, pp. 151–155.

**James, P.T.** (1992) Psychological dimensions of chronic pain. In: S.P. Tyrer (ed.) *Psychology, Psychiatry and Chronic Pain.* Butterworth-Heinemann, Oxford, pp. 25–43.

**Jensen, J.** (1988) Life events in neurologic patients with headaches and low back pain in relation to diagnosis and persistence of pain. *Pain* **32**, 47–53.

**Johnston, M.** (1980) Anxiety in surgical patients. *Psychological Medicine* **10**, 145–152.

**Kaiko, R.F.** (1980) Age and morphine analgesia in cancer patients with postoperative pain. *Clinical Pharmacology and Therapeutics* **28**, 823–826.

**Kaiko, R.F., Wallenstein, S.L., Rogers, A.G. & Houde, R.W.** (1983) Sources of variation in analgesic responses in cancer patients with chronic pain receiving morphine. *Pain* **15**, 191–200.

**Katz, R. & Wykes, T.** (1985) The psychological difference between temporally predictable and unpredictable stressful events: evidence for informational control theories. *Journal of Personality and Social Psychology* **48**, 781–790.

**Khun, S., Cooke, K., Collins, M., Jones, J.M. & Mucklow, J.C.** (1990) Perceptions of pain relief after surgery. *British Medical Journal* **300**, 1687–1690.

**Koh, P. & Thomas, V.J.** (1994) Patient controlled analgesia: does time saved by PCA improve patient satisfaction with care? *Journal of Advanced Nursing* **20**, 61–70.

**Kosambi, D.D.** (1967) Living pre-history in India. *Scientific American* **216**(2), 105–114.

**Lazarus, R.S.** (1966) *Psychological Stress and the Coping Process.* McGraw Hill, New York.

**Lim, A.T., Edis, G., Kranz, H., Mendleson, G., Selwood, T. & Scott, D.F.** (1983) Postoperative pain control: contribution of psychological factors and transcutaneous electrical stimulation. *Pain* **17**, 179–188.

**Lipton, J. & Marbach, J.** (1984) Ethnicity in pain experience. *Social Science and Medicine* **19**(12), 1279–1298.

**Loo, R.** (1979) Note on the relationship between trait anxiety and Eysenck personality questionnaire. *Journal of Clinical Psychology* **35**, 110.

**Mandler, G.** (1972) Helplessness: theory and research in anxiety. In: Spielberger, C.D. (ed.) *Anxiety: Current Trends in Theory and Research.* Academic Press, New York, pp. 93–105.

**Mandler, G. & Watson, D.L.** (1966) Anxiety and the interruption of behaviour. In: Spielberger, C.D. (ed.) *Anxiety and Behaviour.* Academic Press, New York, pp. 263–288.

**Martinez-Urrutia, A.** (1975) Anxiety and pain in surgical patients. *Journal of Consulting and Clinical Psychology* **43**, 437–442.

**Maruta, T., Swanson, D. & Swenson, W.** (1976) Pain as a psychiatric symptom: comparison between low back pain and depression. *Psychosomatics* **17**, 123–127.

**Mather, L.E.** (1983) Pharmacokinetic and pharmacodynamic factors influencing the choice, dose and route of administration of opiates for acute pain. *Clinics in Anaesthesiology* **1**(1), 17–40.

**McCaffery, M.** (1972) *Nursing Management of the Person in Pain.* J.B. Lippincott, Philadelphia.

**Melzack, R. & Wall, P.D.** (1989) *The Challenge of Pain.* Penguin Books, Harmondsworth.

**Miller, J.F. & Shuter, R.** (1984) Age, sex, race affect pain expression. *American Journal of Nursing* August, 981.

**Nayman, J.** (1979) Measurement and control of postoperative pain. *Annals of the Royal College of Surgeons* **61**, 419.

**Pavlov, I.P.** (1927) *Conditioned Reflexes.* Humphrey Milford, Oxford.

**Peck, C.L.** (1986) Psychological factors in acute pain management. In: Cousins, M.J. & Phillips, G.D. (eds) *Acute Pain Management.* Churchill Livingstone, Edinburgh, pp. 251–274.

**Pilowski, I.** (1988) Affective disorders and pain. In: Dubner, R., Gebhart, G. & Bond, M. (eds) *Pain Research and Clinical Management,* Vol. 3. Elsevier, Amsterdam.

**Pilowski, I. & Bassett, D.** (1982) Individual dynamic psychotherapy for chronic pain. In: Roy, R. & Tunks, E. (eds) *Chronic Pain: Psychosocial Factors in Rehabilitation.* Williams and Wilkins, Baltimore.

**Romano, J.M. & Turner, J.A.** (1985) Chronic pain and depression: does the evidence support a relationship? *Psychology Bulletin* **97**, 18–34.

**Roy, R.** (1992) *The Social Context of the Chronic Pain Sufferer.* University of Toronto Press Inc., Toronto.

**Schaffer, C., Donlon, P. & Bittle, R.** (1980) Chronic pain and depression: a clinical and family history. *American Journal of Psychiatry* **137**, 118–120.

**Scott, L.E., Clum, G.A. & Peoples, J.B.** (1983) Preoperative predictors of postoperative pain. *Pain* **15**, 283–293.

**Seers, C.J.** (1987) *Pain, Anxiety and Recovery in Patients Undergoing Surgery.* Unpublished Ph.D. thesis, Kings College, University of London.

**Seligman, M.E.P** (1975) *Helplessness.* Freeman Press, San Francisco.

**Smith, T., Follick, M. & Ahern, D.** (1985) Life events and psychological disturbance in chronic low back pain. *British Journal of Clinical Psychology* **24**, 207–208.

**Sofaer, B.** (1992) *Pain: A Handbook for Nurses,* 2nd edn. Chapman & Hall, London.

**Spielberger, C.D.** (1972) Theory and research on anxiety. In: Spielberger, C.D. (ed.) *Anxiety: Current Trends in Theory and Research.* Academic Press, New York, pp. 3–20.

**Spielberger, C.D., Auerbach, S.M., Wadsworth, A., Dunn, T.M. & Taulbee, S.M.** (1973) Emotional reactions to surgery. *Journal of Consulting and Clinical Psychology* **40**, 33–38.

**Streltzer, J. & Wade, T.C.** (1981) The influence of cultural group on the undertreatment of postoperative pain. *Psychosomatic Medicine* **43**, 397.

**Taenzer, P.A, Melzack, R. & Jeans, M.E.** (1986) Influence of psychological factors on postoperative pain, mood and analgesic requirements. *Pain* **24**, 331–342.

**Thomas, V.J.** (1991) *Personality Characteristics and the Effectiveness of Patient Controlled Analgesia.* Unpublished Ph.D. thesis, Goldsmiths' College, London University.

**Thomas, V.J. & Rose, D.** (1991) Ethnic differences in the experience of pain. *Social Science and Medicine* **32**, 1063–1066.

**Thomas, V.J., Heath, M.L. & Rose, F.D.** (1990) Effect of psychological variables and pain relief system on postoperative pain experience. *British Journal of Anaesthesia* **64**, 388–389.

**Thomas, V.J., Heath, M., Rose, D. & Flory, P.** (1995) Psychological characteristics and the effectiveness of patient-controlled analgesia. *British Journal of Anaesthesia* **74**, 271–276.

**Tyrer, S.P., Capon, M., Peterson, D.M. et al.** (1989) The detection of psychiatric illness and psychological handicaps in a British pain clinic population. *Pain* **36**, 63–74.

**Violon, A.** (1980) The onset of facial pain. *Psychotherapy Psychosomatics* **34**, 11–16.

**Violon, A.** (1990) The process involved in becoming a chronic pain patient. In: Tunks, E., Bellissimio, A. & Roy, R. (eds) *Chronic Pain: Psychosocial Factors in Rehabilitation*, 2nd edn. Krieger, Melbourne.

**Woodrow, K.M., Friedman, G.D., Siegelbaub, A.B. & Collen, M.F.** (1972) Pain tolerance: differences according to age, sex and race. *Psychosomatic Medicine* **34**, 548–556.

**Zborowski, M.** (1952) Cultural components in responses to pain. *Journal of Social Issues* **8**, 16–30.

**Zborowski, M.** (1969) *People in Pain*. Jossey-Bass, San Francisco.

# Pain and thinking: An introduction to cognitive psychology

The aim of this chapter is to support a detailed and comprehensive understanding of the experience of both short-lived and long-term pain. In
introducing the idea of a psychology of thinking, the focus is upon examining the traditional boundaries between physiology and psychology, and
the equally common distinction between injury and pain. This starting point
enables us to look more closely at a recent model of the way in which the
processing of pain-related information affects the interpretation of bodily
sensations and the way we act upon that interpretation. The important
distinction between acute and chronic pain is remade and the importance
of this distinction for a cognitive psychology of pain is addressed in full.

## ■ MIND–BODY

Physiology and psychology are often written and taught as if they were
wholly separate areas of study. In fact, they are more closely related than
they first appear. It is clear that changes in one's physical state can affect
the way that one thinks. If I am confined to my bed ill, this will not only
affect my body, but my lack of movement and stimulation will affect my
mood, the way I think about myself, my future and those around me.
Similarly, the way that I think can affect my bodily state. This is true in an
indirect way, so that the decisions I make often affect my body, for example,

deciding to smoke, drink, eat, visit the doctor, go bungee jumping, etc. The way that I think can also directly affect my body. For example, if I am worried and nervous about an impending examination, a number of changes occur in various bodily systems: I will begin to sweat more, my stomach will tighten, my muscles contract and my appetite disappears.

Pain is one area of research and clinical practice where it has long been recognized that there is a close relationship between the psychological and physiological domains. Many of the earlier theories of pain place an emphasis on explaining pain by the amount of activity in peripheral and central nervous mechanisms. In other words, a central tenet of these earlier theories is in explaining pain report in terms of the amount of nociception. As we have seen, with the popularity of the Gate Control theory and the more recent discoveries of neuroplasticity comes the recognition that there is also a central role to be played by downward inhibition from the cortex. In other words, the way one thinks affects the amount and quality of pain felt and how disabling it is (Price, 1988; Melzack, 1989, 1993; Wall, 1994).

Before going into more detail concerning the role of thinking in pain perception, it is worth reflecting further on the relationship between injury (physical trauma) and reported pain. Although there are many examples of when trauma will equal pain (if I drop a suitcase on my foot from a great height, I will not be surprised to experience pain), there are also many occasions we can think of from our own experience, personal or professional, when an expected response to presumed or actual tissue damage has been missing. Although we generally understand pain to be associated with tissue damage, this relationship is not always so straightforward. Consider the following examples of when the amount of damage does not equal the amount of pain experienced:

- Pain without apparent physical injury. A common example is that of persistent chronic low back pain.
- Pain can also persist after an injury has healed. Again a common example is of wisdom tooth extraction where postoperative healing has occurred but pain persists.
- Injury can occur without pain being experienced. A common example is skin changes owing to exposure to the sun.
- Injury can occur in tissue distant from where the pain is felt, a phenomenon known as 'referred pain', e.g. pain associated with a myocardial infarction which refers pain to the left arm.
- The relationship between pain and injury is a highly variable one. Injury can occur that is serious such that we would expect severe pain but only low-intensity tolerable pain is reported. Similarly, objectively minor tissue damage can produce an experience of high-intensity intolerable pain.

■ Innocuous stimuli can produce pain. Similarly, we can be unclear as to whether some stimuli are neutral, painful or pleasurable.

■ It is also possible to feel pain in a limb which no longer exists. Eighty per cent of all amputees will report detailed sensations associated with the lost limb. Many amputees will lose these sensations in recovery but a proportion will continue to have the sensations of the lost limb. Many of these so-called 'phantom limbs' can be painful.

The idea, then, that there is a simple relationship between pain and physical trauma is difficult for us to accept given not only current theories of pain processing, but also our own experience.

In clinical practice we often find an erroneous received wisdom that the amount of pain should equal the amount of damage, and further that there is a tendency when this does not occur to resort to psychological explanations of a blaming type. (This understandable tendency is based upon the premise that all symptoms can be physically explained). In the absence of physical explanations, we often then resort to psychological explanations. As Gamsa (1994) points out, this is an error in logic, as one does not define a psychological syndrome by the *absence* of physical symptoms. Not only does this reinforce the idea that one can have a psychological explanation of pain divorced of its biological base, but also it is a circular argument that is impossible to disprove. Importantly, this can also lead us to miss critical clinical information and increases the chances of inappropriate or inadequate care (Chapman and Turner, 1986).

The place of psychology in explaining and understanding pain processing and pain-related suffering is not simply a psychology of the odd or strange patient. What follows should be considered an introduction to a *normal* psychology of pain, rather than an abnormal one. We need to focus upon what influences the further processing of pain and suffering, and what we can do to reduce the suffering associated with pain.

## ■ A NORMAL PSYCHOLOGY OF PAIN

Psychology is often defined as the science of human behaviour. Modern psychology, however, is concerned with the interrelationship between the physiological, cognitive, behavioural and social aspects of experience. It largely adopts what is known as an information-processing understanding of thinking. If we accept that there is activity in the nervous system that is often increased when one's environment changes (e.g. the suitcase drops on my foot), we can understand what happens in the nervous system as a sudden increase in information that travels quickly to the brain where it is decoded, and acted upon. This information in the nervous system is what we call 'nociception', the process of decoding is known as 'cognition', and the acting is known as 'behaviour'. It is these three aspects together that make up a pain experience. It is useful to think of these different areas of study as related as it can help in understanding why all people do not respond in a similar way to the same injury, and why the same person may not respond in the same way to the same injury.

Cioffi (1991) has provided a useful framework for understanding the various influences that combine to produce a painful experience. She stresses the importance of the processes that instantaneously structure one's response to a change in the environment. It is useful to think of these differences as occurring at different stages in the processing of the information. If we go back to the earlier example of dropping a suitcase on my foot: long before the suitcase is dropped a number of things are happening.

First (stage one: sensation), there is a gradual change in my environment as I carry this heavy weight without rest. This weight is causing a great many things to happen within my body without my conscious awareness. For example, the sensory free nerve endings in my hand are sending increased messages of pressure to my brain. Also the muscles in my arm, torso, back and neck will be reacting to this weight and sending messages to my brain. Various proprioceptors will send messages to my brain regarding my balance as I move, and my gait and speed of walking will automatically be adapted.

Second (stage two: attention), one has to assume that the brain is receiving information from all of one's senses. The brain is constantly being bombarded with information from the eyes, nose, ears and body. Much of this information is processed unconsciously. For example, I am able, most of the time, to walk upright and to breathe. I do not, however, have to think about these activities, they proceed normally. I can consciously attend towards them, but this is very time-consuming and inefficient. In order to live it is important that many things can proceed automatically. There are other things I need to attend toward consciously. In this case, there are the meeting I am late for, orienting the traffic and other people. As I move through my environment, I am often distracted by many things that happen. Loud sounds will distract me. If I were to hear someone shout my name, this would distract me. If I see a familiar sign, or a gaudy image, I may be distracted. Similarly, I may be distracted by a thought or by a memory. Another thing that may distract me is the information that my body is sending. If I lose my balance, this will become conscious to me and I will try to right myself. If I am getting very hot, it may distract me. Also as I am walking along I get a sharp pain in my back which distracts my attention. Instead of thinking of the important meeting I am missing, or the memory of the last time I was late, my attention is dragged suddenly to an overwhelmingly noxious sensation. The nociception has become so intense that it has interrupted cognition and distracted my attention to it. It is usually as this point that I will label that sensation, that I will call it 'pain'.

Third (stage 3: attributions), when this happens one looks for an explanation for what might have caused the pain to happen. Here, one might well assume that the explanation is readily sought in the carrying of the suitcase. However, it is not always clear what will have caused the pain to occur. In trying to make sense of changing experience, of sudden pain, I will try to 'attribute' the cause of that pain to something and I will also consider the consequences of that pain. Here a large number of psychological factors come into play, including the following:

- My beliefs about what caused back pain
- My expectations
- My styles of thinking
- How much control I think I have over my health
- What recent information I have about back pain
- How anxious I am
- How depressed I am

Some of these factors will be explained below. With our example, we could consider two of the many possible scenarios. One, I could attribute the cause of the pain to the heavy weight in my hand, or, two, it is possible that I have a history of back pain, and I have a friend who recently had back pain which turned out to be due to a cancer. On the radio this morning I heard a news report that the incidence of testicular cancer is increasing and one of the early signs is sudden back pain. Perhaps I am also given to being anxious about my health, and have recently been very depressed as I have suffered a number of losses. In this scenario my back pain becomes a symptom of a possible malignant medical problem.

Fourth (stage 4: priorities), an important interaction between the sensation, my attending to it, and how I understand it occurs with an evaluation of my current priority. If I appraise the meeting to be of life and death importance, I am more likely to ignore both of the above attributions, bear the pain and continue to walk on carrying the suitcase. If, however, I am not looking forward to the meeting, or I appraise the meeting to be less important than my health, I am more likely to change the priorities I have.

Fifth (stage 5: behaviour), all of the above will lead me to act in a certain way. This could be me dropping the suitcase, placing the suitcase down or trying to ignore the pain in order to make a meeting that is of a higher priority. Pain behaviour is immensely important as it structures the way that other people will react to the person in pain. Importantly, it also structures the way that a person will behave the next time that they are in pain. There is little space to cover in detail this important concept. Those interested are referred to the comprehensive coverage by Fordyce (1976), Rachlin (1985) and Keefe and Lefebvre (1994). Of central focus here is the information

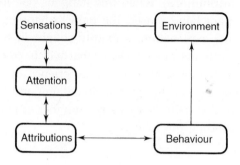

*Figure 3.1. Schematic representation of the process of interpreting bodily sensations.*

processing that occurs in making sense of a pain experience, and how such an approach can further our understanding of pain (e.g. Jerome, 1993).

Caveat: It should be stressed that the above process, which is summarized in Fig. 3.1 is not a linear one. In other words what happens at one stage feeds directly back to the other stages. For example, the way in which I attribute a painful sensation may change the labelling of that sensation. If I feel pain on reactivity, I may attribute this to my getting fitter, stronger and healthier, and decide that this is 'the burn'. It is also important to recognize that this is a constant and not always very transparent process. The way that I behave at the later stage will have an effect upon stage 1. When I drop the suitcase the process will begin again.

Pain perception is, then, a very complex process, and there are many opportunities for information to be processed in any number of ways. Such a complexity can often seem overwhelming and clinically unhelpful as it does not easily lead to ways that we can standardize what we can or should do when people complain of pain. All of the above has been researched in both laboratory and clinical settings and much is known of the cognitive factors that influence pain perception. Before we look at this research in more detail, it is important to make a distinction between acute and chronic pain conditions as the cognitive psychological factors are different in each case.

## ▪ Acute and chronic pain

The word 'acute' is often used to mean severe or in some medical settings to mean immediate. In the pain literature, 'acute' is taken simply to mean 'short-lived', which can be anything up to 6 weeks. Confusingly, the word chronic is also often used to mean severe. In the pain literature, it is taken to mean 'long-lived'. Some writers take long-lived to be of 3 months duration or longer, others take it to mean of 6 months duration or longer.

Psychologically speaking, time is very important as it gives opportunities for the above process to be repeated many times and for different permutations to occur.

For what follows it may be useful to think of the important psychological factors as of two types:

1.  Those that the situation affords or offers. Important factors here include the information that is given to the person in pain by those around him/her, attentional factors in pain control, and the manner and setting in which the pain occurs.

2.  Those that the person in pain brings to the experience. Important factors here are past experience, memory and attentional abilities, styles of thinking, beliefs about health and illness.

For those suffering from acute pain, the first collection of factors are, arguably, of much more importance to understanding the experience of the person in pain and the experience of the person whose primary role it is to relieve that pain. By contrast, with chronic pain one needs an understanding of the cognition of the person who has suffered persistent pain over a long period of time, as this will have changed greatly over that time. In both cases, it is the responsibility of the person helping the patient alleviate or manage the pain to understand how information that is given will be understood and acted upon.

## ■ ACUTE PAIN

Acute pain is a very common part of everyday life, and one that we would not like wholly to disappear as it is one of the ways in which we learn what is dangerous in our environment. It is a central part of our means of survival. Although important, there is an enormous amount of pain that is unnecessary and for which we can offer treatment. Indeed in the acute medical setting, pain control and pain management is often a primary goal for both patient and health professional. Despite this, it is clear that our record of offering pain control has been insufficient to the problem (e.g. Royal College of Surgeons Report, 1990). It is also clear that there is a great deal of unnecessary pain being suffered that we have the skills and techniques to address (Melzack, 1988). Other chapters in this volume deal with some of the developments of interventions for pain control and management, and the changes in practice they predict.

Acute pain problems arise in nearly all areas of medical practice. It is also apparent that many medical procedures routinely carried out can be painful in themselves. In what follows, this area of acute pain will be used as an example of a possible pain experience that is under the control of the health care professional. In clinical settings there are specific parameters associated with certain procedures that will govern the amount of pain reported, such as the age of the patient (e.g. Steine, 1993). It is also clear that for some medical procedures, such as wisdom-tooth extraction, there is a modest but significant positive relationship between tissue damage and reported pain (Levine et al., 1982). However, rather than focus here upon the nociception and its physical parameters, or upon the mechanics of a medical procedure and whether it is commonly painful, we should rather focus upon the wider picture as outlined in the above model of the normal psychology of pain perception. We should first look at the patient's previous experience, the information that is given, the people interacting with the patient, and the place in which pain is experienced and pain relief sought.

## ▪ Previous experience

People have complex and detailed lives. They do not enter clinical situations devoid of ideas and knowledge. We all have ways of understanding what has happened to us and what is about to happen to us. If we take the example of the common cold, there are many theories at large within our culture to help us explain what we should do when we get a cold (Helman, 1978). These theories may not be the same as the dominant medical explanations, but, nonetheless, they are important in making sense of the experience to the patient (Stainton Rogers, 1991). Typically patients will bring these theories to the clinical setting and request further information, or share them with the health professional. Making sense of illness/injury is a primary motivation for most patients in an acute pain setting. Suffering associated with pain is not merely due to the noxious experience, but also due to the fear and anticipation of what it could mean. The person in pain will need to know what the pain 'means'. The person who is about to have a possibly painful medical procedure may need to know the relationship between the procedure and the illness/condition it is aimed at treating (Delvecchio Good et al., 1992).

## ▪ Information

The information one gives about an impending medical procedure, during the procedure and after the procedure, is of primary importance to the experience of pain. When a sensation is ambiguous, it has been demonstrated that pre-labelling it as painful or pleasurable significantly increases the report of the sensation as painful or pleasurable, respectively (Anderson and Pennebaker, 1980). In an experimental pain study, Crombez et al. (1994) found that giving subjects information about the quality of the impending painful event had a positive effect on the judgement of the sensation. The subjects who had this information reported it as less painful than those who did not have that information. Knowing that something will be painful, and what that sensation will be like, can often help in coping with it. Other researchers have found that information about how long the pain would last is also beneficial to the person in pain. Such information does not, of course, always work in this direction. Baron et al. (1993) found that, with a clinical population, the effectiveness of their informational intervention was dependent on whether it matched the pre-existing coping strategies of patients. In other words, if my method for coping with the fear and pain of dentistry is to distract myself and to think of anything else but the pain, giving me detailed information about what it will feel like and how long it will last is more likely to increase the amount of pain experienced, and not decrease it.

Such informational interventions are not new. Childbirth preparation techniques, for example, have been practised for some years. Evidence from this important area also teaches us that suffering is not isolated to the painful experience itself. Leventhal et al. (1989), for example, have demonstrated that preparation can also positively affect other factors such as postpartum fatigue. Related areas of research also demonstrate that one should take account of the meaning that is assigned to any procedure for the effects this can have upon experience. Placebo researchers have noted, for example, that it is possible to produce nocebo effects, or negative changes in bodily systems with a purely informational intervention, either of a subjective nature (e.g. drowsiness, loss of concentration) and/or of an objective nature (e.g. skin rashes, vomiting). Excellent reviews of this topic can be found in Richardson (1989, 1994). Although the mechanism(s) for these changes are poorly understood, they are believed to be cortically generated (e.g. Flor and Birbaumer, 1994).

## ∎ Attention

The amount and type of information given to a patient can affect how likely it is that he or she will experience a pain upon a procedure. It is also true that there are individual differences that structure how likely it is that a person will attend towards what is happening in his or her body. Some people are more likely to attend toward changes in bodily sensation than are others (Ahles et al., 1987; Steptoe and Vogele, 1992). If one has introduced the idea that pain is expected and one has gained information about the way that a patient would normally cope with pain sensations, one can then instruct the patient in either a distraction or an attentionally focusing task.

There is a lot of research concerning the possible effects of such strategies in reducing pain. The majority of these studies are with experimentally induced pain. For example, Dubreuil et al. (1988) asked undergraduate students to undergo a pressure-pain procedure, where they placed a finger in a pressure guillotine. They were interested in both whether focusing upon the pain was better or worse than distracting attention away from the pain, and which strategy worked better for low-intensity pain and which for high-intensity pain. First, they found that both strategies were more effective than not teaching a strategy at all for both high- and low-intensity pain. Second, they found that both strategies were equally effective in reducing low-intensity pain report but the redefinition strategy was more effective for high-intensity pain. Other researchers have, however, found different results. McCaul and Haugtvedt (1982), using a different procedure, found that focusing upon the pain and changing its meaning was more effective than distraction at increasing tolerance to a high-intensity ice-water-induced pain. Although there are methodological difficulties with many of the studies in this field (Eccleston, 1995), there is a number of guidelines that we can give for making attention-based interventions effective in positively affecting pain perception. Strategies work best when the task chosen:

- Is interesting and meaningful to the person in pain
- Is detailed and complex
- Involves switching between different mental processes (e.g. memory and attention)
- Is consonant with the strategies a patient would normally adopt
- Is introduced in a confident and assured manner

Details of such therapies can be found in other texts. The most comprehensive expositions are those by Turk et al. (1983) and McCaffery (1979). It is clear that such strategies are effective in reducing acute pains in medical settings. They should not, however, be thought of as alternative to more traditional pharmacological and counterstimulation methods of pain control, but thought of as useful in conjunction with such methods. By the same token, one can also forcibly argue that failure to offer such pain relief is akin to failure to offer pharmacological pain relief. It is effectively accepting unnecessary pain.

## ∎ Setting and therapist

We know from placebo research that 'the provider's warmth, friendliness, interest, sympathy, empathy, prestige, and positive attitude toward the treatment are associated with positive effects of placebos as well as active treatments' (Turner et al., 1994, p. 1611). If a clinician does not believe in the efficacy of a treatment, then this has been shown to reduce the amount of pain relief reported by the patient (Gracely et al., 1985). This is not a conscious process. Both physicians' and patients' beliefs about the power of a therapy have been clearly demonstrated to produce both perceptual and physiological change. As ever, we should be careful not to overgeneralize from these findings. It is certainly not the case that all settings are able to support such effects. There is a danger, for example, that being overenthusiastic about a treatment merely serves to exacerbate a patient's feelings of being unheard or misunderstood. It can also serve to fuel worry and anxiety if an overpromised result is not achieved. The message is simply that the setting in which someone is reporting pain, and the setting in which pain relief is given, has the power to exacerbate or diminish the suffering associated with that pain, and to ignore it, or treat it, as peripheral to the experience is likely to increase suffering and pain report.

## ▪ Resultant behaviour

Once a procedure has been performed or pain relief provided, this is not the end of the care. Although the importance of resultant health behaviours cannot be given in detail here, one should be clear that these have a strong effect in structuring the way a procedure is delivered and received. In situations where acute pains are delivered regularly (e.g. debridement), each episode is extremely important in predicting how much suffering will occur in the next episode. Experience that is repeated is open to pronounced learning effects which structure the next learning situation. Chapman and Turner (1986), for example, warn that acute pain may become chronic if psychological and environmental factors such as the above are not addressed.

## ▪ CHRONIC PAIN

Pain of long duration is very common and may arise for known or unknown reasons. Common examples are pain associated with chronic diseases and disorders, such as rheumatism and arthritis, pain associated with malignancies or with injuries that take a long time to heal, such as burns, and intermittent pains that recur regularly, such as migraine and dysmenorrhoea. A further category of chronic pain is that which is non-malignant in nature. Much of this is believed to be musculoskeletal in origin but commonly fails to respond to interventionist treatments. The incidence of chronic low back pain alone has grown enormously in recent years (Mason, 1994) and new treatment guidelines have been recently published to address this growth (Clinical Standards Advisory Committee for Back Pain, 1994). Many of these chronic pain sufferers enter the health care system because they fail to cope adequately with the experience of persistent pain. When pain has failed to respond to the traditional interventions, a different approach has to be adopted for the care and management of the patient. The importance of adopting a different approach will be addressed later in this volume. Here, it is important to explore what it means in psychological terms to be a person who has had pain for 6 months or longer, although realistically this is often a matter of many years.

As outlined above, with the prolonged experience of pain, it is more important to focus upon the cognition of the patient reporting pain, including the patient's understanding of what the pain means, the styles of maladaptive and punishing thinking that can develop, the ways in which such cognitions exacerbate and prolong pain, and the disability associated with it.

## ∎ Chronic pain experience

Chronic pain has no survival value. It makes no sense. It is often not associated with current tissue damage, and it does not inform the person of possible or imminent danger. The experience of persistent pain is a very distressing one. However, what is also distressing is that the way in which the pain is responded to will often increase pain and disability. The prevalent model we hold about pain is that it must be related to some damage and that, when that damage has healed, the pain will abate. If I have severe pain I will put into practice means of achieving pain relief, such as visiting a doctor, taking time off work, resting, taking analgesics, being cared for by those people close to me, etc. It is unfortunate, however, that the measures I adopt for an acute pain are not merely ineffective for chronic non-malignant pain but are counterproductive. Prolonged rest, prolonged analgesic consumption, time away from activities, and reduced exercise all conspire to support physical disuse (Bortz, 1984). This in turn creates more pain. Similarly, my theory of pain has proved to be ineffective and I search for some meaning of the pain (Kleinman, 1988). This will often mean more visits to practitioners, more diagnoses and more treatments. Eventually such trips to the doctor will become frustrating as the treatment options are exhausted. Many such interactions will become blaming and my mental health will be questioned, as will my willingness to be well. My home situation may well have adapted to support my disability, and I may have lost my job and income. I will probably withdraw from many social activities as I cannot predict how I will feel, I am dependent upon others and I cannot pay for myself. Such isolation will fuel my depression and my worry for my uncertain future.

## ∎ Cognitive status

Given the above and the issues discussed in Chapter 2, it should come as no surprise that many chronic pain patients become depressed (Romano and Turner, 1985). Many patients also report increased anxiety levels (Craig, 1994) and can suffer from feelings of hostility and anger (Fernandez and Turk, 1995). In addition, the prolonged experience of pain and depression can also affect cognitive abilities. Dufton (1989), for example, found that chronic pain patients made a large number of cognitive errors. Taking this work further, Kewman et al. (1991) also reported that of the 73 chronic pain patients they tested, 32% had pronounced cognitive impairment. Specifically, they had memory and attentional difficulties. These impairments are believed to be due to the interruptive and distracting effects of the pain and of the affective (or emotional) aspects of a pain experience. It is known that acute pain affects one's abilities to perform difficult and complex tasks (Walker, 1971). In chronic pain populations, high pain intensity has been demonstrated to disrupt central attentional abilities. In an experimental study with adult chronic pain sufferers I have explored the effects of pain intensity upon performance of demanding cognitive tasks (Eccleston, 1994). When in intense pain, the attention that would normally be used for planning, for decision-making, for accessing memories and for maintaining conversation, is severely affected by pain. Such a loss in cognitive abilities can add to the depression, and often fuels the fears and anxieties about how symptomatic of a possible illness such losses may be.

Recent evidence has suggested that the experience of chronic pain can also affect the way that pain-related and mood-related information is processed. The priority given to some information in the environment will be changed. Using a memory task, in which chronic pain patients were asked to remember lists of pain-related and non-pain-related words, Pearce et al. (1990) and Edwards et al. (1992) demonstrated that in comparison with non-pain control subjects, pain patients recalled more pain information. Pincus et al. (1994) also reported an elegant experiment which demonstrated that chronic pain patients are more likely to interpret ambiguous words in a pain-related manner than the control subjects who did not suffer pain. One may well assume that this is merely another way of describing what it means to be a pain patient. However, in information processing terms this is very important because it shows that patients are biased toward continually processing pain information which will serve to maintain suffering and disability.

## ▪ Cognitive style

In addition to the above largely unconscious changes in cognition that affect the processing of information, it is also apparent that there are more recognizable effects of the experience of chronic pain including changes in:

- ▪ Inappropriate labelling of other bodily sensation
- ▪ The appraisal of new situations
- ▪ The appraisal of threat
- ▪ The appraisal of self
- ▪ Beliefs about one's abilities to change the situation

Prolonged pain changes the perception and judgment of bodily sensations. Chronic low back pain patients, for example, report an increased number of other physical symptoms (Bacon et al., 1994). As Fordyce (1988) points out, this is a wholly understandable cognitive change and one that is particularly fuelled when a patient has been given no diagnosis or an ambiguous diagnosis. In trying to make sense of a changing experience, in trying to give meaning to the pain, a patient will search for more information. One effect of increasing information is that it increases the possibility of interpreting bodily sensations in line with that information. This is not a tendency that is specific to chronic pain patients. This is a very common occurrence in health care students. For example, Kellner et al. (1986) reported that medical students commonly report fears and beliefs of medical complaints of which they have recently been informed. More information and here salient information increased the likelihood that such information will be considered in self-diagnosis.

One should not infer from this that information should be withheld from the patient but that one should explore further the way in which the information is being interpreted. In other words, one should address the patient's cognition.

An increase in awareness of bodily sensations, and the labelling of such changes as of importance to one's health, can often fuel anxiety and fear. One's physical being can be seen to be a threat to well-being. The appraisal of a possible threat is an important part of the chronic pain experience. A marked style of thinking that is believed to be important in exacerbating chronic pain is that known as 'catastrophizing' or 'awfulizing'. As these names suggest, this way of thinking is characterized by an unrealistic, exaggerated and negative appraisal of current and future situations. For example, a typical catastrophizing way of thinking may be:

> This pain is just too much, I don't think I can cope any longer, where will it all end. It is going to get worse, I know it is. I will have to be in a wheelchair and I will never work again. My wife is bound to leave me, nobody can put up with this forever, and then what will I do . . .'

Although all of us are given to catastrophizing (Heyneman et al., 1990), this is exacerbated in chronic pain populations. Rosentiel and Keefe (1983) and others have isolated this as a particularly important pattern of thinking that serves to further disable chronic pain patients from making changes. Coughlan et al. (1995) have also found that catastrophizing is a major factor in accounting for patient relapse after rehabilitation. Importantly, Vlaeyen et al. (1995) have suggested that this catastrophizing should be seen as central to an analysis of why chronic pain is maintained (see also Philips, 1987).

Chronic pain patients are, as suggested above, very often depressed. A central aspect of this experience is the effect it has upon a patient's sense of identity. As Wall and Jones (1991) point out, to be in chronic pain affects all parts of the patient's life. The patient becomes a pain person. The sense of who we are, which is supported by the many roles that we play (as providers, carers, parents, sons, friends, etc.), has changed dramatically. Much of what was important has been lost. As a consequence a pattern of self-denigration may emerge. Patients often have low self-esteem and low self-worth, which fuel difficulties in making changes. Such a negative appraisal of both self and of situations will directly affect suffering, and is an important focus point in rehabilitation (Turk and Meichenbaum, 1994).

One important aspect of the changes in appraisal that occur is a person's appraisal of his/her ability to cope effectively and to bring about change. Psychologists call this 'self-efficacy' (Bandura, 1977). This is not a personality trait in the sense that it is unchanging. In many situations we have the power to make changes; however, we do not always appraise ourselves as being capable of making those changes. With pain, one has to remember that the actions we put into place when pain is acute are largely passive. We give over responsibility and control to other people, we seek expert advice and we often do as these powerful others command of us. It is perhaps unsurprising then, if this pattern is established, together with the above factors of depression, low self-worth and increased awareness and appraisal of threat, that we can lose the belief in our own abilities to make changes. Litt (1988) has shown tolerance to experimental pain to be reduced with low self-efficacy. Also, in an excellent study, Dolce et al. (1986) have demonstrated that the fear of re-movement and exercise that is common in chronic pain is at least partially mediated by low self-efficacy. As self-efficacy increased in a behavioural rehabilitation programme, so exercise increased.

## ▪ Resultant behaviour

The patterns and habitual ways of thinking are of central importance to an integrated understanding of the patient who has suffered long-term pain. In seeking explanations for the way in which patients act or fail to act, an explanation based upon physiology alone is most likely to be at best insufficient. The above cognitive factors are part of the explanation for why the suffering associated with chronic pain can be so pronounced and seemingly intractable. Perhaps more important than in the acute pain case is the role of chronic pain behaviour. Again, space is inadequate to the task of fully elucidating the processes by which the responses to pain behaviour, and the environment in which we behave, structure and maintain future pain behaviour and suffering. This material is fully covered in Fordyce (1976), Vlaeyen (1991) and Keefe and Lefebvre (1994).

## ■ SUMMARY AND CONCLUSION

Physiology and psychology are not far removed from each other. If we adopt a view of the individual as an active interpreter of both the environment and the physical body that interacts with that environment, it makes sense for us to look at both the body that is seen to be the site of injury, and the person who is suffering from the actual or presumed harm. In clinical practice, we should be careful to avoid solely physiological or solely psychological explanations for a person's suffering. In accounting for the relative importance of different interpretative or cognitive factors in pain, we should also be mindful that the importance of these characteristics is often dependent upon whether the pain is acute or chronic. Research evidence has shown that we cannot afford to ignore the ameliorative effects of psychological methods of pain relief. They can be useful where pharmacological pain relief is impossible, and they can be used to enhance the effects of other treatments. Nurses and therapists have a powerful tool for creating the relief from acute pain. With chronic pain, we similarly cannot afford to focus only on the physical presentation of the patient. The experience of long-lasting persistent pain is one that changes one's interpretation and appraisal in life, one's family, home and work life, and one's sense of identity. In both assessment and treatment, we should account more fully for the patient's understanding of the cause, course and meaning of the pain.

## ■ REFERENCES

**Ahles, T.A., Cassens, H.L. & Stalling, R.B.** (1987) Private body consciousness, anxiety and the perception of pain. *Journal of Behaviour Therapy and Experimental Psychiatry* **18**, 215–222.

**Anderson, D. & Pennebaker, J.** (1980) Pain and pleasure: alternative interpretations of identical stimulation. *European Journal of Social Psychology* **10**, 207–212.

**Bacon, N.M.K., Bacon, S.F., Hampton Atkinson, J., Slater, M.A., Patterson, T.L., Grant, I. & Garfin, S.R.** (1994) Somatization symptoms in chronic low back pain patients. *Psychosomatic Medicine* **56**, 118–127.

**Bandura, A.** (1977) Self-efficacy: toward a unifying theory of behaviour change. *Psychological Review* **84**, 191–215.

**Baron, R.S., Logan, H. & Hoppe, S.** (1993) Emotional and sensory focus as mediators of dental pain among patients differing in desired and felt dental control. *Health Psychology* **12**, 381–389.

**Bortz, W.M.** (1984) The disuse syndrome. *Western Journal of Medicine* **141**, 691–694.

**Chapman, C.R. & Turner, J.A.** (1986) Psychological control of acute pain in medical settings. *Journal of Pain and Symptom Management* **1**, 9–20.

**Cioffi, D.** (1991). Beyond attentional strategies: a cognitive–perceptual model of somatic interpretation. *Psychological Bulletin* **109**, 25–41.

**Clinical Standards Advisory Committee for Back Pain** (1994) *Working Party Report on Producing the 'Management Guidelines for Back Pain'*. Department of Health Publications, HMSO, Bristol.

**Conghlan, G.M., Ridout, K.L., Williams, A.C.D. & Richardson, P.H.** (1995) Attrition from a pain management program. *British Journal of Clinical Psychology* **34**, 471–479.

**Craig, K.D.** (1994) Emotional aspects of pain. In: Wall, P.D & Melzack, R. (eds) *Textbook of Pain*, 3rd edn. Churchill Livingstone, Edinburgh.

**Crombez, G., Baeyens, F. & Eelen, P.** (1994) Sensory and temporal information about impending pain: the influence of predictability on pain. *Behaviour Research and Therapy* **32**, 611–622.

**Delvecchio Good, M.-J., Brodwin, P.E., Good, B.J. & Kleinman, A.** (eds) (1992) *Pain as Human Experience: An Anthropological Experience.* University of California Press, Berkeley, CA.

**Dolce, J.J., Crocker, M.F., Moletteire, C. & Doleys, D.M.** (1986) Exercise quotas, anticipatory concern and self-efficacy expectancies in chronic pain: a preliminary report. *Pain* **24** 365–372.

**Dubreuil, D.L., Endler, N.S. & Spanos, N.P.** (1988) Distraction and redefinition in the reduction of low and high intensity experimentally induced pain. *Imagination, Cognition and Personality* **7**, 155–164.

**Dufton, B.** (1989) Cognitive failure and chronic pain. *International Journal of Psychiatry in Medicine* **19**, 291–297.

**Eccleston, C.** (1994) Chronic pain and attention: a cognitive approach. *British Journal of Clinical Psychology* **33**, 535–547.

**Eccleston, C.** (1995) The attentional control of pain: methodological and theoretical concerns. *Pain* **63**, 3–10.

**Edwards, L., Pearce, S.A., Collett, B.-J. & Pugh, R.** (1992) Selective memory for sensory and affective information in chronic pain and depression. *British Journal of Clinical Psychology* **31**, 239–248.

**Fernandez, E. & Turk, D.C.** (1995) The scope and significance of anger in the experience of chronic pain. *Pain* **61**, 165–175.

**Flor, H. & Birbaumer, N.** (1994) Basic issues in the psychobiology of pain. In: Gebhart, G.F., Hammond, D.L. & T.S. Jensen (eds) *Proceedings of the VIIth World Congress on Pain*. IASP Press, Seattle.

**Fordyce, W.E.** (1976) *Behavioral Methods for Chronic Pain and Illness*. C.V. Mosby Company, St Louis.

**Fordyce, W.E.** (1988) Psychological factors in the failed back. *International Journal of Disability Studies* **10**, 29–31.

**Gamsa, A.** (1994) The role of psychological factors in chronic pain: a half century of study. *Pain* **57**, 5–15.

**Gracely, R.H., Dubner, R., Deeter, W.R. & Wolskee, P.J.** (1985) Clinicians' expectations influence placebo analgesia. *Lancet* **43**.

**Helman, C.G.** (1978) 'Feed a cold and starve a fever'. Folk models of infection in an English suburban community, and their relation to medical treatment. *Culture, Medicine and Psychiatry* **2**, 107–137.

**Heyneman, N.E., Fremouw, W.J., Gano, D., Kirkland, F. & Heiden, L.** (1990) Individual differences and the effectiveness of different coping strategies for pain. *Cognitive Therapy and Research* **14**, 63–77.

**Jerome, J.** (1993) Transmission or transformation? Information processing theory of chronic human pain. *American Pain Society Journal* **2**, 160–171.

**Keefe, F.J. & Lefebvre, J.C.** (1994) Behaviour therapy. In: Wall, P.D. & Melzack, R. (eds) *Textbook of Pain*, 3rd edn. Churchill Livingstone, Edinburgh.

**Kellner, R., Wiggins, R.G. & Pathak, D.** (1986) Hypochondriacal fears and beliefs in medical and law students. *Archives of General Psychiatry* **43**, 487–489.

**Kewman, D.G., Vaishampayan, N., Zald, D. & Han, B.** (1991) Cognitive impairment in musculoskeletal pain patients. *International Journal of Psychiatry in Medicine* **21**, 253–262.

**Kleinman, A.** (1988) *The Illness Narratives: Suffering, Healing and the Human Condition*. Basic Books, New York.

**Leventhal, E.A., Leventhal, H., Shacham, S. & Easterling, D.V.** (1989) Active coping reduced reports of pain from childbirth. *Journal of Consulting and Clinical Psychology* **57**, 365–371.

**Levine, J.D., Gordon, N.C., Smith, R. & Fields, H.L.** (1982) Post-operative pain: effect of injury and attention. *Brain Research* **234**, 500–504.

**Litt, M.** (1988) Self-efficacy and perceived control: cognitive mediators of pain tolerance. *Journal of Personality and Social Psychology* **54**, 149–160.

**Mason, V.** (1994) *The Prevalence of Back Pain in Great Britain*. OPCS, HMSO, London.

**McCaffery, M.** (1979) *Nursing Management of the Patient with Pain*. J.B. Lippincott Company, Philadelphia.

**McCaul, K.D. & Haugtvedt, C.** (1982) Attention, distraction, and cold-pressor pain. *Journal of Personality and Social Psychology* **43** 154–162.

**Melzack, R.** (1988) The tragedy of needless pain: a call for social action. In: Dubner, R. Gebhart, G.F. & Bond, M.R. (eds) *Proceedings of the Vth World Congress on Pain*. Elsevier, Amsterdam.

**Melzack, R.** (1989) Phantom limbs, the self and the brain (The D.O. Hebb Memorial Lecture). *Canadian Psychology* **30** 1–16.

**Melzack, R.** (1993) Pain: past, present and future. *Canadian Journal of Experimental Psychology* **47**, 615–629.

**Pearce, S., Isherwood, S., Hrouda, D., Richardson, P., Erskine, A. & Skinner, J.** (1990) Memory and pain: tests of mood congruity and state dependent learning in experimentally induced and clinical pain. *Pain* **43**, 187–193.

**Philips, H.C.** (1987) Avoidance behaviour and its role in sustaining chronic pain. *Behaviour Research and Therapy* **25**, 273–279.

**Pincus, T., Pearce, S., McClelland, A., Farley, S. & Vogel, S.** (1994) Interpretation bias in responses to ambiguous cues in pain patients. *Journal of Psychosomatic Research* **38**, 347–353.

**Price, D.D.** (1988) *Psychological and Neural Mechanism of Pain*. Raven Press, New York.

**Rachlin, H.** (1985) Pain and behavior. *The Behavioral and Brain Sciences* **8**, 43–53.

**Richardson, P.** (1989) Placebos: their effectiveness and modes of action. In: Broome, A.K. (ed.) *Health Psychology: Processes and Applications*. Chapman and Hall, London.

**Richardson, P.** (1994) Placebo effects in pain management. *Pain Reviews* 15–32.

**Romano, J.M. & Turner, J.A.** (1985) Chronic pain and depression: does the evidence support the relationship? *Psychological Bulletin* **97**, 18–34.

**Rosentiel, A.K. & Keefe, F.J.** (1983) The use of coping strategies in chronic low back pain patients: relationship to patient characteristics and current adjustment. *Pain* **17**, 33–44.

**The Royal College of Surgeons** (1990) *The College of Anaesthetists, Commission of the Provision of Surgical Service, Report on the Working Party on Pain After Surgery.* The Royal College of Surgeons of England, London.

**Stainton Rogers, W.** (1991) *Explaining Health and Illness: An Exploration of Diversity.* Harvester Wheatsheaf, New York.

**Steine, S.** (1993) Will it hurt, doctor? Factors predicting patients' experience of pain during double contrast examination of the colon. *British Medical Journal* **307**, 100.

**Steptoe, A. & Vogele, C.** (1992) Individual difference in the perception of bodily sensations: the role of trait anxiety and coping style. *Behaviour Research and Therapy* **30**, 597–607.

**Turk, D.C. & Meichenbaum, D.** (1994) A cognitive-behavioural approach to pain management. In: Wall, P.D. & Melzack, R. (eds) *Textbook of Pain*, 3rd edn. Churchill Livingstone, Edinburgh.

**Turk, D.C., Meichenbaum, D. & Genest, M.** (1983). *Pain and Behavioral Medicine: A Cognitive-Behavioral Approach.* The Guilford Press, New York.

**Turner, J.A., Deyo, R.A., Loeser, J.D. Von Korff, M. & Fordyce, W.E.** (1994) The importance of placebo effects in pain treatment and research. *JAMA* **271**, 1609–1614.

**Vlaeyen, J.W.S., Geurts, S.M., Kole-Snijders, A.M.J., Schuerman, J.A., Groenman, N.H. & Van Eck, H.** (1990) What do chronic pain patients think of their pain? Towards a pain cognition questionnaire. *British Journal of Clinical Psychology* **29**, 383–394.

**Vlaeyen, J.W.S., Kole-Snijders, A.M.J., Boeren, R.G.B. and van Eck, H.** (1995) Fear of movement in chronic low back pain and its relation to performance. *Pain* **62**, 363–372.

**Walker, J.** (1971) Pain and distraction in athletes and non-athletes. *Perceptual and Motor Skills* **33**, 1187–1190.

**Wall, P.D.** (1994) Introduction to the edition after this one. In Wall, P.D. & Melzack, R. (eds) *Textbook of Pain*, 3rd edn. Churchill Livingstone, Edinburgh.

**Wall, P.D. & Jones, M.** (1991) *Defeating Pain: The War against a Silent Epidemic.* Plenum Press, New York.

# Ethical issues in pain management

Pain caused by disease or accident is a natural phenomenon. Pain caused or allowed to continue as the result of human attitudes and practices, or as the result of human value judgements in the absence of other proportionate human values, becomes a matter of ethics. Pain control, as an ethical issue, touches the very centre of clinical practice as it is where the two goals of health care (prolonging life and alleviating suffering) come into conflict most dramatically (Lisson, 1987). The nurse's effectiveness in the management of the patient's pain comes from assessment of the pain experience *and* an increasing awareness of those aspects of pain management which clearly support the values that underlie ethically defensible responses, action and nursing care (Copp, 1985).

Ethics have been said to be the conversation between society and its members that results in expected standards of behaviour (Winslow, 1989, cited in Omery 1991). Over the past five years a plethora of material has emerged in both the British and American literature. Ethics means 'moral philosophy' and is generally a core curriculum subject in nurse education, but many nursing students find this an awesome and difficult subject (Jolley and Brykczynska, 1992). Although it may appear a dry and complex subject, the teaching of the tools of philosophy, that is, of analytical thought and rational argument, are imperative because these form the framework for ethical decision-making. Pain management is intimately linked with clinical decision-making, since nurses must decide, for instance, whether to give medication, how much, how often and by which route (Ferrell et al., 1991).

Pain control in hospitals and community settings has long been criticized, yet it continues to remain a problem, for many patients continue to suffer inhumane and unrelieved pain, with up to 75% of patients treated for pain retaining moderate to severe levels of pain (Shimm et al., 1979; Coyle, 1985). It is a subjective phenomenon, difficult to measure and sometimes invisible to the onlooker, and yet advances in pharmatherapeutics and related therapies have not significantly altered or reduced the extent of the problem. That suffering is permitted to continue begs an exploration of pain management within an ethical framework. It is the purpose of this chapter to explore the facets of ethical enquiry in relation to pain management, which will consequently heighten awareness and cause the practitioner to reflect upon his/her practice in a new light.

## ■ ETHICAL PRINCIPLES AND PAIN CONTROL

The United Kingdom Central Council Code of Professional Conduct (UKCC, 1992) notably defines itself as a 'code of professional conduct' rather than a code of ethics. Codes of ethic do exist, for instance, the Canadian Nurses Association support the Canadian Code. For a more detailed exploration of the differences refer to Chadwick and Tadd (1992). Accountability is a fundamental part of the code, which states:

> 'As a registered nurse, midwife or health visitor, you are particularly accountable for your practice and, in the exercise of your professional accountability, . . .'
>
> UKCC (1992)

The clauses that follow are then underpinned by the ethical principles, which centre on autonomy, beneficence, non-maleficence and justice. Each of these as well as veracity (truth telling) are explored, in relation to the management of pain.

## ■ RESPONSIBILITY AND ACCOUNTABILITY

Accountability can been seen as being personally *responsible* for the outcome of one's own professional actions. One can see that the two principles are implicitly linked together; by being accountable one is also held responsible. Within nursing, one has a legal accountability, which has arisen out of the training a person has had and relates to a position held. It was in 1974 that Strauss and colleagues asserted that staff were not accountable for the information they provided and the actions they took with regard to the patient in pain. They suggested that, until staff became genuinely accountable for their pain work, there would be little improvement in the care of patients and that change would only occur when pain became a matter of collective concern and organizational accountability. Twenty years on some of their vision has emerged, maybe within terminal care and chronic pain, but there is little evidence to suggest accountability has been fully acknowledged. Somerville (1986) explores 'pain and suffering' as it relates to medicine and the law, and she discusses the implications for hospitals that fail to take reasonable steps to offer adequate pain-relief treatments. She suggests that unless patients have reasonable access to pain relief treatment, hospitals could be liable for negligence in the nature of 'systems negligence'.

In exploring ethical reasoning utilized by doctors and nurses, Uden et al. (1992) suggested that physicians may be better developed in their ethical attitudes than nurses, as they use a 'more principled ethical reasoning'. Perhaps this response is enhanced by the need to avoid litigation. The rationale for this is that physicians take an individual responsibility for their decisions and actions. However, Stauffer (1993) suggests that, in the USA, the responsibility for decision-making is shifting from the physician and nurse towards the patient and family with a more shared approach. It would seem logical with the recent changes in the National Health Service that the UK would start to move towards the latter. For this to become a reality, the patient and the family need to have access to information upon which informed decisions can be made.

## ■ AUTONOMY

> *'Freedom for the professional to practise their profession in accordance with his/her professional training.'*
>
>                                                                    Engel (1970)

The concept of autonomous decision-making can be related to the examination of informed consent, informed refusal and many other forms of decision-making (Beauchamp and Childress, 1989). Firstly, let us consider the nurse. For decision-making to enable autonomous choice then knowledge must be the core element. To what extent do nurses have the knowledge upon which a course of action can be taken? A course of action is usually taken after consideration of knowledge available to that person. However, the literature on nurses' and doctors' levels of knowledge of pain control reflects that this is often inadequate (Charap, 1978; Myers, 1985; Watt-Watson, 1987). Although Griepp (1992b) suggests that individual nurses must take the moral and ethical responsibility for self-assessment of knowledge, there must also be a professional responsibility to ensure appropriate education is included in pre-registration courses and opportunities are available for further education. Ferrell et al. (1991) carried out a survey to elicit common clinical decisions related to pain, barriers to providing optimum pain relief, and ethical/professional conflicts in pain management. It was of concern that, as in many surveys of nursing knowledge, they too found that there was unfounded concern about addiction (expressed by 22% of nurses) and respiratory depression (33%). For several years the risk of such addiction has been cited as being less than 1% (American Pain Society, 1989), yet this unrealistic fear of addiction held by doctors and nurses impairs potential pain relief for the patient, and results in an ethical conflict for the nurse. Even when the nurse does have adequate knowledge about pain relief, there may be frequent and difficult decisions to be made.

There is, of course, autonomy related to the client and McCaffery and Beebe (1994, p. 11) believe the patient has various pain rights which include:

'To decide the duration and intensity of pain he is to tolerate, to be informed of all possible methods or to choose which method he wishes to try, and to choose to live with or without pain'.

The role and function of informed consent include preservation of autonomy, self-determination, inviolability, privacy and respect for the person (Somerville, 1986, p. 311). By 'informed consent' we usually mean where the patient is given all the information (including consequences and risks of proposed medical treatment and its alternatives, as well as the option of abstaining from treatment) and that the patient consents freely to the course of action taken. Faden and Beauchamp (1986) suggest that informed consent must be sought whenever a procedure is intrusive, whenever there are significant risks, and whenever the purposes of the procedure may be questionable.

The aim of informed consent has been viewed as a way of reducing suffering because informed refusal of treatment which the physician perceives as inflicting pain may at the same time reduce the suffering from the patient's point of view (Somerville, 1986). This cogent paper also explores the nature of informed consent and suffering when one is dealing with a person who has impaired cognitive functions and also when the physician fails to share information about the uncertainty of the treatment outcome. The requirements of obtaining informed consent may encourage health professionals to view each person as an individual and not as a member of a homogeneous group, which may emphasize the uniqueness of each patient and their own individual desires.

The patient in pain needs information to make an informed choice about the management of their pain; should they have an epidural or would intravenous patient-controlled analgesia be preferable? To make a decision they need to be aware of other treatments available, understand the procedure to place the epidural and be aware of the associated risks. Uncontrolled pain can have physiological and social implications beyond those perceived by the patient. If the patient lacks that information (e.g. abdominal pain may reduce the quality of respirations and predispose him to a chest infection, which could have serious implications), then once more the choice not to ask for pain relief is not freely given and patient autonomy is being violated (Omery, 1991).

Pain destroys autonomy as the patient is afraid to make the slightest movement. All choices are focused on either relieving the present pain or preventing future pain (Lisson, 1987), and ending their suffering. Cassell (1991) suggests that people frequently report 'suffering' from pain when pain is chronic, when the source of pain is unknown and when they feel out of control. Some types of pain (e.g. cancer) can exhibit all of these features, which results in helplessness and depression.

For these reasons, patients who have pain are vulnerable to any form of pain relief, hoping that it will remove the unpleasant sensation. Their autonomy is further threatened because as health care develops and treatments become more advanced, patients may become less informed and consequently leave decisions regarding their treatments to others, notably physicians (Whedon and Ferrell, 1991).

The fear of unacceptable pain laid the foundation to requests for doctor-assisted death (Helig, 1988) and pain control is so important to American cancer patients that 69% stated that they would consider suicide if their pain was not effectively controlled (Levin et al., 1985). Cain and Hammes (1994a, b) believe that the ethical dimensions of pain management must be considered with the same degree of diligence as the clinical and pharmacological dimensions. Severe unrelieved pain is a major infringement on the patient's ability to make choices regarding care, and ethically compels the health care practitioner to restore autonomy and beneficence by efficient pain control.

There are threats to a patient's autonomy that can emerge owing to a conflict of interests associated with pain treatment. In America, where hospitals purchase large numbers of patient-controlled analgesia (PCA) pumps, nurse clinicians have reported incidences where they have been instructed to seek all patients who could use the pumps, in order to generate revenue. Decisions based on revenue may conflict with patient autonomy (Pellegrino, 1982).

There is one further consideration that needs to be raised. Do all patients want to be autonomous in their pain management? If we are to consider each person as an individual, we must respect the fact that each is different, and insisting that a person exercise their autonomy could cause them stress or conflict. There are occasions when patients will not want autonomy, and look to the nurse or physician to decide. These wishes should be recognized and respected.

## ■ BENEFICENCE

'*Beneficence is the duty to do good and help others when we can at minimal risk to self.*'

Beauchamp and Childress (1989)

Beneficence can suggest acts of mercy, kindness or charity, but in its most general form the concept is not limited to these only. It also asserts an obligation to help others further their important and rightful interests (Beauchamp and Childress, 1989).

Encompassing the notion that we do good or try to help others with minimal risk to self, this principle would seem to be ignored when one considers the high incidence of the undertreatment of pain with narcotic analgesics. Common threats to beneficence for the patient in pain include undermedication, misconceptions about the nature of pain, and failure of the professions to provide adequate pain education in schools of nursing or medicine. Knowledge about appropriate pain management has advanced to such an extent that, for example, the use of meperidine for chronic pain has been classified as malpractice and, as a result, a court case following the case of a patient who was forced to die in pain has raised this possibility to a reality (Whedon and Ferrell, 1991).

## ■ NON-MALEFICENCE

'*In its simplest form nonmaleficence relates to the notion of not inflicting harm and is often viewed as the fundamental principle of the Hippocratic tradition in medical ethics.*'

Beauchamp and Childress (1989)

The principle of non-maleficence states that a nurse should avoid causing harm and strive to protect the patient from harm. However, pain treatments may decrease pain intensity but cause unpleasant side-effects, such as urinary retention, nausea, vomiting and pruritus, resulting in a decrease in the quality of life (Ferrell et al. 1989).

Nurses and doctors have been found to be overly concerned with addiction and respiratory depression when using narcotic analgesia, and may withhold them or reduce the dose through fear of causing the patient harm.

Through these discussions regarding the possibility of harmful side-effects when using opiates for the relief of pain, one may realize this principle is ignored when we consider that the sequela of uncontrolled pain can result in pulmonary complications, deep vein thrombosis and the deleterious consequences of immobility. Nurses must work with patients and physicians to achieve effective client analgesia, but there are times when nurses may meet physicians who maintain that providing pain relief actually violates the principles of non-maleficence (Omery, 1991). In discussing clients with peripheral vascular disease, Omery remarks that the physicians believe negative consequences result from the physiological–pharmacological effects of pain medications in those patients where a line of ischaemic demarcation is being determined prior to surgery. However, allowing the patient to suffer pain violates both the principles of beneficence and non-maleficence. Somerville (1993a) suggests that there should be limits to what health care professionals may do to relieve suffering, saying that:

> 'the provision of all reasonably necessary treatment or the relief of pain or other symptoms of serious physical distress are ethically and legally acceptable.'

However, physician-assisted suicide and euthanasia are not ethically and legally acceptable, and highlight that the 'middle' approach between the two is difficult to establish and maintain. It is the situation where to act will have undesirable consequences and not to act will also have undesirable consequences, resulting in what is often termed the 'double effect' (Rumbold, 1986). In making decisions where either course of action could be harmful, four criteria should be met. These are:

1. The act itself must be morally good or at least neutral.
2. The purpose must be to achieve good consequence, the bad consequence being only a side-effect.
3. The good effect must not be achieved by way of the bad, but both must result from the same act.
4. The bad result must not be so serious as to outweigh the advantage of a good result.

In pain management this principle emerges quite obviously. Consider the scenario where a patient is dying from cancer and is experiencing severe pain. The doctor knows that to increase the dose of narcotic to relieve the pain will also hasten the patient's death. In this case death could be described as a side-effect of the treatment but it is clearly the doctor's duty to try to alleviate the pain. To leave the patient in pain would not be ethically defensible. A similar argument operates when the medical staff attempt to withhold adequate pain relief for fear of causing addiction. Although this judgement may be based on faulty knowledge (as previously mentioned), there is a question to be asked: 'Does it really matter if the terminally ill patient becomes addicted?'. The goal for the relief of suffering must be paramount.

Somerville (1986) considers the legal issue, which is raised when there is inadequate treatment of pain in the hospitalized patient. Namely, is it lawful to give pain relief treatment when this may shorten life? The issues raised are clarified by considering 'patient variables', such as terminally ill patients, non-terminally ill patients, non-terminally ill patients with severe chronic pain and consent to pain treatment. When considering the patient suffering from terminal illness, then failure to give pain relief treatment (which may potentially shorten life) may constitute a breach of duty and result in negligence. In contrast, the non-terminally ill patients whose life may be shortened by having pain-relief treatment, especially where the pain is of a short duration, is unacceptable and should be forbidden. The harm avoided–benefit conferred/harm inflicted–benefit lost assessment of each possible course of action must conclude with an overall positive balance in favour of benefit.

## ■ JUSTICE

*'The common definition that relates to justice has been attributed to the writings of Aristotle who suggested that equals must be treated equally, and unequals must be treated unequally.'*

(Beauchamp and Childress, 1989, p. 259).

This also pertains to the distribution of resources, in that they should be distributed fairly and individuals should have equal access to care. The ability to act with equality and impartiality when managing a patient's pain is not supported by the literature when one considers patient variables, such as age, sex and social class. There are numerous examples where patients' suffering and pain have been found to be attributable to patient characteristics. For instance, Burke and Jerrett (1989) found that student nurses' perceptions of the best management strategy for people with acute pain varied, depending on the age of the client. In general, more options were selected by the students for persons of their own age group (adolescents and adults) than those who were younger or older. As already highlighted in Chapter 2, the literature of gender and pain relief is inconclusive. Disturbingly, Morgan (1988, cited in Oden, 1989) reviewed the charts of 106 patients having cholecystectomy and found that less medication was given to those patients who did not have private insurance and those who were non-White.

There is little current literature which has costed the consequences of high-technology pain management, but it is unlikely to be long before such data are available. Common costs associated with pain-relief technology include epidural catheters, infusion devices and supplies. Current costs of PCA infusion pumps are in excess of £2000 and several models require special tubing and cassettes. Owen et al. (1988) have argued that, by giving 'high-risk' patients PCA, hospital costs can be reduced. The evidence does suggest that PCA can be cost-effective by saving time in drug administration (Ready, 1990; Thomas, 1991).

There is a need to consider the principle of justice in pain management. The judgements that are made in the process of assessing pain and the subsequent nature of the action taken also require more careful consideration. As pain technology advances, there will be an increasing need to take into account the ethical and clinical concerns and particularly their relationship to justice.

## ■ VERACITY

The four moral principles that have previously been discussed are drawn upon and applied to establish rules of veracity (to tell the truth, not to lie or deceive others), confidentiality and privacy. It is the rule of veracity which is of particular concern when we consider the patient who has pain. In contrast to the previously mentioned codes, the code of medical ethics generally ignores the rules of veracity, although it is commonly agreed that we have an obligation to veracity (Beauchamp and Childress, 1989). Are we truthful when we give an intramuscular injection and we say 'this won't hurt'? In the face of administering painful treatments (debriding wounds, removing packs or sutures) are nurses truthful to the patient about the amount of pain they are likely to experience? Whilst one would not wish to frighten patients, surely they have a right to know the truth? Equally important is believing the patient.

How much pain should be endured in the name of therapy? The responsibility for acquainting the patient with the facts of undesirable side-effects of radiation or chemotherapy may be assumed by the physician, but it is the nurse who will support the patient hour after hour in their pain. The responsibility for management of untoward symptoms associated with therapies is often assumed by the nurse, and the physician is spared confrontation of the facts, feelings and issues; the ethical dimension may go unrecognized (Copp, 1985).

## ■ A MODEL OF ETHICAL DECISION-MAKING

The ethical decision-making process is the core element that encompasses health care practice, yet its nature and complexity have changed dramatically owing to major advances in technology, scientific progress, economic constraints and the consumer's higher expectations (Grundstein-Amado, 1993). Griepp (1992a) designed a model of ethical decision-making to

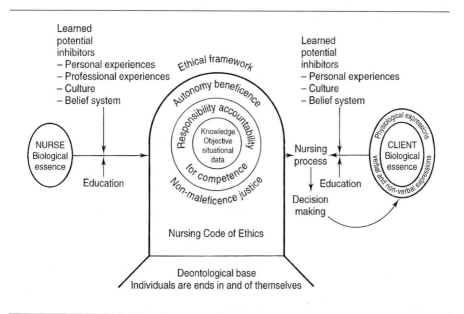

*Figure 4.1.* Griepp's model of ethical decision-making. (Reproduced from Griepp (1992a) with kind permission of Blackwell Science Ltd.)

illustrate an overall conception of the interaction between the nurse and the client within an ethical framework. The underlying theory of the model is systems theory and is compatible with the extensive work done by Leininger and her theory of transcultural nursing (Leininger, 1978).

Griepp (1992b) has applied her model to decision-making and pain management, and considers not only the ethical principles already discussed but relates the 'learned potential inhibitors' of both the nurse (as these can influence the decision) and the patient. Learned potential inhibitors are defined as the nurse's and patient's psychosocio-cultural variables that may enhance the person's interactions with others, relative to pain experiences (Griepp, 1992a). Importantly she suggests that the model will generate further scientific enquiry by identifying breakdown in ethical decision-making for and by patients experiencing pain. By framing pain management in an ethical context, positive change may be facilitated in clinical practice. Figure 4.1 is an illustration of Griepp's model applied to pain management.

The model starts on the left-hand side by considering the nurse and the influence of the learned potential inhibitors. These inhibitors are powerful as they enlighten or bias the nurse as caregiver, as well as shape the patients' pain responses and behaviours. From the literature there is ample empirical evidence supporting the influence of these variables on pain assessment, which will now be discussed.

# ■ THE NURSE AND PATIENT: LEARNED POTENTIAL INHIBITORS

The personal experiences of the nurse have been shown to influence his/her assessment of the patient's pain and inference of suffering (Davitz and Davitz, 1981). Holm et al. (1989) conducted a study to determine the effects of nurses' personal pain experiences on the assessment of their patients' pain. Their findings support the notion that nurses who have experienced intense pain are more sympathetic to the patient in pain. Griepp (1992a) considers all of an individual's pain experiences, from birth to the present, as influencing their pain. The study by Walmsley et al. (1992) exploring patients' expectations of postoperative pain, found that the two variables that correlated significantly with pain expected post-surgically were: (1) a single item from the interview schedule 'pain is to be expected after surgery even with medicine'; and (2) the total of the global ratings of past pain experiences (the sum of global surgical pain, global trauma pain, global childbirth pain, chronic pain and other pain). The latter finding supports Griepp's predictions. However, there is a paucity of research in this important area.

Being pain-free is analogous to being comfortable and, according to Schunior (1994), providing comfort is the *raison d'être* of nursing. In spite of their substantial power to enhance comfort, nurses have by and large availed themselves of this authority only partially and inconsistently (Schunior, 1994). With respect to managing pain, they relinquish the control to physicians and yet historically the management of pain has been given greater priority in nursing than medicine. The failure to recognize that pain control lies within the nursing domain stems from the devaluation of practice disciplines (Benner and Wrubel, 1989). In general, nurses are motivated to provide the 'best' nursing care and consequently experience great frustration when the care environment does not permit this (Benner and Wrubel, 1989). Research on clinical decision-making and pain identified inadequate pain relief as the most frequent ethical/professional conflict that nurses experience, whilst undermedicating the patient was the second most common (Ferrell et al., 1991).

Nurses' decisions regarding pain control have significant outcomes, some of which have deleterious (for example, respiratory depression) consequences. Nurses make mental cost–benefit analyses in their daily management of pain, which can represent a barrier to effective pain relief. The main problem with nurses undertaking such analyses is that they are frequently carried out without involving the patient. This behaviour reflects a paternalism, which is at odds with sharing information that will allow patients to make their own decisions if they so wish.

Professional experiences may also affect the nurse's assessment of pain; negative experiences can precipitate negative attitudes (Lisson, 1987) and experience does not always protect the practitioner from making faulty clinical decisions. Although the amount of information a person has increases their confidence in their decision-making (Oskamp, 1965, cited in Lander, 1990), confidence has been negatively related to accuracy in judgement.

Perhaps this poor relationship between experience and confidence stems from the already mentioned devaluation of nursing as a practice discipline. Benner and Wrubel (1989) have argued that giving status and legitimization to the clinical judgement inherent in skilled practice is essential to an accurate valuation of nursing care. This, in turn, will ensure that patients benefit, through having the diagnostic and monitoring abilities of the nurse endorsed by physicians and other health care professionals (Benner and Wrubel, 1989).

When culture is considered, as a nurse variable, the classic work by Davitz and Davitz (1980), described in Chapter 2, illuminates clearly how the social and cultural background of both the patient and the nurse influenced a nurse's assessment of the degree of pain a patient was feeling.

In the UK where patients come from a variety of cultures, nurses should be aware of their own values and biases, and the ways in which they affect their interaction with patients who are culturally different. Although some values and biases cannot be changed or modified, being aware of their existence and their effects can help to monitor any prejudices (Pedersen, 1988). It is extremely important for nurses to recognize and accept that there are differences, since it is impossible for them to adapt themselves to every value system with which they interact.

Diversity in human beings brings life, vibrancy and colour to society (Kareem, 1992). However, as the late Jafar Kareem (1992) has argued, diversity can sometimes cause tension and mistrust, but this is a concern for *all* humans (my italics).

The belief system is the basic set of values and assumptions, which the person holds to be true regarding pain, suffering, treatment and analgesia, which may or may not be based on fact (Griepp, 1992b). Many studies have clearly demonstrated that the nurse may hold erroneous beliefs about the nature of the patient's pain. Attitudes towards pain were essentially learned responses, which reflected the values and beliefs of the nurse's own background (Weis et al., 1983; Dudley and Kolm, 1984; Ketovuori, 1987). As stated above, being aware of our biases is an important initial step in rectifying this learned inhibitor.

For the patient the belief system and its influence on pain can be very powerful. Patients may believe that to suffer pain is good for them and they may view it as necessary to their recovery. If the patient believes that pain builds character, this may influence their pain behaviour (Weis et al., 1983). Illogical beliefs that reduce the patient's opportunity to have effective pain relief need to be explored and where appropriate dispelled. Nurses, therefore, have important roles in providing information and evidence to refute these views.

The value of this model to the nurse is that it holds the essential ethical principles within the centre of the model, whilst clearly defining relevant variables on both the nurse and client side. These factors have often appeared in the literature as contributing to poor pain management but have not, to date, been brought together collectively in a framework that connects them so logically and emphasizes their crucial influence on the decision-making process.

## ■ CONCLUSION

It has been the intention of this chapter to bring together the ethical principles within the context of pain and to consider how our decision-making can be influenced by an ethical framework. Pain is a critical ethical issue because of its capacity to dehumanize, and complicated by the fact that it is a subjective, qualitative experience being treated in an objective, empirically focused health care environment (Lisson, 1987).

Margaret Somerville (1993a) identifies trust as one of the basic obligations for relieving pain. Trust is essential for the formation of all good relationships and, in nursing, the ability to establish trust is the hallmark of good nursing. However, when we talk of trust we may not mean the same thing. Somerville (1993b) distinguishes between 'blind trust', which she describes as paternalistically based, and 'earned trust' that is based on an egalitarian relationship. Blind trust is established on differentials in role, power and status, and is manifest in the unspoken communication of 'You should trust me because I know what is best for you and will act only in your best interest'. In contrast, earned trust makes no use of role, power and status, and is reflected in the statement 'You can trust me because I will show you that you can trust me'.

Somerville (1993b) suggests that the theory of trust that we uphold will influence our approach to caring for the person in pain. Control of pain reduces suffering and restores 'sanity'. Since humans have a tendency towards self-enhancement (Eiser, 1986), it is reasonable to assume that nurses and other health care professionals believe that they utilize the 'earned trust' approach in their management of pain. However, an important point to make is that, when we leave our patients in pain, we are in effect demanding their trust (i.e. using a blind trust perspective), we are not earning their trust. Somerville believes that failure to relieve pain is counter to establishing earned trust.

Reflecting on the literature pertaining to pain management, one repeatedly finds studies illuminating inappropriate attitudes, knowledge and practices. Despite advances in pain management technology, such as PCA, one cannot help feeling concern that health care professionals are not utilizing the already available knowledge in their practice. Discussing pain within an ethical framework may coerce practitioners to consider anew the implications of their actions, which in turn may lead to a genuine reappraisal of our central role in pain and suffering.

# ■ REFERENCES

**American Pain Society** (1989) *Principles of Analgesia Use in the Treatment of Acute Pain and Chronic Cancer Pain*, 2nd edn. American Pain Society, Stokie, IL.

**Beauchamp, T.L. & Childress, J.F.** (1989) *Principles of Biomedical Ethics*. Open University, Milton Keynes.

**Bellville, J.W., Forrest W.H., Miller, E. & Brown, B.W.** (1971) Influence of age on pain relief from analgesics. *JAMA* **217**, 1835–1841.

**Benner, P. & Wrubel, J.** (1989) *The Primacy of Caring: Stress and Coping in Health and Illness*. Addison-Wesley, Menlo Park, CA.

**Burke, S.O. & Jerrett, M.** (1989) Pain management across age groups. *Western Journal of Nursing Research* **11** (2), 164–180.

**Cain, J.M. & Hammes, B.J.** (1994a) Ethics and pain management: respecting patient wishes. *Journal of Pain and Symptom Management* **9**(3), 160–165.

**Cain, J.M. & Hammes, B.J.** (1994b) Ethics and pain management for cancer patients: case studies and analysis. *Journal of Pain and Symptom Management* **9**(3), 166–170.

**Calvillo, E.R. & Flaskerud, J.H.** (1993) Evaluation of the pain response by Mexican Americans and Anglo American women and their nurses. *Journal of Advanced Nursing* **18**, 451–459.

**Cassell, E.J.** (1991) *The Nature of Suffering and the Goals of Medicine*. Oxford University Press, Oxford.

**Chadwick, R. & Tadd, W.** (1992) *Ethics and Nursing Practice: A Case Study Approach*. Macmillan Education, London, pp. 3–16.

**Charap, A.D.** (1978) The knowledge, attitudes and experiences of medical personnel treating pain in the terminally ill. *The Mount Sinai Journal of Medicine* **45**(4), July–August, 561–580.

**Copp, L.A.** (1985) Pain, ethics and the negotiation of values. In: *Perspectives on Pain. Recent Advances in Nursing* Vol. 11. Churchill Livingstone, Edinburgh, pp. 137–150.

**Coyle, N.** (1985) Symptom management: pain – an overview of current concepts. *Cancer Nursing* 1 (Suppl.), 44–49.

**Davitz, L.L. & Davitz, J.R.** (1980) *Nurses' Response to Patients' Suffering*. Springer-Verlag, New York.

**Davitz J.R. & Davitz, L.J.** (1981) *Influences on Patients' Pain and Psychological Distress*. Springer-Verlag, New York.

**Dudley, S.R. & Holm, K.** (1984) Assessment of the pain experience in relation to selected nurse characteristics. *Pain* **18** (2), 179–186.

**Eiser, R.** (1986) *Social Psychology: Attitudes, Cognition and Social Behaviour*. Cambridge University Press, Cambridge.

**Engel, G.** (1970) Professional autonomy and bureaucratic organisation. *Administration Sciences Quarterly* **15**, 12–21.

**Faden, R.R. & Beauchamp, T.L.** (1986) *A History and Theory of Informed Consent.* Oxford University Press, New York, pp. 288–336.

**Ferrell, B.R., Wisdom, C. & Wenzl, C.** (1989) Quality of life as an outcome variable in the management of cancer pain. *Cancer* **63**, 2257–2265.

**Ferrell, B.R., Eberts, M.T., McCaffery, M. & Grant, M.** (1991) Clinical decision making and pain. *Cancer Nursing* **14** (6), 289–297.

**Griepp, M.E.** (1992a) Griepp's model of ethical decision making. *Journal of Advanced Nursing* **17**, 734–738.

**Griepp, M.E.** (1992b) Undermedication for pain: an ethical model. *Advances in Nursing Science* **15** (1), 44–53.

**Grundstein-Amado, R.** (1993) Ethical decision-making processes used by health care providers. *Journal of Advanced Nursing* **18**, 1701–1709.

**Helig, S.** (1988) The San Francisco Medical Society Euthanasia Survey: results and analysis. *San Francisco Medicine* **61**, 24–34.

**Holm, K., Cohen, F., Duda, S., Medema, P.G. & Allen, B.** (1989) Effect of personal pain experiences on pain assessment. *IMAGE: Journal of Nursing Scholarship* **21** (2), 72–75.

**Jolley, M. & Brykczynska, G.** (eds) (1992) *Nursing Care: The Challenge to Change.* Edward Arnold, London.

**Kareem, J.** (1992) The Nafsiyat Intercultural Therapy Centre: ideas and experience in intercultural therapy. In: Kareem, J. & Littlewood, R. (eds) *Intercultural Therapy: Themes, Interpretations and Practice.* Blackwell Scientific Publications, Oxford, pp. 14–37.

**Ketovuori, H.** (1987) Nurses' and patients' conceptions of wound pain and the administration of analgesics. *Journal of Pain and Symptom Management* **2**(4), 213–218.

**Lander, J.** (1990) Clinical judgements in pain management. *Pain* **42**, 15–22.

**Leininger, M.** (ed.) (1978) *Transcultural Nursing: Concepts, Theories and Practices.* John Wiley & Sons, New York.

**Levin, D.N., Cleeland, C.S. & Dar, R.** (1985) Public attitudes towards cancer. *Cancer* **56**, 2337–2339.

**Lisson, E.L.** (1987) Ethical issues related to pain control. *Nursing Clinics of North America* **22**(3), 649–659.

**McCaffery, M. & Beebe, A.** (1994) *Pain: Clinical Manual for Nursing Practice.* Mosby, St Louis.

**Myers, J.S.** (1985) Cancer pain: assessment of nurses' knowledge and attitudes. *Oncology Nursing Forum* **12**(4), 63–66.

**Oden, R.V.** (1989) Acute postoperative pain: incidence, severity and the etiology of inadequate treatment. *Anaesthesiology Clinics of North America* **7**(1), 1–5.

**Omery, A.** (1991) Culpability and pain management: control in peripheral vascular disease using the ethics of principles and care. *Critical Care Nursing Clinics of North America* **3**(3), 551–558.

**Owen, H., Mather, L. & Rowley, K.** (1988) The development and clinical use of patient controlled analgesia. *Anaesthesia and Intensive Care* **16**(4), 437–447.

**Pedersen, P.** (1988) In: Alexandria, V.A. (ed.) *A Handbook of Developing Cultural Awareness.* American Association for Counselling Development.

**Pellegrino, E.D.** (1982) The clinical ethics of pain management in the terminally ill. *Hospital Formulary* **17**(7), 1493–1496.

**Ready, L.B.** (1990) The economics of patient controlled analgesia. In: Ferrant, F.M., Ostheimer G.W. & Covino B.G. (eds), *Patient Controlled Analgesia.* Blackwell Scientific Publications, Boston, pp. 191–197.

**Rumbold, G.** (1986) Ethics in Nursing Practice. *Balliere Tindall, London.*

**Schunior, C.E.** (1994) Patient comfort: the nurse's imperative. In: Funk, S.G., Tornquist, E.M., Champagne, M.T., Copp, L.A. & Weise, R.A. (eds) *Management of Pain Fatigue and Nausea.* Macmillan Press, Basingstoke, pp. 312–316.

**Shimm, D.S., Logue, G.L. & Malbie, A.A.** (1979) Medical management of chronic cancer pain. *JAMA* **241**, 2408–2412.

**Somerville, M.A.** (1986) Pain and suffering at interfaces of medicine and law. *University of Toronto Law Journal* **36** (3), 286–317.

**Somerville, M.A.** (1993a) Pain, suffering and ethics. Paper presented at the *7th World Congress on Pain*, August 22–27, Paris, France. International Association for the Study of Pain Publications, Seattle.

**Somerville, M.A.** (1993b) Death of pain. In: Gebhart, G.F., Hammond, D.L. & Jensen, T.S. (eds) *Proceedings of the 7th World Congress on Pain: Progress in Pain, Research and Management*, Vol. 2. IASP Publications, Seattle, pp. 41–58.

**Stauffer, G.M.** (1993) Janforum. Ethical decision-making: the patient's right. *Journal of Advanced Nursing* **18**, 1854.

**Strauss, A., Fagerhaugh, S.Y. & Glaser, B.** (1974) Pain: an organisational-work-interactional perspective. *Nursing Outlook* **22**(9), 560–566.

**Taenzer P., Melzack, R. & Jeans, M.E.** (1986) Influence of psychological factors on postoperative pain, mood and analgesic requirements. *Pain* **24**, 331–342.

**Thomas, V.J.** (1991) *Personality Characteristics of Patients and the Effectiveness of Patient Controlled Analgesia.* Unpublished Ph.D. thesis, Goldsmiths' College, University of London.

**Uden, G., Norberg, A., Lindseth, A. & Marhaug, V.** (1992) Ethical reasoning in nurses' and physicians' stories about care episodes. *Journal of Advanced Nursing* **17**(9), 1028–1034.

**United Kingdom Central Council for Nursing, Midwifery and Health Visiting (UKCC)** (1992) *Code of Professional Conduct*, 3rd edn. UKCC, London.

**Walmsley, P.N.H., Brockopp, D.Y. & Brockopp, G.W.** (1992) The role of pain experience and expectations on postoperative pain. *Journal of Pain and Symptom Management* **7**(1), 34–37.

**Watt-Watson, J.H.** (1987) Nurses' knowledge of pain issues: a survey. *Journal of Pain and Symptom Management* **2**(4), 207–211.

**Weis, O.F., Sriwatanakul, K., Alloza, J.L., Weintraub, M. & Lasagna, L.** (1983) Attitudes of patients, housestaff, and nurses towards postoperative analgesia care. *Anaesthesia and Analgesia* **62**, 70–74.

**Whedon, M. & Ferrell, B.R.** (1991) Professional and ethical considerations in the use of high-tech pain management. *Oncology Nursing Forum* **18**(7), 1135–1143.

# The assessment of pain

## ■ INTRODUCTION

A major obstacle to accurate assessment of pain is the subjective nature of
the experience. Describing pain is a very complex task and the fact that
people use different words to describe their pain adds to the complexity.
The language used by a patient to describe his/her pain may convey a
different message from that which is intended because the patient and the
nurse use language in different ways owing to their individual experiences
and perspectives. For these reasons pain can only be assessed indirectly
(Turk and Melzack, 1992). The effects of analgesic drug therapies can be
assessed and improved only if some form of measurement of the effects is
made.

Within the clinical practice of acute postoperative pain control, the routine
use of measurement of analgesic efficacy is very rare (Mitchell and Smith,
1989). Instead there is a reliance on subjective assessments made by nursing
staff, which have been shown to be inaccurate (Seers, 1987). Pain cannot be

properly controlled if it is not assessed. Objective assessment techniques have relied upon biochemical indices such as the changes in plasma concentrations of hormones, but these tend to be inaccurate, expensive and not applicable in clinical practice (Mitchell and Smith, 1989), although simple respiratory function tests may be a useful indicator of pain severity after abdominal and thoracic surgery (Chapman, 1989). Posture and facial expression can be observed and are part of the behavioural aspects of acute pain. Although an experienced observer may be able to use these indicators to make a rough estimate of the degree of pain suffered by the patient, it is widely accepted that the amount of suffering can only be assessed by the individual concerned (Reading, 1984; McCaffery and Beebe, 1989; Barker and Hughes, 1990; Green, 1990).

In recent years some advances have been made in the clinical measurement and evaluation of pain. A huge area of research has been devoted to the development of assessment tools, which are aimed at enhancing the person's verbal expression of their suffering so that they can convey their subjective experience.

The nursing assessment of pain is vital if effective management is to be achieved, and yet Carr (Chapter 10) and King (Chapter 15) have presented substantial evidence which demonstrates that nurses are poor assessors of pain. McGuire (1984) has suggested that nurses' assessment and pain management skills are limited because they rarely use assessment tools which reflect the multidimensional nature of pain. This has resulted in a recommendation for education initiatives which would instruct nurses in the assessment of psychophysiological factors (Dalton, 1989). Education is of vital importance because the evidence does suggest that experienced nurses provide more detailed and accurate pain assessments (see Chapter 15).

## ■ THE PROCESS OF PAIN ASSESSMENT

McGuire (1993) suggests that pain assessment is synonymous with surveillance. She suggests that surveillance implies a 'constant watchfulness to anticipate or predict so that early interventions may be initiated'. A surveillance framework helps to establish objectives and priorities, and allows planning and structure in the delivery of care (McGuire, 1993).

Therefore the main reasons for assessing pain are to assist in establishing a baseline, to select appropriate interventions and to evaluate the patient's response to treatment. This demands that patients are actively involved in their own care. McGuire (1993) suggests that the chief benefit of pain assessments for patients is that the pain is legitimized, described and quantified. In undertaking pain assessment, nurses also benefit because they obtain a better understanding of the nature of pain as well as taking more responsibility and accountability for pain management (McGuire, 1993).

Accurate pain assessment requires effective communication skills and Meinhart and McCaffery (1983) have suggested that, during pain assessments, nurses should gather the following pain information:

1. Location
2. Quality
3. Pattern
4. Intensity
5. Factors that increase the pain
6. Verbal statements about the pain
7. Non-verbal expression
8. Associated symptoms

During assessment the communication process will be effective if nurses can also ascertain from the person in pain what pain means to him/her, what goals he/she wishes to achieve and the types of relief methods he/she finds acceptable and useful. Communication is a two-way process so nurses should not just extract information from patients, they ought to provide information for the patients as well. This is especially useful in acute pain settings, such as the surgical and coronary care settings. In these situations fear and anxiety are high so nurses have the important role of providing information in order to reduce distress. As the classic work Information: Prescription against Pain by Hayward (1975) has shown, accurate information allows patients to interpret and understand their circum-stances, removing uncertainty, reducing helplessness and enhancing their sense of personal control over their environment. Research has shown that both procedural information, which includes details of an impending operation (Miller et al., 1989) and sensory information about what the patient will see, feel and hear (Johnson et al., 1978), are important sources of information for sharing with patients.

Patients experiencing pain display a wide range of observable behaviour, which communicates to others that they are in pain. Therefore the assessment of non-verbal communication cues is also an important part of pain assessment. However, as Carroll (1993) points out, nurses should not rely on non-verbal cues as the primary index. Non-verbal pain cues include restlessness, facial expressions and vocal signals, such as sighing or crying. Fordham and Dunn (1994) suggest that measurements of pulse and blood pressure are useful observations to make in conjunction with the assessment of non-verbal cues, and these are of paramount importance in the management of children's pain (see Chapter 9 for an account of the barriers which hinder effective assessment and management of pain in children).

# ■ ASSESSING CHILDREN'S PAIN

In the absence of language, pain assessment must depend on the physiological and behavioural parameters of pain. Effective management of children's pain therefore requires skilful knowledge concerning children's responses. Elevated heart rate and blood pressure, poor oxygenation and palm sweating are good physiological indices, but observation of behaviour is the principal assessment method for the pre-linguistic child and is an adjunct to assessment in children with language. Facial expressions (Izard and Dougherty, 1982), body movement (Davis and Calhoon, 1994; Mills, 1994) and crying behaviour (Fuller et al., 1994) have been evaluated, and found to be reliable indices of pain and infant distress.

## ▪ Facial expressions of pain in young children

According to Craig et al. (1992), infants' facial response is the most obvious behavioural evidence of pain. Support for this suggestion comes from Johnson and Strada (1986), who reported that the facial response to injection pain was more consistent across infants than were cry patterns, heart rate or body movements. The Neonatal Facial Coding System (NFCS) provides an objective and detailed approach for studying infants' reaction to painful stimuli. Using this measure, Grunau and Craig (1987) were able to classify a relatively stereotypical pattern of facial display. Craig et al. (1992) suggest that this is comprised of lowered brow, squeezed shut eyes, deepened nasolabial furrow (a line that begins adjacent to the nostrils and extends down and out beyond the lip), an opened mouth, and a taut, cupped tongue. The authors suggest that the remarkable similarity between the newborn and adult facial response to pain provides ample evidence that the newborn infant has a capacity to experience and to communicate pain when subjected to invasive procedures. Comparisons have been made of the facial expressions of pain in full-term and pre-term infants (Craig et al., 1991; cited in Craig et al., 1992) and the findings indicate that the general pattern of facial activity in pre-terms was essentially the same as full-term infants (see Craig et al., 1992, for details of this measure and a thorough discussion).

## ▪ Crying behaviour

Crying is the most obvious and insistent way the child has of conveying levels of discomfort. According to Fuller et al. (1994), vocal measures of pain are very useful because they draw the carer's attention to the infant, and this in turn influences the infant–carer relationship. In addition crying involves complex neurophysiological mechanisms providing subtle cues about the child's biological status. Early research found that differences in acoustic tenseness of an infant's cry is a useful way of differentiating infants' hunger-induced cries from pain-induced cries (Wasz-Hockert et al., 1968, cited in Fuller et al., 1994) and Johnston (1989) has found that a tense, high-pitched cry is characteristic of very stressed states.

Fuller et al. (1994) investigated tenseness (high voice energy and frequency) and pitch as acoustic indices of pain during circumcision in children aged from 2 to 6 months. The results indicated that crying associated with non-physical trauma (restraint and betadine cleansing) gave rise to crying with increased tenseness whereas physical trauma gave rise to crying characterized by increases in both tenseness and pitch. The authors suggest that these indices are cues that paediatric nurses could learn in order to differentiate between combinations of tenseness and other cues in children's cries when assessing pain.

In addition to crying, observation of infants and young children's physical movements can provide valuable information about pain. In an attempt to document acute pain behaviour in children, Mills (1994) studied 32 infants and toddlers ranging from birth to 3 years in age. A summary of the results is presented below, revealing interesting and marked differences between the age groups, which was primarily a function of the developmental or maturational processes (see Mills, 1994, for a detailed account of the findings).

## ∎ Pain behaviour in infants

### Birth to 3 months

The physical extremities movements ranged from mild wriggling and kicking of arms and legs to flailing, thrashing and hard kicking associated with loud crying. Clenched fists were a common feature, and infants' cries ranged from brief mild crying and grunting to sustained intense crying. Facial expressions varied from neutral to frowning or grimacing. Infants interacted less with parents when they were in pain than when they were pain free. After surgery, babies who moved normally a few times cried out in pain and thereafter quickly learned to move less often.

### Infants 3–6 months

Movements in the extremities were the same as those of younger infants but Mills reported that there was a greater level of control. Squirming, writhing and frequent jerking were common body movements. Jerking prevented children from sleeping well at night. Pain medication reduced the frequency of jerking but did not abolish it. Infants' communications consisted of moans, whimpers and restrained cries. Crying became vigorous and prolonged if the children coughed or were moved suddenly. Infants were not interested in playing and were inclined to cling to mothers. They were able to console themselves by putting a pacifier in their own mouths. During times of severe pain, infants lost control and parents' attempts at consoling were usually ineffective.

### Infants 6–9 months

New movements in this age group included hand wringing, pinching or biting themselves or rubbing a body part. Children with burns screamed during dressing changes and made attempts to escape burn debridement. Children also cried as a response to non-painful events, such as being moved to the treatment room, seeing nurses wearing masks and when parents were leaving. Aggressive behaviour towards staff was displayed during procedures. Playing with a toy brought brief distraction for some children.

### Infants 9–12 months

Children were observed to move a nurse's hand away. Crying was prolonged and children cried out for mummy during procedures. Infants responded to nurses' verbal cues such as 'almost done' or 'all done' by becoming quiet. Some children wore angry expressions and exhibited aggressive behaviour during painful procedures.

### Toddlers 12–18 months

Much more sophisticated avoidance behaviour is evident in this age group. For example, one child fought to take a wash cloth from a nurse and to push her away. Children cried at the sight of their own blood, when they saw syringes or scissors, and when wounds were being checked. Toddlers were more wary and vigilant than younger children and the memory of earlier painful procedures contributed to this vigilance. Children resisted nurses by kicking them. Toys were useful in providing brief distraction.

### Toddlers 18–24 months

The major changes in this age range came from their improving ability to communicate linguistically. New words included 'ow', 'hurts' and 'burns'. Children were now much more able to comprehend and complied willingly with nurses' requests. Play with parents was common but this was sometimes interrupted by cries from muscle spasms.

### Toddlers 24–36 months

Toddlers in this age group became increasingly more articulate, expressing their pain to nurses by saying 'yes it hurts', 'my hurt' and 'I am mad'. They requested information such as 'why' and are you 'done'. Verbal resistance such as 'no bath' was now common and delaying tactics featured in the form of 'I want to go to bed', or putting on a pouting facial expression. As language skills increased so did the degree of sophistication displayed. There was an increase in the amount of anger and aggression displayed towards parents and nurses. Toddlers commonly attributed blame, especially among the 30–36 months age group, when children were sometimes observed to refuse help to get up or being turned by saying to nurses or parents 'no! you hurt me'.

It is evident from Mills' research that children are capable of displaying many pain behaviours, which caregivers can use as reliable measures of pain and distress.

## ▪ Pain assessment scales for assessing children's pain

There are now a wide range of qualitative and quantitative instruments for measuring the sensory and emotional aspects of children's pain. These include projective methods, in which children's attitudes or perceptions of pain are inferred from their selection of colours, their drawing, or their interpretation of cartoons and stories (Unruh et al., 1983; Kurylyszyn et al., 1987) and self-report measures, which directly describe their pain and rate its intensity (Hester, 1979; Abu-Saad, 1984; McGrath and Unruh, 1987; Varni et al., 1987; Aradine et al., 1988; Tesler et al., 1988; McGrath, 1990; Wilkie et al., 1990). A brief description of some of the commonly used self-report pain assessment tools will be presented here, but the reader is referred to McGrath et al. (1993) for a more comprehensive coverage.

### Rating scales

There are a number of rating scales commonly used to measure pain in the clinical situation. These vary according to the nature and number of anchor points supplied, and include numbers, words or the presentation of visual analogue lines. Visual analogue scales (VASs) consist of a straight line, with numerical, verbal or pictorial anchors and the ends representing the extreme limits of pain. The child makes a mark on the line appropriate to the level of pain he or she is experiencing (see Figs 5.1, 5.2 and 5.3). VASs are particularly valuable in children with limited language skills and among non-English-speaking adults.

VASs provide valid and reliable pain measurements and correlate highly with parents' and nurses' pain ratings (Varni et al., 1987). Although Ross and Ross (1988) have suggested that verbal rating scales (VRSs) may be difficult for children to interpret, their successful use naturally depends on the cognitive and educational level of the child (Wilkie et al., 1990).

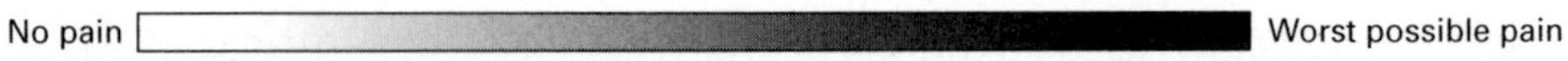

No pain ⎡_____⎤ Worst possible pain

*Figure 5.1. Visual analogue scaling. This scale should normally be 10 cm in length.*

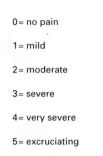

0 = no pain

1 = mild

2 = moderate

3 = severe

4 = very severe

5 = excruciating

*Figure 5.2. The verbal rating scale.*

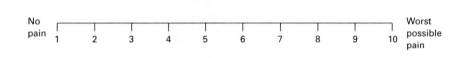

*Figure 5.3. The numeric pain intensity scale (from Jeans, 1993).*

### The Poker Chip Tool

This is a measure that uses real poker chips, where children are asked to rate the intensity of their pain by choosing poker chips to represent 'pieces of hurt' (Hester, 1979). McGrath et al. (1993) suggest that this measure is especially useful in children between the ages of 4 and 8 years. This tool has been found to correlate well with parents' and nurses' ratings of children's pain (Hester et al., 1990).

### The Oucher

The Oucher is one of the many varieties of pictorial scales which make use of happy and sad faces. It was developed by Beyer (1984) to assess pain intensity in children aged between 3 and 12 years. It consists of a numerical scale ranging from 0 to 100 for children who are numerate and a six-picture scale for those who cannot use numbers. The picture scale is scored from 0 to 5 (see Fig. 5.4).

Beyer (1994) suggests that nurses should familiarize children with the Oucher by giving them the opportunity to remember and rate past painful

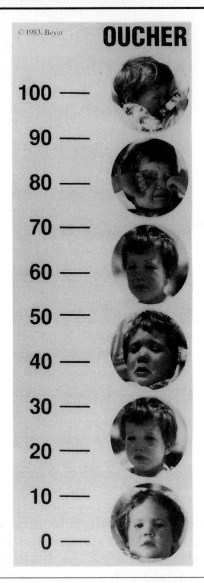

*Figure 5.4.* *The Caucasian version of the Oucher, developed and copyrighted by Judith E. Beyer, RN, PhD, 1983, currently at the University of Missouri Kansas City, USA.*

experiences on the scale. This provides an opportunity for the nurse to ascertain the child's level of understanding as well as to provide an explicit representation of pain for the child. In an attempt to assess whether the sequencing of pictures was in the right order, Beyer and Aradine (1986) used children to act as expert judges and the results revealed this to be a valid measure.

According to Beyer (1994), the nurse should explain that the bottom picture represents 'no hurt', whilst the top means 'the biggest hurt you could ever have'. The Oucher has been shown to have excellent concurrent validity, correlating highly with VAS (100 mm vertical line) and Hester's Poker Chip as well as showing discriminant validity. It is also able to differentiate between fear and pain (Beyer and Aradine, 1988).

Beyer developed the Oucher scale using photographs of a white child and so she suggests that research to test the content validity and acceptability of the Oucher to other ethnic groups is crucial (Beyer, 1994). Therefore, research has been undertaken to assess validity and acceptability among Hispanics and African American children and is currently available for these groups (Beyer et al., 1992) (see Figs 5.5 and 5.6). The Ouchers are printed and distributed by the Association for Care of Children's Health, 7910 Woodmont Avenue, Suite 300, Bethesda, MD 20814, USA.

Picture scales, which are also used among adult pain populations, were first developed by Frank et al. (1982). The scale consists of eight line drawings of human faces experiencing different levels of pain. The drawings are presented randomly and the patient is asked to choose which represent their present pain (see Frank et al., 1982, for scoring details). This technique has the advantage that the patient need not be verbally fluent and therefore it is suitable for children and patients from non-Western cultures.

### Eland Colour Tool

The Eland Colour Tool (Eland, 1981) was developed to assess pain in children aged between 4 and 10 years, and can also be used for adults with learning disability (Eland, 1994). Children are asked to choose colours from a selection of red, orange, yellow, brown, blue, black, purple and green crayons to colour front and back body outlines (Eland, 1994). These crayons are presented in a random order and the child is asked to choose the colours that represent the hurt he/she is experiencing. Red and black indicate pain of strong intensities. The full protocol for using the Eland Colour Tool is outlined in Eland (1994). This tool is very reliable and is widely used to assess children's pain in a variety of cultures (Hester, 1979; Lee, 1986; Zavah, 1986, cited in Eland, 1994).

### ▪ Pain drawings

In the absence of any of the above tools, nurses can ask children to represent their pain in drawings. McGrath et al. (1993) suggest that children are typically asked to draw pictures to depict the intensity of their pain. Unruh et al. (1983) have shown that drawings can be classified according to content and dominant colours: the colours black and red seem to be commonly used by children to indicate the intensity of their pain (Eland and Anderson, 1977; Eland, 1994; Unruh et al., 1983; Kurylyszyn et al., 1987).

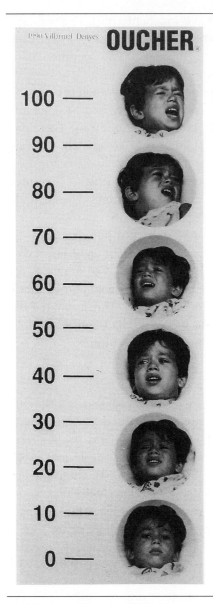

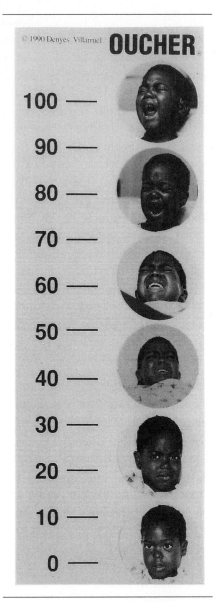

**Figure 5.5.** The Hispanic version of the Oucher, developed and copyrighted by Antonia M. Villarruel, RN, PhD (University of Pennsylvania) and Mary J. Denyes, RN, PhD (Wayne State University), 1990.

**Figure 5.6.** The African-American version of the Oucher, developed and copyrighted by Mary J. Denyes, RN, PhD (Wayne State University) and Antonia M. Villaruel, RN, PhD (University of Pennsylvania), 1990. Cornelia P. Porter, RN, PhD, and Charlotta Marshall, RN, MSN contributed to the development of this scale.

# ■ TOOLS FOR ASSESSING PAIN IN ADULTS

The rating scales described above (VRS, VAS and numeric intensity scale) are also useful for assessing pain in adults. They are simple and easy to use and therefore they have a special place in acute pain settings (Jeans, 1993).

However, these unidimensional rating scales do not reflect the complexity of the pain experience and Reading (1984) suggests that, over repeated trials, patients may use the same single scales to reflect different components of their pain. Attempts have been made to overcome this problem in two ways: the development of questionnaire scales and psychosocial assessment techniques, which reflect the acceptance of pain as a multidimensional phenomenon. These more comprehensive measures are most commonly used for the assessment of chronic pain (see also Chapter 12 for assessment tools which are of particular value in the management of cancer pain).

## ■ Questionnaire methods

The McGill Pain Questionnaire (MPQ) (Melzack and Torgerson, 1971) was developed from work demonstrating high agreement among patients, students and physicians on the meaning attached to pain adjectives. It consists of 78 adjectives arranged into groups. The questionnaire is intended to reflect three dimensions: sensory, affective and evaluative, with three remaining groups reflecting a sensory miscellaneous category. Words such as flickering, flashing, burning and stabbing refer to sensory qualities in terms of temporal, spatial, thermal, pressure and other properties. The affective qualities of tension, fear, punishment and autonomic properties are conveyed through terms such as exhausting, frightful, punishing and sickening. Evaluative words such as miserable, annoying and unbearable summarize the total experience. Distinctive constellations of these descriptors characterize pain associated with different clinical conditions (Graham et al., 1980) (see Fig. 5.7).

The MPQ yields a number of indices: a pain rating index based on two types of numerical values that can be assigned to each word descriptor; the number of words chosen; and the present pain intensity based on a 1–5 intensity scale. The mean scale values of these words are equidistant and represent equal scale intervals, and therefore act as 'anchors' for description of overall pain intensity. Good correlations have been shown between all the pain indices.

Since its introduction, the MPQ has been used extensively and experience suggests that it provides precise information on the sensory, affective and evaluative aspects of pain experience as well as being able to discriminate between different pain problems (Melzack, 1975). The extent and rigour to which this assessment tool has been tested is remarkable. Researchers from various countries have translated it and tested its reliability and validity.

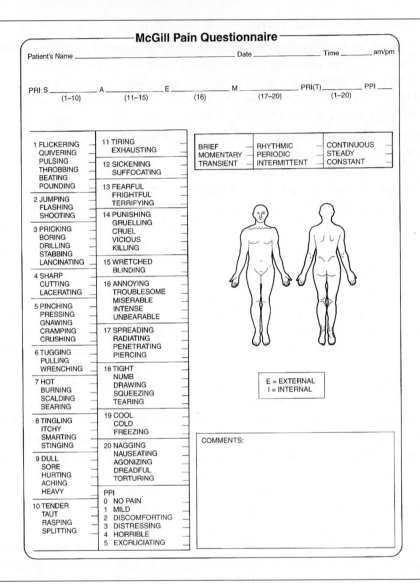

*Figure 5.7.* The McGill Pain Questionnaire (reproduced with permission by Roland Melzack).

For example, it is available in Italian (Maiani and Sanavio, 1985), Dutch (Vanderiet et al., 1987), Arabic (Harrison, 1988), French (Boureau et al., 1984), German (Kiss et al., 1987), Japanese (Satow et al., 1990), Norwegian (Strand and Wisnes, 1991) and Polish (Sedlack, 1990). These are cited in Melzack and Katz (1992), so the reader is referred to this source for a more comprehensive list of translations of the MPQ (see also the discussion about culture and language which follows later).

Davis (1988) studied the MPQ's ability to discriminate between a sample of 30 patients with acute pain and 30 with chronic pain. The results showed that the MPQ was able to measure and discriminate between chronic and acute pain. The McGill is also of value in adolescents and children as young as 8 years (Tesler et al., 1988; Abu-Saad, 1990). Nevertheless, the MPQ has not been without its critics. For example, Holroyd et al. (1992) conducted a multicentre factor analysis evaluation of the MPQ (involving 1700 chronic pain patients) and concluded that the MPQ did not demonstrate either discriminant validity or clinical utility. According to Gracely (1992), these criticisms concerning lack of discriminant validity stem from the erroneous assumption that the MPQ can be analysed in a manner similar to other commonly used psychological assessment scales. Gracely suggests that most psychological scales assess dimensions that are theoretically distinct and empirically unrelated. The sensory, affective and cognitive components of pain are all interrelated and Gracely likens the relationship between these dimensions to height and weight. Since taller people are generally heavier, height and weight will be highly correlated and it would make little sense to consider one without taking the other into account. He believes that the sensory, affective and cognitive components of pain experience share a common variance in a similar manner to height and weight. Lack of discrim-inant validity is therefore not a valid criticism.

A shortened form of the MPQ (SF-MPQ) has been developed more recently (Melzack, 1987) for use in the clinical and research situations which require a more rapid acquisition of data than the standard MPQ. The data obtained with the SF-MPQ provide information on the sensory, affective and overall intensity of pain.

The Joint Colleges Commission report on pain after surgery (Royal College of Surgeons and Royal College of Anaesthetists, 1990) suggests that post-operative pain is best assessed by a subjective unidimensional scale such as VAS or VRS because of ease and simplicity of use. However, the SF-MPQ is of immense value because it provides sensory, affective and evaluative as well as overall intensity information about pain, and yet it is simple and quickly administered within the acute surgical setting.

## ■ CULTURAL ISSUES IN THE LANGUAGE OF PAIN

Language offers an important medium through which much cultural knowledge is acquired. As we have seen in Chapter 2 cultural variables strongly influence the way in which pain is communicated. The range of the vocabulary used to refer to pain varies considerably between cultures. Garro (1990) has posed the question of whether a limited pain vocabulary reflects a cultural tendency to be non-demonstrative about pain. However, the answer to this question is not clear-cut, since anthropologists working in two cultures described as having an impassive response to pain have presented contrasting views.

For example, Sargent (1984) found that talk about pain among the Bariba of Benin focuses on stoical values of honour and courage in the face of pain. On the other hand, Landar (1967) found an extensive and rich vocabulary for communicating pain among the Navajo (cited in Garro, 1990). These contrasting views of talking about pain are also reflected in the language used to describe pain. For example, in English there are several basic pain terms – 'pain', 'hurt', 'sore' and 'ache' (Fabrega and Tyma, 1976). In Thai, there are more than a dozen distinct basic pain terms (Diller, 1980), whilst the Japanese have a single comprehensive term for pain, which can be qualified by optional descriptors (Diller, 1980; Fabrega and Tyma, 1976). Garro (1990), in her review of the literature, highlights the complexity of cultural differences in the report of pain. She suggests that a Thai speaker, using one of the basic pain terms, may convey information about the location or cause of pain. Two examples are words which have been translated as 'to suffer focused abdominal pain' and 'to feel irritated by skin abrasion'. In Thai language, pain is not treated like a subject, which means that the level of intensity and other features of sensory pain experience routinely communicated by English speakers through descriptive qualifiers (e.g. 'I have a stinging pain') does not appear to be given explicit consideration by Thai speakers (Fabrega and Tyma, 1976).

The use of verbal report measures for the assessment of pain in people from different cultures is especially problematic, since particular words denoting alteration in the felt-experience of pain in one language may have no equivalence in another language (Scarry, 1980). In English, there are many descriptive words which serve as descriptive qualifiers and, as we saw from the development of the MPQ, there are 78 adjectives for describing pain. The use of a common multidimensional pain-assessment tool provides a useful means for analysing cross-cultural differences in pain experience and the McGill Pain Questionnaire is probably the most widely used pain questionnaire.

As stated above, the MPQ is available in a variety of languages and, in their attempts to develop different language versions, researchers have used either dictionary translations of the MPQ (Maiani and Sanavio, 1985; Kiss et al., 1987), or reconstructions of the questionnaire using Melzack and Torgerson's (1971) original methodology of having native speakers generate pain words and descriptors, and classifying them in culturally appropriate groupings (De Bennedittis et al., 1988). For an Italian version of the MPQ, two sets of researchers adopted different approaches and developed essentially different questionnaires (Maiani and Sanavio, 1985; De Bennedittis et al., 1988). The dictionary translation version replicates the English MPQ

(Maiani and Sanavio, 1985). For the reconstructed version (De Bennedittis et al., 1988), the major classes of sensory, evaluative and affective were retained, but changes occurred in the composition and type of subclasses. An additional subclass was added to the evaluative group. In the sensory class, several subclasses were eliminated, one was added, and another was subdivided. The 'punishment' subclass was renamed 'negative emotional impact' to reflect the fact that in Italian, the concept of 'punishing' pain is not an appropriate category. Garro (1990) states that the dictionary translation approach is favoured by those wanting to preserve a close structural relationship with the original MPQ in order to facilitate cross-cultural comparisons. However, this approach has been criticized for being over-simplistic, invalid, unreliable and misleading by researchers favouring the reconstruction approach (De Bennedittis et al., 1988; Madjar, 1993).

Within the context of nursing, Madjar (1993) states that caution should be exercised in the use of assessment tools developed by Western (usually English-speaking) researchers, even when these are translated into other languages. The difficulty is that translations of individual words, and even phrases, however accurate in the literal sense, may fail to capture the reality of experience for those whose culture and language have very different roots and orientations. Madjar elaborates her objections by stating that it is not surprising to find that when difficulties in the use of translated tools are encountered, the problems are attributed to the patients, rather than the tool or the underlying rationale, since translations are essentially one way, from the English-speaking to the non-English-speaking cultural groups. To highlight this problem she points to use of the Brief Pain Inventory among Vietnamese cancer patients. Commenting on the researchers' (Cleeland et al., 1988) evaluation that the Vietnamese found various mood words confusing, Madjar suggests that Anglo-American patients would have had similar difficulties if the Brief Pain Inventory had been developed within the Vietnamese culture. Researchers should demonstrate honesty and humility by the admission that some ideas do not translate directly and easily into another language (Arruda et al., 1992).

## ■ Factors to consider when assessing pain in people from different cultures

Madjar (1993) suggests that the recognition of cultural variables should be a significant feature in the assessment of pain. She puts forward the following nursing guidelines for assessing pain in patients from different cultures.

1. First and foremost, effective communication should be established with the person. This is greatly assisted by a trained interpreter who may be invaluable in facilitating adequate assessment of the patient's current pain experience as well as in obtaining a history of past experiences of pain,

preferred modes of coping, cultural and personal values, and preferences in relation to pain management. Self-report remains a crucial component of adequate pain assessment and should not be neglected when language differences create barriers between patients and nurses.

2. Assessment of pain intensity needs to be an ongoing process, and it is also dependent upon establishing good communication. Because of their simplicity and ease of administration, visual analogue scales are particularly useful in cross-cultural settings and, with sufficient coaching in their own language, they can even be used by people with very low levels of educational attainment (Madjar, 1985). On the other hand, terms such as minimal, moderate or intense, which are frequently used by nurses and other health professionals in assessing patients' pain, may be ambiguous or inappropriately utilized with patients who are not in the habit of using such terminology in their everyday communication.

3. Assessing the quality of pain may be particularly difficult in a cross-cultural context. Culture and language affect not only the communication process but also the total experience of pain, since they influence perception, thought and cognition. One way of increasing mutual understanding between patients and nurses is to invite patients to explain what the pain is like, not in the language of assessment tools or charts, but as their own stories, likening the current pain to something that may be imagined and understood by others. Given permission to tell someone what the pain is like, patients will provide vivid and sometimes horrifying images of their experience. Madjar (1981) presents the following examples of patients who had undergone abdominal surgery.

■ Like a screwdriver . . . – turning inside', 'like being torn apart and your insides pulled out' or 'as if I was going to break open'.
■ Similar descriptions are used by patients with sickle cell disease to describe painful crises (see Chapter 11): 'like someone hammering a nail into my bones', 'it is as if someone puts a screwdriver into my bones and slowly turns it inside and sometime, when you least expect, it is yanked out'.

These descriptions not only provide information about intensity but they also provide clues about the affective and evaluative components. For example, from these vivid descriptions, one can get a sense of the fear (affective) and the exhausting (evaluative) nature of the experience. In such situations, we need to listen sympathetically to what the patients are trying to tell us, rather than attempting to 'educate' people from different cultures to present their experience in language that fits our conceptual frameworks and our cultural ideologies (Parsons, 1990).

4. Finally, and most importantly, as nurses we need to recognize the central role of ethics in our practice with those who are ill and in pain. One possible

option is a paternalistic relationship, in which cultural and individual values and practices are overlooked, ignored or discounted, on the basis of the assumption that, as health professionals, we know what is best for the patient. Clinical judgements about a patient's pain and 'need for pain relief' may thus be made on the basis of a medical diagnosis or normative expectations for someone at a particular stage of illness or recovery. One effect of such a stance may be to place on all patients the expectation that they will behave with courage and stoical endurance. The alternative is the ethic of therapeutic partnership, which requires the fostering of a therapeutic alliance based on mutual trust and deep understanding of what the patient is experiencing, what he or she is willing or able to tolerate, and what the nurse has within his/her powers to alleviate. Free expression of pain in such a context is not a sign of cultural inferiority or personal weakness, but an essential component of adequate pain assessment and a sign of trust between the nurse and the patient.

## ■ ASSESSMENT OF PSYCHOSOCIAL CONTRIBUTIONS TO PAIN EXPERIENCE

Perhaps the most common method of psychosocial assessment is the clinical interview, a method with which nurses are very familiar. Interviews with patients and their significant others are a useful way of evaluating the impact of pain on lifestyle.

The Gate Control theory (Melzack and Wall, 1965) was the impetus for the now well-known proposition that mood and cognition influence pain, and indeed pain can affect the psychological state and behaviour of people. Within the context of chronic pain, the importance of psychosocial factors in influencing pain perception has been firmly incorporated in assessment and management strategies for a considerable time. According to Kerns and Jacobs (1992), there are a number of reasons for this development. Firstly, the development of clinical concepts such as 'psychogenic pain' (Engel, 1959) and 'pain behaviour' (Pilowski and Spence, 1975; Fordyce, 1976) have encouraged the point of convergence on psychosocial factors as a prominent feature of pain experience. Secondly, the formulation of operant conditioning (Fordyce, 1976) and cognitive-behavioural appreciation of chronic pain have encouraged psychosocial factors in the development and maintenance of the pain.

Psychologists have been very diligent in the development of a wide variety of standardized questionnaires for the sole purpose of assessing the psychosocial components of pain and their discussion warrants a chapter to itself. These instruments require the expertise of health and clinical psychologists for their appropriate use and interpretation, therefore the intention here is not to present a review of these techniques, but to introduce the reader to the existence of psychosocial assessment tools and the important role that psychologists have in the systematic assessment of pain. The reader is referred to Kerns and Jacobs (1992) for a thorough discussion of psycho-social and behavioural measures for assessing pain.

## ■ CONCLUSION

This chapter has discussed many different methods of pain assessment and some important psychosocial factors that should be taken into account when assessing pain. No one assessment method is superior in all circumstances. Indeed, since the intensity and quality of pain varies from time to time and from person to person, there is no reason to suppose that one ideal method for assessing pain exists. Objective physiological measurements are useful under laboratory conditions where the intensity of the stimulus is known and there is little emotional influence (Green, 1990). However, in the case of pain in clinical settings, the intensity of the stimulus cannot be directly measured and there are usually profound emotional effects altering the perception of pain. In this situation, the subjective assessment tools, which reflect the multidimensional nature of pain, are most appropriate.

## ■ REFERENCES

**Abu-Saad, H.H.** (1984) Assessing children's responses to pain. *Pain* **19**, 163–171.
**Abu-Saad, H.H.** (1990) Toward the development of an instrument to assess pain in children: Dutch study. In: Tyler, D.C. & Krane, E.J. (eds) *Advances in Pain Research and Therapy: Paediatric Pain*. Raven Press, New York, pp. 101–106.
**Aradine, C., Beyer, J. & Tompkins, J.** (1988) Children's perception before and after analgesia: a study of instrument construct validity. *Journal of Paediatric Nursing* **3**, 11–23.
**Arruda, E.N., Larson, P.J. & Meleis, A.I.** (1992) Comfort: immigrant Hispanic cancer patients' views. *Cancer Nursing* **15**, 387–394.
**Barker, M. & Hughes, B.** (1990) Using a tool for pain assessment. *Nursing Times* **86** (24), 50–52.
**Beyer, J.** (1984) *The Oucher: A User's Manual and Technical Report*. The Hospital Play Equipment Co., Evanston, IL.
**Beyer, J.** (1994) The Oucher: a pain intensity scale for children. In: Funk, S.G, Tornquist, E.M., Champagne, M.T., Copp, L.A. & Weise, R.A. (eds) *Management of Pain, Fatigue and Nausea*. Macmillan Press, Basingstoke, pp. 65–71.
**Beyer, J. & Aradine, C.** (1986) Content validity of an instrument to measure young children's perceptions of the intensity of their pain. *Journal of Paediatric Nursing* **1**, 386–395.
**Beyer, J. & Aradine, C.** (1988) The convergent and discriminant validity of a self report measure of pain intensity. *Children's Health Care* **16**, 274–282.
**Boureau, F., Luu, M. Doubrere, J.F. & Gay, C.** (1984) Elaboration d'un question-naire d'auto-evaluation de la douleur par liste de qualicatifs (Development of a self-evaluation questionnaire comprising pain descriptors). *Therapie* **39**, 119–129.

**Carroll, D.** (1993) Pain assessment. In: Carroll, D. & Bowsher, D. (eds) *Pain: Management and Nursing Care*. Oxford, Butterworth-Heinemann, pp. 16–27.

**Chapman, C.R.** (1989) Assessment of pain. In: Nimmo, W.S. & Smith, G. (eds) *Anaesthesia*. London, Blackwells, pp. 1149–1165.

**Cleeland, C.S., Ladinsky, J.L., Serlin, R.C. & Thuy, N.C.** (1988) Multidimensional measurement of cancer. Comparisons of US and Vietnamese patients. *Journal of Pain and Symptom Management* **3**, 23–27.

**Craig, K.D., Prkachin, K.M. & Grunau, R.V.E.** (1992) The facial expression of pain. In: Turk, D.C. & Melzack R. (eds) *A Handbook of Pain Assessment*. The Guildford Press, New York, pp.257–276.

**Dalton, J.A.** (1989) Nurses' perceptions of their pain assessment skills, pain management practices and attitudes towards pain. *Oncology Nursing Forum* **16**(2), 225–231.

**Davis, D.H. & Calhoon, M.** (1994) Do pre-term infants show behavioural responses to painful procedures? In: Funk, S.G, Tornquist, E.M., Champagne, M.T., Copp, L.A. & Weise, R.A. (eds) *Management of Pain, Fatigue and Nausea*. Macmillan Press, Basingstoke, pp. 35–45.

**Davis, G.C.** (1988) Measuring the clinical outcome of chronic pain. In: Waltz, C.F. & Strickland, O.L. (eds) *Measurement of Nursing Outcomes*, Vol. 1: *Measuring Client Outcomes*. Springer, New York, pp. 160–184.

**De Bennedittis, G., Massei, R., Nobili, R. & Pieri, A.** (1988) The Italian Pain Questionnaire. *Pain* **33**, 53–62.

**Diller, A.** (1980) Cross-cultural pain semantics. *Pain* **9**, 9–26.

**Eland, J.M.** (1981) Minimizing pain associated with pre-kindergarten intramuscular injections. *Issues in Comprehensive Pediatric Nursing* **5**, 361–372.

**Eland, J.M.** (1994) The effectiveness of TENS with children experiencing cancer pain. In: Funk, S.G., Tornquist, E.M., Champagne, M.T., Copp, L.A. & Weise, R.A. (eds) *Management of Pain, Fatigue and Nausea*. Macmillan Press, Basingstoke, pp. 87–100.

**Eland, J.M. & Anderson, J.E.** (1977) The experience of pain in children. In: *Pain: A Source Book for Nurses and Other Health Professionals*. Little, Brown and Company, Boston, pp. 453–473.

**Engel, G.** (1959) Psychogenic pain and the pain prone patient. *American Journal of Medicine* **26**, 899–918.

**Fabrega, H. & Tyma, S.** (1976) Language and cultural influences in the description of pain. *British Journal of Medical Psychology* **49**, 349–371.

**Fordham, M. & Dunn, V.** (1994) *Alongside the Person in Pain: Holistic Care and Nursing Practice*. Baillière Tindall, London.

**Fordyce, W.E.** (1976) *Behavioural Methods for Chronic Pain and Illness*. Mosby, St Louis.

**Frank, A.J.M., Moll, J.M.H. & Hort, J.F.** (1982) A comparison of three ways of measuring pain. *Rheumatology and Rehabilitation* **21**, 211–217.

**Fuller, B.F. Yoshiyuki, H. & Conner, D.** (1994) Vocal measures in infant pain. In: Funk, S.G., Tornquist, E.M., Champagne, M.T., Copp, L.A. & Weise, R.A. (eds) *Management of Pain, Fatigue and Nausea*. Macmillan Press, Basingstoke, pp. 46–51.

Garro, L. (1990) Culture, pain and cancer. *Journal of Palliative Care* **6**(3), 34–44.

Gracely, R.H. (1992) Evaluation of multi-dimensional pain scales. *Pain* **48**, 297–300.

Graham, C., Bond, S.S., Gerkovich, M.M. & Cook, M.R. (1980) Use of the McGill Pain Questionnaire in the assessment of cancer pain: replicability and consistency. *Pain* **8**, 377–387.

Green, C.P. (1990) The evaluation of pain in man. Frontiers of *Pain* **2**(2), 4–6.

Grunau, R.V.E. & Craig, K.D. (1987) Pain expressions in neonates: facial action and cry. *Pain* **28**, 395–410.

Harrison, A. (1988) Arabic pain words. *Pain* **32**, 239–250.

Hayward, J. (1975) *Information: Prescription Against Pain*. The Study of Nursing Care Project Report Series 2, no. 5. Royal College of Nursing, London.

Hester, N. (1979) The preoperational child's reaction to immunisation. *Nursing Research* **28**, 250–254.

Hester, N., Foster, R. & Kristensen, K. (1990) In: Tyler, D.C. & Krane, E.J. (eds) *Advances in Pain Research and Therapy: Paediatric Pain*. Raven Press, New York, pp. 79–84.

Holroyd, K.A., Holm, J.E., Keefe, F.J., Turner, J.A., Bradley, L.A., Murphy, W.D., Johnson, P., Anderson, K., Hinkle, A.L. & O'Malley, W.B. (1992) A multi-centre evaluation of the McGill Pain Questionnaire: results from 1700 chronic pain patients. *Pain* **48**, 301–312.

Izard, C.E. & Dougherty, L.M. (1982) Two complementary systems for measuring facial expressions in infants and children. In: Izard, C.E. (ed.) *Measuring Emotions in Infants and Children*. Cambridge University Press, Cambridge, pp. 97–126.

Jeans, M.E. (1993) The management of acute pain. *IASP Refresher Course Syllabus: Pain Issues Relevant to Nursing*. International Association for the Study of Pain Publications, Seattle, pp. 165–171.

Johnson, J.E., Rice, V.H., Fuller, S.S. & Endress, M.P. (1978) Sensory information, instruction in coping strategy and recovery from surgery. *Research in Nursing and Health* **1**(3), 4–7.

Johnston, C.C. (1989) Pain assessment and management in infants. *Pediatrician* **16**, 16–23.

Johnston, C.C. & Strada, M.E. (1986) Acute pain response in infants: a multidimensional description. *Pain* **24**, 373–382.

Kerns, R.D. & Jacobs, M.C. (1992) Assessment of the psychosocial context and the experience of pain. In: Turk, D.C. & Melzack, R. (eds) *A Handbook of Pain Assessment*. The Guildford Press, New York, pp. 235–256.

Kiss, I., Muller, H. & Abel, M. (1987) The McGill Pain Questionnaire – German Version. A study of cancer pain. *Pain* **29**, 195–207.

Kurylyszyn, N., McGrath, P.J., Capelli, M. & Humphreys, P. (1987) Children's drawings: what can they tell us about intensity of pain? *Clinical Journal of Pain* **2**, 155–158.

Landar, H. (1967) The language of pain in the Navajo culture. In: Hymes, D.H. & Bittle, W.H. (eds) *Studies in South Western Ethnolinguistics: Meaning and History in Language of the American Southwest*. Mouton & Co., The Hague, Netherlands, pp. 117–144.

**Lee, C.** (1986) Korean Children's Painful Reaction. Unpublished master's thesis, University of Iowa, Iowa City.

**Madjar, I.** (1981) The experience of pain in surgical patients: a cross cultural study. Unpublished MA thesis, Massey University, New Zealand.

**Madjar, I.** (1985) Pain and the surgical patient: a cross cultural perspective. *Australian Journal of Advanced Nursing* **2**, 29–33.

**Madjar, I.** (1993) Cultural issues in pain assessment. *IASP Refresher Course Syllabus: Pain Issues Relevant to Nursing.* International Association for the Study of Pain Publications, Seattle, pp.161–163.

**Maiani, G. & Sanavio, E.** (1985) Semantics of pain in Italy: the Italian version of the McGill Pain Questionnaire. *Pain* **22**, 399–405.

**McCaffery, M. & Beebe, A.** (1989) *Pain: Clinical Manual for Nursing Practice.* C.V. Mosby, St Louis.

**McGrath, P.A.** (1990) *Pain in Children: Nature, Assessment and Treatment.* Guildford, New York.

**McGrath, P. & Unruh, A.M.** (1987) *Pain in Children and Adolescents,* Vol. 1: *Pain Research and Clinical Management.* Elsevier, Amsterdam.

**McGrath, P.J., Richie, J.A. & Unruh, A.** (1993) Paediatric pain. In: Carroll, D. & Bowsher, D. (eds) *Pain Management and Nursing Care.* Butterworth Heinemann, Oxford, pp. 100–123.

**McGuire, D.B.** (1984) The measurement of clinical pain. *Nursing Research* **33**(3), 152–156.

**McGuire, D.B.** (1993) Comprehensive and multidimensional assessment and measurement of pain. *IASP Refresher Course Syllabus: Pain Issues Relevant to Nursing.* International Association for the Study of Pain Publications, Seattle, pp. 135–159.

**Meinhart, N.T. & McCaffery, M.** (1983) *Pain: A Nursing Approach to Assessment and Analysis.* Appleton-Century-Crofts, New York.

**Melzack, R.** (1975) The McGill Pain Questionnaire: major properties and scoring methods. *Pain* **1**, 277–299.

**Melzack, R.** (1987) The short-form McGill Pain Questionnaire. *Pain* **30**, 191–197.

**Melzack, R. & Katz, J.** (1992) The McGill Questionnaire: appraisal and current status. In: Turk, D.C. & Melzack, R. (eds) *Handbook of Pain Assessment.* The Guildford Press, New York, pp. 152–168.

**Melzack, R. & Torgerson, W. S.** (1971) On the language of pain. *Anaesthesiology* **34**, 50–59.

**Melzack, R. & Wall, P.D.** (1965) Pain mechanisms: a new theory. *Science* **150**, 971–979.

**Miller, S.M., Coombs, C. & Stoddard, E.** (1989) Information, coping and control in patients undergoing surgery and stressful procedures. In: Steptoe, A. & Appels, A. (eds) *Stress, Personal Control and Health.* Wiley and Sons, Chichester, pp. 107–129.

**Mills, N.** (1994) Acute pain behaviour in infants and toddlers. In: Funk, S.G., Tornquist, E.M., Champagne, M.T., Copp, L.A. & Weise, R.A. (eds) *Management of Pain, Fatigue and Nausea.* Macmillan Press, Basingstoke, pp. 52–59.

**Mitchell, R.W.D. & Smith, G.** (1989) The control of postoperative pain. *British Journal of Anaesthesia* **63**, 147–158.

Parsons, C. (1990) Cross-cultural issues in health care. In: Reid, J. & Trompf, P. (eds) *The Health of Immigrant Australia*. Harcourt, Brace, Jovanovich, Sydney, pp. 108–153.

Pilowski, I. & Spence, N.D. (1975) Patterns of illness behaviour in patients with intractable pain. *Journal of Psychosomatic Research* **19**, 279–287.

Reading, A.E. (1984) Testing pain mechanisms in persons in pain. In: Wall, P.D. & Melzack, R. (eds) *Textbook of Pain*. Churchill Livingstone, Edinburgh, pp. 195–206.

Ross, D. & Ross, S.A. (1988) *Childhood Pain: Current Issues, Research and Management*. Urban & Schwarzenberg, Baltimore.

Royal College of Surgeons (RCS) & Royal College of Anaesthetists (RC Anaes) (1990) *Commission on the Provision of Surgical Services. Report of the Working Party on Pain after Surgery*. RCS and RCAnaes, London.

Sargent, C. (1984) Between death and shame: dimensions of pain in Bariba culture. *Social Science and Medicine* **19**, 1299–1304.

Satow, A., Nakatani, K., Taniguchi, S. & Higashiyama, A. (1990) Perceptual characteristics of electrocutaneous pain estimated by the 30 word list and visual analogue. *Japanese Psychological Review* **32**, 155–164.

Sedlack, K. (1990) A Polish version of the McGill Pain Questionnaire. *Pain* (Suppl. 5), S308.

Seers, C.J. (1987) Pain, Anxiety and Recovery in Patients Undergoing Surgery. Unpublished Ph.D. thesis, King's College, London.

Strand, L.I. & Wisnes, A.R. (1991) The development of a Norwegian pain questionnaire. *Pain* **46**, 61–66.

Tesler, M.D., Savedra, M., Ward, M. et al. (1988) Children's language of pain. In: Dubner, R., Gebhart G.F. & Bond, M. (eds) *Proceedings of the 5th World Congress on Pain*. Elsevier, Amsterdam.

Turk, D.C. & Melzack, R. (1992) The measurement of pain and the assessment of people experiencing pain. In: Turk, D.C. & Melzack, R. (eds) *A Handbook of Pain Assessment*. The Guildford Press, New York, pp. 3–12.

Unruh, A., McGrath, P.K., Cunningham, S.J. & Humphreys, P. (1983) Children's drawing of their pain. *Pain* **17**, 385–392.

Vanderiet, K., Adriaensen, H., Carton, H. & Vertommen, H. (1987) The McGill Pain Questionnaire constructed for the Dutch language (MPQ-DV). Preliminary data concerning reliability and validity. *Pain* **30**, 395–408.

Varni, J.W., Thomspson, K.L. & Hanson, V. (1987) The Varni/Thompson paediatric pain questionnaire: 1, Chronic musculo-skeletal pain in juvenile arthritis. *Pain* **28**, 27–38.

Wasz-Hockert, O., Lind, J., Vourenkoski, V., Partanen, T. & Valanne, E. (1968) *The Infant's Cry: A Spectographic and Auditory Analysis*. Clinics in Developmental Medicine, Vol. 29. Spastics International Medical Publications, Lavenham.

Wilkie, D.J., Holzemer, W.L., Tesler, M.D., Ward, J.A., Paul, S.M. & Savedra, M.C. (1990) Measuring pain quality: validity and reliability of children's and adolescent pain language. *Pain* **41**, 151–159.

Zavah, M.F. (1986) Ice as a Pain Relief Measure after Subcutaneous Injection. Unpublished master's thesis, State University of New York, Buffalo.

# The use of pharmacology in pain management

## ■ INTRODUCTION

The relief of pain, as opposed to the imposition of unconsciousness, has received remarkably little academic attention until the last few years. It seems barely credible that when I became a consultant anaesthetist in 1969 I was regarded as very peculiar in my insistence on perioperative analgesia for children undergoing such operations as tonsillectomy.

In this chapter the principal agents available for managing pain will be described. In general, only examples of each class of drug will be used. The British National Formulary (BNF) is the place to look for succinct therapeutic information; it can be used to place other drugs in the correct category and note specific properties, interactions or contraindications. Locally developed formularies can also be helpful as they contain good general guidance and clear information on the restricted range of drugs chosen by the hospital or practice. It is essential that anyone prescribing or administering a drug with which they are not personally familiar should check the basic information on which safe action depends. It is equally important to obtain the same information on all drugs that a patient is taking to avoid incompatibility, and to take a careful history of allergies.

The various strategies for administration and management will also be outlined. Some of these will be treated in more detail in other chapters.

## ■ AN ANATOMICAL AND NEUROPHYSIOLOGICAL BASIS FOR PAIN

An understanding of the generation of painful stimuli and their transmission routes to the central nervous system (CNS), comprising the brain and the spinal cord, forms an essential map on which to place an appreciation of the factors that can act at various points. These factors can come from within the individual or from outside.

Although dealt with in more detail in Chapter 1, the key points (obviously much simplified) are illustrated again in Fig. 6.1. Specific pain-sensitive nerve endings on the skin and mucous membranes or within organs will respond to noxious stimulation by sending impulses via sensory and autonomic nerves to the spinal cord. On entering the spinal cord, several types

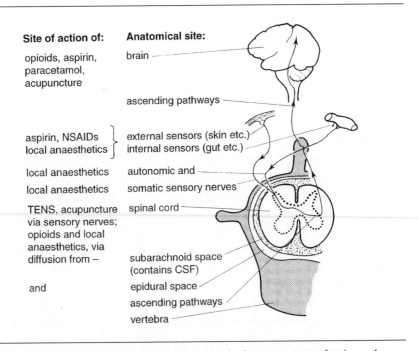

**Figure 6.1.** *Schematic representation of the principal components of pain pathways and the sites at which various drugs may act.*

of response will occur simultaneously and these responses can be modified by neural activity from higher and lower centres. It is important to grasp the fact that such neural activity may be excitatory/facilitatory or inhibitory. All this means that the 'telephone switchboard' analogy for the CNS is unhelpfully restrictive. Drugs and different physical stimuli can act at any of these sites and action at two or more sites (morphine, for instance, can act within the spinal cord as well as in the brain) has often led to problems of understanding. The sites of action of the main pain relief techniques and drugs are indicated.

## ■ METHODS OF TREATING PAIN

The principal methods of treating pain can be classified as psychological, physical and pharmacological – 'three Ps for the big P.' It should be very rare for any significant pain not to be treated by a combination of at least two of these methods. However, psychological aspects are dealt with extensively in other parts of this book and will not be further considered here, although I have to re-emphasize that, whenever drugs or other techniques are used, the absolute minimum must be to provide information (both about the condition being treated and the treatment plan) and reassurance.

## ■ PHYSICAL TECHNIQUES

These range from the simple (but often neglected) components of physical comfort – warmth, position, massage, appropriate lighting and ventilation – to specific methods such as transcutaneous electrical nerve stimulation (TENS) and acupuncture.

## ▪ TENS

Transcutaneous electrical nerve stimulation works by bombarding the pain pathways with non-painful stimuli at the same level in the spinal cord that is receiving the impulses from the painful area. This induces sufficient inhibitory activity to prevent the passage of the pain 'message' up to the brain. It is possible that endogenous opioids are produced locally as well as neurotransmitters. A small battery-operated pack generates stimuli, which are connected by fine wires to electrodes, like electrocardiograph (ECG) electrodes. The electrodes are stuck to the skin in the area served by the same nerves as the source of pain. The frequency and pattern of the electrical impulses are initially set by the prescriber but are then adjusted by the patient (usually just short of discomfort), and relief will typically commence within ten minutes or so. The patient is encouraged to experiment with all aspects of the treatment – electrode position, impulse pattern and strength, length and frequency of treatment periods – to obtain the results that suit him or her the best. Certain types of pain (particularly musculoskeletal) respond better than others.

## Acupuncture

Acupuncture is the insertion of fine needles into specific points on the surface of the body, often penetrating fairly deeply. Some stimulus is usually then applied, either mechanically, by rotating the needles, or electrically. A variant is acupressure, when very firm pressure is applied to the point over some minutes. The points have been discovered, mapped and systematized over a very long time period by Chinese traditional medicine, and the effects can be sufficiently striking to allow major surgery to be undertaken; this is rarely done in the UK. Sceptics are inclined to attribute placebo effects and hypnotic augmentation, but many well-designed studies have demonstrated the reality of the benefits. It has also been used successfully for operations on horses (Richardson and Vincent, 1986; Schoen, 1994).

Acupuncture points may be close to the origin of the pain but many are far removed: dental pain may be treated from a point on the hand. The effects are probably mediated by central neural modulation and by the release of endogenous opioids.

Acupuncture can often be unpleasantly painful in its own right, but will frequently produce lasting or repeatable benefit in conditions where other treatments have less acceptable side-effects. As long as equipment is properly cleaned and sterilized, the potential for serious harm is almost negligible, which contrasts powerfully with drug treatments (Anonymous, 1992).

## PHARMACOLOGICAL TECHNIQUES

Pain treatment that involves drugs requires an appropriate level of knowledge and understanding from everyone concerned, especially the patient. Anyone ordering medication for another person must take responsibility for the identity of the drug, precise instructions as to the dose, route and frequency, and the limits of any discretion allowed in these areas as well as any special precautions, such as observation and monitoring. In addition, the prescriber must ensure (or reasonably assume) appropriate knowledge and understanding for the patient or other person administering the drug. Where self-medication takes place using OTC (over the counter, i.e. available without prescription) drugs, some of these responsibilities fall to the supplier.

## Drugs available

These vary in effectiveness, site of action, incidence of side-effects (unwanted effects not necessarily restricting use), toxicity (dangerous effects usually dose related) and adverse events (serious unwanted effects occurring in a few patients sometimes mediated by the immune system). The doses given here are illustrative and must not be relied on as a source of prescribing information. In particular, prescribing for children, the elderly and those with limited organ function requires especial care.

## ▮ Simple analgesics

These are normally given orally but are available as suppositories. They are useful for mild pain and as adjuncts to more powerful drugs when they can have a dose-sparing effect.

Paracetamol is the most commonly used analgesic. Although it can cause severe liver damage in overdose, in normal doses it is safe and effective for mild pain. It is contraindicated in renal or hepatic failure. The adult dose is two 500 mg tablets with a maximum of eight tablets in 24 hours. It reduces pain perception centrally in the brain. Unfortunately, it rarely acts for longer than 4 hours and therefore continuous pain can cause a problem, since only 16 hours will be covered. Patients can be helped by fixing a dose schedule that fits the pattern of the pain, for instance, ensuring a dose at bedtime where sleeping has been disturbed by pain. Aspirin also lasts for about 4 hours, is an effective simple analgesic, but has many relative contraindications, most of which relate to its complex effects on thrombotic regulation. It shares many properties with non-steroidal anti-inflammatory drugs (NSAIDs) including hypersensitivity reactions, which may exacerbate severe asthma. On the other hand, it can be very effective in musculoskeletal pain and should not be forgotten. It must not be given to children because of its association with Reye's syndrome, which may be fatal and is untreatable (Anonymous, 1986).

## ▮ NSAIDs

The non-steroidal anti-inflammatory agents will act as analgesics in many conditions in which there is an inflammatory component. Apart from the rheumatic and musculo-skeletal problems, such as osteoarthritis, for which they were primarily developed, it has been increasingly recognized that they are very helpful for perioperative pain control, since the trauma of surgery causes an inflammatory response which they reduce (Dahl and Kehlet, 1992). Since the drugs act peripherally at the site of trauma, they complement the central actions of opiate drugs and can thus improve pain control without increasing the side-effects (e.g. respiratory depression) associated with them.

However, they are contraindicated in patients with renal impairment and have the potential to cause acute renal failure in situations where renal blood flow is compromised, e.g. severe perioperative hypotension. There is also some evidence that they reduce new bone formation and should not therefore be used in patients having non-cemented joint replacements. They can cause gastrointestinal bleeding and hypersensitivity/asthmatic reactions and should not be given to patients who are allergic to aspirin, since cross-sensitivity is common. These reactions are mainly associated with long-term use and the incidence of problems when NSAIDs are used for acute conditions, such as postoperative pain, seems to be low.

Ibuprofen (200–400 mg, 2–4 times daily) is the safest but others (e.g. diclofenac 50 mg, three times daily) may be more effective. Slow release and rectal preparations are available and make these drugs easy and convenient to use in a variety of situations. There are injectable formulations of some NSAIDs, but they seem to offer few advantages and some are painful.

The long-term use of these drugs in arthritic conditions is only symptomatic and does nothing to reduce the underlying disease process. Serious reactions are commoner in the elderly and can be fatal. It is therefore very important to reassess at intervals whether they cannot be replaced by simpler drugs, such as paracetamol, given regularly (March et al., 1994).

### ∎ Weak opioid drugs and combinations

Several drugs related to morphine are used in an attempt to increase analgesia via the oral route without producing respiratory depressant or addiction problems. Codeine, dihydrocodeine and dextropropoxyphene are in this category. Some are available on their own, but they are most often used in combination with aspirin or paracetamol. The prefix co- in a name indicates 'combination', not necessarily codeine! It is important to check the precise content to avoid substances to which the patient is allergic or reacts badly in some way. In general the 'weakness' of these drugs refers to their analgesic power; they are unfortunately equally capable of causing severe constipation. Similarly, they are capable of producing respiratory depression in overdose and the combination with paracetamol is then particularly dangerous, since hypoxia will potentiate the hepatotoxicity (Proudfoot, 1984).

The main uses of this group of preparations is as a 'step-up' or 'step-down' treatment in the management of changing situations, either when simple analgesics cease to be effective in a progressive condition or where the degree of pain (e.g. postoperatively) no longer requires strong opioids. Patients often express strong preferences between different preparations that could be expected to have very similar effects and it is usually better to respect their views rather than your own. They tend to be longer acting than simple analgesics and this may be part of why they are often found to be more effective by patients. Dosages and limits should be checked individually.

### ∎ Strong opioids

Drugs such as morphine and diamorphine (heroin) have stood the test of time in their effectiveness in severe pain. Despite all the problems they bring with them, the relief that they can afford a person suffering overwhelming pain cannot be overvalued. These drugs act at specific receptors of which there are several different types. These receptors have been identified only relatively recently and active research is constantly updating our under-standing of them. The discovery of specialized opiate receptors indicated that some similar compounds must be present normally and have a physi-ological function (Basbaum and Besson, 1991); in due course, endogenous opioids – the endorphins – were discovered in the central nervous system (Pleuvry, 1991). Their roles are proving difficult to unravel, but they give us some basis for understanding the enormous variation in dosage require-ments for administered opioids between individuals and at different times. Since they are produced in response to neural activity, it is clear that the levels, production and inactivation of endogenous opioids will interact in a complex fashion with administered drugs and with the neurological state of a person.

Morphine acts centrally by diffusion from the blood into the pain-sensing areas of the brain. The intensity of its action will therefore depend on blood levels but the effects will be balanced by the intensity of the painful stimuli reaching the brain. It also acts on centres in the spinal cord and these actions will predominate when morphine is put near to the spinal cord (by spinal or epidural techniques), since higher local concentrations will be reached. The duration of action depends on the method of administration and will be considered in more detail under this heading (see page 103).

## ▮ Side-effects

### Respiratory depression

The analgesia produced will be accompanied by variable degrees of side-effects of which the most dangerous is respiratory depression. Morphine depresses the respiratory centre in the brain, making it less sensitive to carbon dioxide ($CO_2$) which is the normal stimulus to respiration.

#### *Monitoring*

The rate of respiration is usually decreased more than the depth but this is so variable that respiratory rate is not a good indicator of respiratory depres-sion. The most useful aspect of monitoring respiratory rate is to ensure that the patient receives regular overall assessment. In the absence of significant sedation, slow breathing is not an indication for reducing morphine dosage, if pain relief is still required.

There is increasing use of pulse oximetry as a patient monitor post-operatively, and it is important to understand not only what the machine measures but also how it works, otherwise interpretation of the readings can be faulty. Briefly, oximeters depend on sensing pulsatile blood flow and comparing the relative absorption of two wavelengths of light, since oxygenated and deoxygenated haemoglobin behave differently. If the sensor is incorrectly placed, the machine is unable to interpret the absorption pattern and the readings may be too high or too low. To check this, all machines display a pulse rate (the better ones also display a pulse wave form that gives more confidence to interpretation). If the displayed rate differs from the patient's pulse rate (measured either by an ECG trace or by palpation) by more than a few beats the sensor should be repositioned. On compound monitors (where ECG, pulse oximetry, blood pressure, etc. are displayed simultaneously), the true rate will be labelled 'heart rate' and measured from the ECG, and the rate measured by the oximeter will be labelled 'pulse rate'.

Having thus checked that the machine is giving a true reading, the significance of the reading must be interpreted. The normal value is between 98% and 100% indicating that the blood has been fully oxygenated whilst passing through the lungs. The relative levels of $CO_2$ and $O_2$ in air and blood, and the design of the lungs means that they are better at oxygenating the blood than at getting rid of $CO_2$, consequently oxygenation may be maintained even when ventilation is depressed. Adding oxygen to the inspired air accentuates this – under anaesthesia it is possible for a patient to stay fully oxygenated for many minutes without any ventilation, since oxygen will diffuse down the tracheal tube as it is used up; however, $CO_2$ will rise to dangerous levels.

It is clear, therefore, that a normal pulse oximeter reading does not exclude respiratory depression – a most important fact for patient safety. Conversely, a reduced saturation reading shows that the patient's blood is not carrying as much oxygen to the tissues as it should. There are many possible reasons for this, including respiratory depression, possibly combined with other abnormalities such as shunting of venous blood through collapsed areas of lung. A degree of desaturation may have to be accepted. The important rule is that written instructions should define what are acceptable limits for any parameter that is being monitored and the appropriate action to be taken when these limits are passed must be clearly stated.

### Treatment of respiratory depression

Naloxone is an effective antagonist of all the actions of morphine and will therefore reverse the analgesic as well as the respiratory depressant effects of morphine by competition at the receptors. It should be immediately available whenever morphine or related drugs are being given by injection but should only be used in life-threatening respiratory depression, since it may have serious side-effects (Andree, 1980). A suitable initial dose for an adult is 100–200 µg given slowly intravenously. Its action is shorter than that of morphine and treatment that is initially effective may need to be repeated or followed up with an infusion.

## Cough suppression

This action of morphine is shared by diamorphine and codeine, but less by other opiates. It is not closely related to respiratory depression. Patients should be encouraged to cough and breathe deeply regularly. Their ability to cooperate is increased by good pain relief and this is a more effective way of protecting respiratory function.

## Gastrointestinal problems

Nausea, vomiting and constipation are also common and unwanted accompaniments, which can seriously impede recovery and are extremely unpleasant for the patient. Anti-emetics should be freely administered up to the prescribed limits and, if ineffective, the prescription should be reviewed.

Metoclopramide 10–20 mg or prochlorperazine 12.5 mg are usually the first-line drugs. Although both may cause unpleasant muscle spasms, these are not common, and doses that approach those used as prophylaxis for emesis induced by cytotoxic drugs suggest that it would be reasonable to give much larger or more frequent doses of metoclopramide in certain cases. Cyclizine may be effective and the recently introduced ondansetron is justified for persistent vomiting, despite its high cost. When constipation is a problem during morphine treatment, particularly of prolonged pain, a stimulant laxative such as senna may be indicated.

## Mood elevation, addiction and dependence

Morphine can cause euphoria and this is related to its addictive potential. However, this action is virtually confined to administration in the absence of pain. There is no good evidence that the use of morphine to relieve severe acute pain ever results in addiction in the absence of other precipitating factors. Fear of causing addiction is commonly cited as a reason for not giving needed pain relief; this is totally unfounded and unacceptable.

When used for the treatment of chronic pain, it is common for dosage requirements to increase and dependence (characterized by serious withdrawal symptoms on cessation) may occur. Its use in chronic painful conditions is therefore normally reserved for palliation of incurable disease and the benefits are carefully weighed against the likely length of the course of the disease and the problems that may ensue.

## Hypotension

When used intra- and postoperatively, it is common to see minor degrees of hypotension, caused by reduction in vascular tone. This can become important when the patient is vasoconstricting to compensate for fluid depletion. One of the most common areas of mismanagement of postoperative care is the attribution of significant hypotension to pain relieving agents and to respond by reducing them rather than increasing fluid administration. If correction of this common error appears to result in a higher general level of perioperative fluid replacement, I believe that this is because under-replacement has been endemic in the past but inadequately relieved pain has tended to conceal it. Fear of overloading the circulation has been fuelled by the occasional case where replacement of known fluid losses in a shocked and severely vasoconstricted patient has led to pulmonary oedema. This is paradoxically more common in young healthy patients whose ability to vaso-constrict is immense. Vasoconstriction, from whatever cause, requires time to undo even when no longer appropriate. Good pain relief will assist the process.

## ▪ Other strong opiates

These will be mentioned only briefly.

Pethidine is an effective analgesic but has a shorter period of action than morphine. It appears to relieve smooth muscle spasm rather than increase it. It is unsuitable for prolonged use because toxic metabolites may accu-mulate.

Diamorphine has some advantages over morphine because it diffuses more rapidly and therefore its actions may be apparent more rapidly. It is widely regarded as more addictive than morphine.

Pentazocine, phenoperidine, buprenorphine and meptazinol are synthetic drugs that have been introduced in an attempt to improve on some aspects of morphine. Any advantages tend to have been balanced or outweighed by disadvantages.

Alfentanil and fentanyl are relatively short-acting opiates that are mainly used intraoperatively. They are also used specifically for infusions where blood levels can be changed frequently and the effects thus titrated to patients' needs in an intensive therapy situation. Close monitoring is mandatory.

## ▪ Local anaesthetic agents

Drugs such as lignocaine and bupivacaine are used to interrupt transmis-sion of painful impulses by nervous tissue. Their sites of action can therefore be at peripheral nerve endings (infiltration anaesthesia), on somatic or auto-nomic nerves (nerve blocks), or within the spinal cord and nerve roots (spinal and epidural anaesthesia). They are deposited as near to their required site of action as possible, but require transformation and diffusion before they act and therefore (depending on site) delays in the order of 20 minutes may be encountered. If they reach the brain in significant concentrations, very serious toxic reactions occur including convulsions and cardiorespiratory depression. They are unusually toxic drugs in that the safety margin between the effective and toxic doses is much less than for most drugs. They have virtually no side-effects (as opposed to toxic effects).

The pain relief afforded by local anaesthetics tends to be an all-or-nothing phenomenon: either nervous transmission is blocked or it is not, although partial diffusion can lead to patchy blocks with some areas pain free but others with full sensation. The absoluteness of the lack of sensation often needs careful explanation to the patient with reassurance that they have not actually lost sensation (or the leg itself!) for good. Care must also be taken in managing the wearing off of a block, since, if the source of pain is still present and no systemic analgesia has been provided, the effects will be felt as a catastrophic onset of pain. This may not be a simple phenomenon, since adaptation of the central nervous system will also have been interfered with.

Local anaesthetic drugs also affect autonomic nerves and therefore will abolish normal vasoconstrictor tone in blood vessels. If this occurs over a wide area, then a degree of hypotension may result. In normal circumstances, since blood flow is unimpaired, this is of little consequence and merely requires a little extra fluid to fill the increased intravascular space. As with opiate pain relief, it is vital to recognize and treat hypovolaemia due to blood loss or fluid depletion, rather than ascribing it automatically to the effects of nerve block.

### ▪ Clonidine

This drug stimulates alpha-2-adrenoreceptors and is used to treat hypertension. However, it also has analgesic actions when given epidurally or spinally, presumably by blocking transmission in the dorsal horn of the spinal cord (Mendez et al., 1990). It is widely used in veterinary practice and is being evaluated in man. It may find a place as an adjuvant drug.

## ▪ ROUTES OF ADMINISTRATION

There are some points specific to pain treatment that need to be appreciated when considering possible methods of administering drugs. In addition, specialized techniques have been developed to improve the quality of pain management.

### ▪ Oral route

This implies that the patient will swallow the drug and that it will then be absorbed from the gastrointestinal tract (which must therefore be functioning normally) into the blood, and from there diffuse to its site of action. Ease of swallowing can be a very important feature from the patient's point of view and may account for some of the preference for particular formulations (e.g. co-proxamol). Appropriate allowance needs to be made for absorption time when devising a dosage schedule and explaining it to the patient. Slow-release preparations are helpful as they can avoid resurgence of pain during sleep.

## ▪ Rectal preparations

The suppository is probably an underused device in the UK. Absorption of drugs such as NSAIDs, paracetamol and some antiemetics is rapid, and can avoid using injections in nauseated patients. Although widely used as a routine during anaesthesia to smooth pain relief during recovery, the general public are largely unaware of this and need to be informed pre-operatively by the anaesthetist as part of the explanation of anaesthetic/analgesic management.

## ▪ Surface action

EMLA cream (eutectic mixture of local anaesthetics) will effectively anaesthetize intact skin if applied under an occlusive dressing for 90 minutes. The recommended time of one hour is insufficient in a substantial number of cases. It has revolutionized paediatric practice and should be used more widely in adults, at least 10% of whom are needlephobic and regard injections as the worst part of any procedure.

A gel preparation of amethocaine has recently been introduced (Ametop) and seems likely to offer advantages in terms of speed of action and venodilation.

Patch medication, in which drugs are held in special formulations allowing diffusion across the skin, is being developed for many drugs and has been used successfully for antiemesis using hyoscine. It is likely to find a place in the field of daycase surgery (Bailey et al., 1990).

Some drugs such as fentanyl and buprenorphine are also well absorbed from the buccal or nasal mucosa from tablets or sprays, and these routes may merit further investigation.

## ▪ Intermittent injections

The use of injections is hallowed by tradition and some patients (and professionals) undoubtedly regard this route as the most important and effective. Absorption from muscle tissue can be rapid but there is mounting evidence of substantial variability, both between patients and between different sites (Austin et al., 1980). The increasing prevalence of obesity probably results in many 'intramuscular' injections landing in subcutaneous fat, from which absorption will be slow and particularly susceptible to reduced blood flow in postoperative states. With respect to opiates, the enormous variability in dose requirements between patients makes it impossible to ensure an effective but safe dose until the response of a particular patient has been evaluated. To some extent, the anaesthetist is able to do this during and immediately after an operation, and is in a good position to select an appropriate range of dose and minimum time interval for an intramuscular regimen. This opportunity is not taken up often enough.

For children and the many adults who dislike injections, the use of indwelling subcutaneous or intramuscular cannulae is a substantial advance. It has been shown recently that prescribing a minimum dose interval of one hour (rather than the traditional four) allows nurses to manage a flexible dosage scheme to produce excellent results (Gould et al., 1992). The knowledge that a second dose can be given soon if the first is not effective allows a cautious approach. It could be said that a dose that actually provides pain relief for 4 hours is probably too large and one that does not is clearly inadequate.

Using the intravenous route ensures rapid feedback and small increments (e.g. 2 mg morphine every 3–4 minutes) will get on top of acute pain rapidly and safely. Titrating a patient to comfort in this way makes it relatively easy to judge appropriate dosage of opiate by whatever regimen is chosen.

## ▪ Continuous infusions

Intravenous infusions of opiates are often used in the intensive care unit where monitoring is at a high level and patients are often ventilated. On the general ward it is difficult to select an appropriate rate and patient-controlled analgesia (PCA) is almost always to be preferred.

The epidural route, using local anaesthetics alone or in combination with opiates, is more predictable, but requires a higher level of monitoring than is common on postoperative wards. The local anaesthetic blocks nerve and spinal cord function, including the sympathetic nerves that maintain blood vessel tone. The number of segments blocked depends on the balance between the rates of infusion and of inactivation of the block. The aim is to block the segments transmitting pain impulses from the operation site without affecting those responsible for respiratory muscle function or too many of those maintaining vascular tone. The height of the block needs to be checked frequently and the rate of infusion adjusted to maintain good pain relief without respiratory embarrassment or excessive hypotension. Pulse, BP and respiratory rate must be checked and recorded at least every 15 minutes. Continuous monitoring of the oxygen saturation and (preferably) respiratory rate with clear protocols that allow immediate treatment of respiratory problems is  mandatory.

Staff responsible for such patients must understand the monitors, check the alarm settings against those ordered and ensure that alarms are never cancelled (unless automatic reset occurs within one minute). Special training is required and care must not be entrusted to untrained staff. The possibility of migration of the epidural cannula into the subarachnoid (spinal) space, where small amounts of drugs will produce catastrophic nerve blockade and respiratory arrest, is ever present. In addition, epidural and spinal opiates migrate unpredictably within the cerebrospinal fluid and can cause delayed, severe respiratory depression centrally. The intensity of anaesthesia can lead to patient immobility and special care is needed to avoid pressure damage.

Nerve blocks, whilst excellent for some procedures, are rarely suitable for repeated or prolonged use, although some indwelling cannula techniques have been developed, for example, the paravertebral approach for blocking pain from fractured ribs where it is desirable to avoid any respiratory depression from opiates.

## ▮ Patient-controlled analgesia

The majority of patients can and should control their own pain relief. This is common with oral preparations outside hospital and should be extended to in-patients. A daily supply of drugs with instruction and intermittent checking and encouragement would improve patient care and reduce nursing workload. The 'as required' regimen for intramuscular injections should be an example of PCA but delays and inhibitions are built in. The term PCA is normally reserved for systems that allow the patient to administer small amounts (bolus doses) of intravenous or epidural drugs (PCEA) directly. The apparatus is programmed to deliver a dose selected by the prescriber who also specifies a lockout period – a time interval during which the full effects of the bolus can be expected and the machine will not administer another dose. Management protocols, patient information and staff training are necessary but the system is inherently safe, since excessive dosage will result in sedation and the patient will not activate the machine. It is the best way to compensate for inter-patient variability and varying pain levels, and has led to improved patient satisfaction and recovery.

## ■ REFERENCES

**Andree, R.A.** (1980) Sudden death following naloxone administration. *Anesthesia and Analgesia* **59**, 782–788.

**Anonymous** (1986) CSM update: Reye's syndrome and aspirin. *British Medical Journal* **292**, 1590.

**Anonymous** (1992) Hepatitis B associated with an acupuncture clinic. *Communicable Diseases Report Weekly* Nov 27, **2**(48), 219.

**Austin, K.L., Stapleton, J.V. & Mather, L.E.** (1980) Multiple intramuscular injections: a major source of variability in analgesic response to meperidine. *Pain* **8**, 47–62.

**Bailey, P.L., Streisand, J.B., Pace, N.L., Burbers, S.J.M., East, K.A., Mulder, S. & Stanley, T.H.** (1990) Transdermal scopolamine reduces nausea and vomiting after outpatient laparoscopy. *Anesthesiology* **72**, 977–980.

**Basbaum, A.I. & Besson, J.M.** (eds) (1991) *Towards a New Pharmacotherapy of Pain.* John Wiley, Chichester.

**Dahl J.B. & Kehlet, H.** (1992) Non-steroidal anti-inflammatory drugs: rationale for use in severe postoperative pain. *British Journal of Anaesthesia* **66**, 703–712.

**Gould, T.H., Crosby, D.L., Harmer, M., Lloyd, S.M., Lunn, J.N., Rees, G.A.D. et al.** (1992) Policy for controlling pain after surgery: effect of sequential changes in management. *British Medical Journal* **305**, 1187–1193.

**March, L., Irwig, L., Schwarz, J. et al.** (1994) n Of 1 trials comparing a non-steroidal anti-inflammatory drug with paracetamol in osteoarthritis. British Medical Journal **309**, 1041–1045.

**Mendez, R., Eisenach, J.C. & Kashtan, K.** (1990) Epidural clonidine analgesia after Cesarian section. *Anesthesiology* **73**, 848–852.

**Pleuvry, B.J.** (1991) Opioid receptors and their ligands: natural and unnatural. *British Journal of Anaesthesia* **66**, 370–380.

**Proudfoot, A.T.** (1984) Clinical features and management of distalgesic overdose. *Human Toxicology* **3**, 853.

**Richardson, P.H. & Vincent, C.A.** (1986) Acupuncture for the treatment of pain: a review of evaluative research. *Pain* **24**, 15–40.

**Schoen, A.M.** (ed.) (1994) *Veterinary Acupuncture, Ancient Art to Modern Medicine.* American Veterinary Publications Inc., Goleta.

## ■ FURTHER READING

These are all relatively short, practically oriented books:

**Diamond, A.W. & Coniam, S.W.** (1997) *The Management of Chronic Pain* (2nd edn) Oxford University Press, Oxford.

**Heath, M.L. & Thomas, V.J.** (1993) *Patient Controlled Analgesia.* Oxford University Press, Oxford.

**Park, G. & Fulton, B.** (1991) *The Management of Acute Pain.* Oxford University Press, Oxford.

This useful, very brief, booklet helps with particular problem situations:

**Forrest, J.B.** (1993) *Postoperative Pain Management in the At-risk Patient.* Adis, Chester.

# Psychological techniques in the management of pain

## ■ MIND OVER MATTER?

We all use psychological techniques in managing incidental mild to moderate pains, and we may try to help others to mobilize the same techniques when they are in pain. However, pain and associated emotions are far from simple, and severe or chronic pains are not accessible to the same everyday methods. To a certain extent, we can divide discussion of psychological techniques into those processes which are part of any successful treatment, and those psychological techniques which have been developed for use alone or in combination with other specific techniques, such as relaxation.

Before doing so, it would be useful to refer back to the models described in Chapter 1, in order to appreciate that psychological aspects of pain are not a secondary response to an unambiguous stimulus, but a fully integrated part of the pain system from the first synapse. In the Gate Control model (Melzack and Wall, 1965), descending fibres from many parts of the brain (not only from the cortex) are part of 'setting the scene' in the nervous system of the organism about to receive a stimulus, which may ultimately be experienced as pain. Previous experience (whether learned from single or repeated painful instances), current state, mood, alertness and expectations all play a part in the effect of a potentially painful stimulus on that system. We know from animal research that dogs reared in isolation withdraw from pain as expected, but learn neither to avoid it, nor to show other behaviour to which we are accustomed, whimpering and wincing. We learn about pain in a social context, and it is presumably highly adaptive in evolutionary terms that we convey painful experience in a clear way in order that others may avoid it and (if necessary) help us.

If our brains play such an important part in pain, why can we not exercise more control over it? There are extraordinary circumstances in which this seems to occur: in some religious and ecstatic states, for instance, and perhaps in 'emergency analgesia' in battle and sports injuries, but it is far from the norm. More prosaically, dealing effectively with stress may attenuate or prevent stress-related headache. However, in a sense, psychological techniques have been a disappointment in pain control, particularly those with more mystique, such as hypnosis. We have no 'off switch' at the gate which we can operate by thinking the right thing. What is certainly clear, however, is that negative emotions, which often accompany pain of any significance, can be addressed by psychological methods, and that the reduction in suffering brought about by these methods is found to be worthwhile by the sufferer.

Whether enhanced control, reduced anxiety or comfort should be described as reducing pain is probably not a helpful question, since pain is a multidimensional experience, and emotions and beliefs concerned with the pain are important dimensions of it. Gracely (1992) expressed the relationship between sensory and cognitive–affective dimensions of pain using the analogy of height and weight. For some purposes, we can usefully combine the two into the notion of size, but neither height nor weight adequately substitutes for size, and although they are to some extent correlated, it is usually the relationship between the two that we are interested in. This is certainly a more helpful model than that of trying to assign percentages of the total pain experience to emotion, beliefs or any other of the multiple interacting dimensions.

## ■ PSYCHOLOGICAL ISSUES ACCESSORY TO PHYSICAL TREATMENTS

The expectations on the part of the person being treated and those of the person or team delivering the treatment are important components of the still incompletely understood placebo phenomenon, and are not covered here. The reader is referred to a general review by Richardson (1995), and to papers concerning placebo phenomena in pain by Richardson (1994) and by Peck and Coleman (1991). Placebo response is not, as commonly believed, a fixed characteristic of a gullible person. In one person, it can vary across substances, across time for the same substance and even across measures on the same occasion. It appears not just in self-report (such as of analgesia), but in processes not under conscious control, such as blood pressure or swelling. It tends to be greater where the treatment is more serious or impressive, with an 85% response rate in fake surgery for angina. (In the placebo condition, patients were anaesthetized, an incision made and sutured, but no other surgery done. Unfortunately for placebo researchers, such experiments are no longer ethically acceptable.) It can also be greater where the therapist has higher status, and where he/she believes strongly in the treatment, and shows considerable interest in the patient and the effects of treatment. Such effects in a range of therapies are explored in a fascinating book by Frank and Frank (1991).

No single process can account for placebo response, but anxiety reduction, conditioning and various cognitive processes can all contribute. Pain relief by a saline injection provides no information about the quality or quantity of pain, nor about the patient's personality. It is most emphatically not a test of the 'reality' of the pain, and it is unethical to use it in this way. More commonly, psychological effects which militate against analgesia are induced by systematic undermedication (Morgan, 1989; Royal College of Surgeons and College of Anaesthetists, 1990), often through irrational fears of addiction (Morgan, 1989; Portenoy and Payne, 1992). The term 'pseudoaddiction' (Weissman and Haddox, 1989) has been used to describe the addict-like behaviour of the anxious, distressed patient whose analgesia is delayed and restricted. He or she starts to exaggerate the pain and to anticipate it, to counteract the delays and restrictions. Staff become suspicious and more restrictive; the patient may try to obtain illicit supplies and to hoard and lie. The alternative is clear: patients given adequate analgesia recover faster, are less distressed, and are easier for staff to manage. Under patients' own control (see Chapter 10 on post-operative pain) good analgesia can make a very significant difference to psychological and physical recovery. Patients' expectations of good pain relief can be mobilized when they are given genuine information about analgesic options, with discussion about how they can best be used in relation to sleep, daytime function, and concern about short- or long-term adverse effects. Nursing staff are well placed to elicit and to answer patients' questions and doubts, and to enhance patients' confidence in and adherence to treatment.

# ■ PSYCHOLOGY-BASED TREATMENTS

The psychological techniques described and discussed here are biofeedback and hypnosis, cognitive strategies and the pain management approach for chronic pain. Relaxation, an important intervention for both, is covered in a separate chapter in this volume (Chapter 13), but will be referred to here, since, like enhanced sense of control, it describes a process by which some interventions appear to be effective.

The techniques that follow are not separate processes but are discussed separately for the sake of clarity. It is tempting to try to develop linear models in which a sequence of stages leads towards the outcome – in this case, reduced pain – but such oversimplification is not helpful. Instead the focus here has been on points or routes of intervention demonstrated to be of some help. So while some researchers suggest that whatever the treatment modality, functional improvement always requires cognitive change, this is hard to prove or disprove, and it is more useful just to recognize that any intervention, however apparently simple and concrete, may be associated with a sense of enhanced control, of hope, of gratitude for help, of relief that the pain is recognized by another person who provided help, or conversely of disappointment at being unable to manage without help, of anxiety about adverse effects, and so on.

# ■ BIOFEEDBACK

Biofeedback describes any technique where a biological process of which the individual does not usually have direct awareness is indicated by some means (usually an auditory or visual signal) which brings it to awareness. It is used to enable the individual to develop control over that process: blood flow in migraine and in peripheral neuropathy, muscle tension in headache and musculoskeletal pain. It is little used in the UK and is unfamiliar as a medical technique, although increasingly gyms and chemists provide means of measuring and displaying heart rate, and alpha-wave monitors have a small following. However, several reviews (Turk et al., 1979; Turner and Chapman, 1982a; Jessup and Gallegos, 1994) have found it no more effective than well-taught relaxation, which can also reduce muscle tension, modify blood flow, etc. Relaxation is one of the means by which biofeedback brings about effective change; it also gives individuals a sense of control, which is helpful in itself. One review (Turner and Chapman, 1982a) attributed its popularity largely to aggressive marketing by manufacturers, and advertisements certainly make much greater claims than have ever been substantiated by properly conducted studies. One of the major problems is that there is very little association between muscle tension and pain in the area of tension, so that gaining considerable control over tension levels in those muscles may make no difference to pain. In fact, reversing the feedback so that patients learn to increase tension is as effective in relieving pain! Another problem is that patients can find it hard to transfer the skills of awareness and relaxation into everyday situations, having learned them wired up to a machine, which, certainly initially, may have added credibility to what is otherwise a very 'low-tech' treatment.

However, it may be that the simple chronic muscle tension model, rather than biofeedback, is at fault. Work in which tension increases in the low back were monitored and shown to be responsive to personally relevant stresses, with a very slow return to baseline, has shown long-term benefits of muscle activity biofeedback over relaxation in reducing chronic rheumatic back pain (Flor et al., 1985, 1986). This occurred perhaps because patients effectively learned stress management skills, and because those who had learned to relax with biofeedback continued to practise more frequently than those who had learned without. There is also some evidence that patients develop dysfunctional muscle tension patterns on movement, but measuring and recording these complex sequences is technically very difficult.

## ■ HYPNOSIS

Hypnosis is not easily defined or measured, nor can a brief section here explore all the issues. The chapter by Spanos et al. (1994) is strongly recommended to interested readers. Laboratory studies, in which volunteer subjects immerse a hand in ice-water for as long as they can tolerate it, show impressive increases in tolerance under hypnosis. However, similar increases occur when patients are given the same instructions without being hypnotized, or when they are instructed in the use of certain cognitive strategies. In clinical studies, results are not so clear, and there is often no check on whether, in fact, the patient is in a hypnotic state. In headaches it can provide brief relief; in dental procedures, burn dressing, and postoperative pain, it provides better pain relief than no treatment, but where it is compared with instruction in coping with pain, it does not show clear benefit. Although physiological changes have been shown under hypnosis, comparison with the same instructions without hypnosis was not made. Hypnotic pain relief (like placebo pain relief) appears to rely on relaxation, plus a mixture of psychological processes which have barely been studied in the context of hypnosis, but which include a range of cognitive strategies such as relabelling and reduced catastrophizing, and social pressures to do (and feel) as instructed (Turner and Chapman, 1982b; Spanos et al., 1994). (As some popular television programmes demonstrate, apparently sensible members of the general public do not require hypnosis, only persuasive instruction, to perform extraordinary behaviours.) Self-hypnosis, while not arousing the expectations of hypnosis by an 'expert', is an effective version of relaxation. The addition of positive self-statements about sensations and physical state is called autogenic relaxation (Linden, 1990).

## ■ COGNITIVE STRATEGIES

It is possible to use the attention phenomena described in Chapter 3 to manage brief painful episodes, particularly when pain is expected, as in medical procedures such as burn debridement. Cognitive strategies, which require attention to be devoted to them, can be grouped variously: an empirical classification of their dimensions (Fernandez and Turk, 1989) contrasts those which acknowledge the sensation with those which deny it. Examples of those which acknowledge the sensation are those which develop verbal labels or imagery for the pain, and associated sensations which are progressively modified towards less unpleasant versions (burning reduced to warm); and those which build the pain into an imaginal storyline, whether relaxing (lying in the shade under a tree but with an uncomfortable root in one's back) or active (using a sports or adventure 'script'). Strategies which deny the sensation are commonly described as distracting, and may use events or objects in the environment as a focus for concentration, or mental stimuli (from mental arithmetic or recitation of memorized poetry or prose to imaginal storylines or images without incorporating pain). The effectiveness of the strategy in attenuating pain appears to be related to its demands on attention (see Chapter 3). All take practice, and what might be most important for efficacy is that the patient becomes skilled in several, so that he or she can select appropriately, and switch strategies when the current one becomes hard to sustain. Relying on a single cognitive strategy, as many women are taught to do in preparation for childbirth, risks leaving the user feeling that he or she has failed and has no further means to cope if the chosen strategy cannot be sustained.

Behavioural distraction should also be mentioned. Many chronic pain sufferers report that they try to 'keep busy' or 'do something rather than nothing' to engage at least some of their attention. This can be effective in modifying depressed mood (Williams, 1992), in turn easing the experience of pain directly and indirectly. The disadvantage of this method, however, is that in performing the 'something', the pain sufferer may make demands on his or her body for which it is no longer in fit condition (even if only sitting for an hour at a computer), and postural strains and muscle tensions may lead to a punishing build-up of pain, so that the cost in pain of such distraction discourages the patient.

The theme of having control, or believing oneself to have control, runs through the examination of cognitive and behavioural strategies. Sometimes, having control can consist of putting oneself in the hands of someone with superior knowledge and skills, such as a doctor (Skevington, 1990), but more usually, the principle is that improved control over various aspects of life can improve health significantly (Rodin, 1986). Education alone may facilitate the acquisition of skills, but may not be sufficient to engender belief that exercising those skills will exert control. In addition, it is not so easy to teach the early identification of situations in which the skills can bring the user benefit, nor the flexible matching of strategy to situation and demands, which characterizes those who handle substantial pain without significant adverse emotional or intellectual effects (Weisenberg, 1987; Meichenbaum, 1993). Cognitive strategies appear to involve more than just attention diversion (Rybstein-Blinchik, 1979). It does appear that the experience is reformulated so that it is less distressing (Rybstein-Blinchik and Grzesiak, 1979; Thompson, 1981). Belief in one's ability to tolerate pain is directly related to tolerance of experimental pain (keeping one's hand in ice-water), as is attribution of the ability to tolerate painful cold to one's own efforts, since subjects who took a placebo tolerated less pain, and gave higher pain ratings (Dolce et al., 1986).

## ■ INFORMATION

The importance of information (or education, or explanation) in helping to appraise and manage pain has been described by Eccleston in Chapter 3. In the acute situation, preparation and mobilization of personally preferred strategies seems to be important. In the chronic situation, it is perhaps more important that such strategies counteract unhelpful and inaccurate beliefs and the catastrophizing which is often associated with those beliefs. For instance, patients often have a crude understanding of the nervous system in which pain, numbness and tingling all warn of 'something wrong with nerves', leading to inevitable worsening and paralysis. Others, informed that they have 'degenerative' back conditions, understand that to mean that their spines are crumbling with use. It is important to recognize that patients are often acting logically within their conceptualization of their bodies and what is wrong, and that without comprehensible and appropriate information, those conceptualizations will not become any more accurate. Adherence to treatment is also significantly improved by the provision of information about treatment and its effects on the symptoms which trouble the patient (Vandereycken and Meermann, 1988).

Anxiety is an important concomitant of acute and chronic pain. It can be reduced by information. It can also be reduced by other behavioural and cognitive means. Graded exposure to a feared activity or event is a well-established treatment for a variety of fears, and this exposure can take place in the imagination (this is probably one of the functions of worry where it serves to improve eventual coping) or can be observed in another person. This learning by seeing another person cope, modelling, is used formally in helping children to prepare for unpleasant medical procedures (Melamed, 1977), and informally in the solidarity which patients give one another. Gaining and exercising control helps people to cope better with a wide range of stressors, including pain. Reassurance, where it is effective, often consists of appropriate information, plus a statement of confidence in the coping capacity of the recipient of the reassurance.

Chronic pain is strongly associated with depression. It is probably pointless to try to arrive at a statement of prevalence, as it depends crucially on the population studied, on the measure of pain and the measure of depression. For patients, it is associated directly with the pain, and the sense of defeat if they feel unable to control it, and indirectly with the pain through its effects on their lives. These range from everyday concerns about movements and activities, and a wish to conserve both energies and uncertain physical state, to minor and major giving up of work, social and leisure activities. With these changes often come a sense of helplessness and pointlessness, a loss of everyday satisfactions and pleasures in a variety of pursuits, of a sense of health and resilience, and of independence. In extreme cases, of which there are all too many, work loss and reduced income can be followed by loss of home and family break-up.

Unfortunately, added to this is usually a sense of injustice and isolation. Chronic pain sufferers are often disbelieved, by their friends, families, employers and workmates, and by medical personnel. They have no way to prove their pain, and the stereotype invoked is that of a malingerer – someone who is inventing a physical problem or exaggerating a minor one in order to obtain sympathy and attention, a sickness-based income, and psychoactive analgesics. Like many stereotypes, there are odd elements of truth, but the concept is oversimplified and overused to the extent that it is much more damaging than helpful. Patients may be told – and may believe – that it is 'all in the mind' (that is, imagined), and that they should try to ignore it or fight it: that if they wished or exerted themselves, they could control and therefore overcome the effects of the pain on their lives. This implies that patients have either not thought of this or not tried it, suggestions which they understandably find somewhat insulting and rejecting.

Let us for a moment examine what would provide secure foundations for the 'all in the mind' model. We would have to overlook 30 years of impressive research arising from the Gate Control model (Melzack and Wall, 1965) and associated models of neuroplasticity in relation to pain. We would have to assume that medical investigative technology and diagnostic procedures have reached the point where all physical problems can be detected and diagnosed. We would have to be sure that pain can only arise from structural problems identified by such technology and not from changes of function within intact structures. We would have to believe that large numbers of people, many giving powerful impressions of suffering, do in fact find satisfactions ('secondary gains') in being recognized as physically ill or disabled, satisfactions which outweigh the personal, social, vocational and financial losses they experience (usefully contrasted as 'primary loss'). How well does this stand up to scrutiny? Yet the 'mind over matter' model is all too common among health professionals. Psychology would do well to investigate why such models persist, against the evidence. It is certainly easier for the professional faced with a distressed patient to opt for an explanation which blames (and dismisses) the patient, rather than for one which acknowledges the shortcomings of current medical diagnostic systems and treatment techniques, and finds a way, as the patient must do, to bear the uncertainties of our current understandings. There are many worthwhile techniques by which the chronic pain sufferer can be enabled to regain the losses contingent on pain and these are described below.

## ■ DIRECT MODIFICATION OF NEGATIVE AFFECT

Pain can also be attenuated by reducing anxiety and distress directly. In fact, the implied contrast is a false one, since current state and past experience, including affective experience and affect integral to memories of pain and coping, contribute to any pain experience (Weisenberg, 1987). However, as we saw in Chapter 2, it is not uncommon for a pain to be reduced to a trivial discomfort or to disappear altogether when it is explained as indigestion rather than impending heart attack, or minor tissue damage rather than cancer. A vivid example from the author's clinical experience is that of a patient who reported herself to be unable to sit for a few seconds, and when asked to speak her thoughts out loud as she prepared to sit was found to be repeating 'I can't bear it – this is going to kill me'. Since she believed that the stress of intense pain could in fact kill her, the situation was extremely threatening for her, but replacing her statement with 'This cannot harm me – I can cope with the pain', backed up by education both about her physical condition and about stress, resulted in an immediate tenfold increase in her sitting tolerance. This sort of thinking – that only the worst can happen, and is sure to happen – is characteristic of intense anxiety and panic, and is often described as 'catastrophizing'.

The capacity for catastrophizing in imagery has probably been underestimated and there is increasing interest in the use of imagery in cognitive therapy. Many patients use vivid and horrific images of torture, which implies absolute helplessness in the face of malign power. They may also

*Table 7.1* *Cognitive behavioural management of chronic pain*

| Aims | Means |
| --- | --- |
| Improve mobility | Fitness programme |
| Increase activity | Goal setting and placing |
| Improve mood and confidence | Cognitive techniques |
| Cease taking unhelpful drugs | Staff- or patient-controlled gradual reduction |
| Improve sleep | Relaxation and sleep habits |
| Improve social relationships | Communication/negotiation skills |
| Improve understanding of condition | Education and access to information |

use unpleasant similes rarely based on experience, such as of being stabbed. It is possible to modify such images to render them less unpleasant, frightening and hopeless versions, as described for acute pain.

## ■ COGNITIVE-BEHAVIOURAL MANAGEMENT OF CHRONIC PAIN

The term pain management covers quite a wide variety of practices, most compatible with one another and with cognitive and behavioural principles as described in the key texts (Fordyce, 1976; Turk et al., 1983; Philips, 1988), but sometimes unduly influenced by orthodox medical and psychiatric models and practices. The aim of pain management, as distinct from pain relief, is to modify the overall experience of suffering: the components of a typical programme are shown in Table 7.1. Of course, significant pain reduction may also be a realistic goal for some patients, but is a standard goal of treatment only in headache sufferers. The problems arising from having chronic pain have considerable impact in their own right. In the physical domain, the patient becomes unfit, often develops habits of posture and tension (which in the long term exacerbate the problem) and progressively loses flexibility and mobility. In the everyday domain, the patient becomes less able to carry out many tasks and chores, and also to meet work and family responsibilities, and to continue social, sporting and other pleasurable pursuits. When he or she does try to carry on as before, the increase in pain punishes those attempts. He or she may not be able to find any position which is comfortable for long, and suffer disturbed sleep because of the pain.

In the medical arena, the patient is disappointed at the failure of procedures intended to help, and dismayed when the pain is worsened, as it may be by repeated surgery with little indication (Waddell, 1991). Analgesics provide little relief but have unpleasant unwanted effects; psychotropic drugs for mood elevation or for sleep may compound the problems, leaving the patient sedated and with added discomforts such as constipation. Emotionally, the patient may be anxious about the continuing pain and its meaning, depressed by the apparently irreversible losses suffered, bitter about the unfairness of it all, and not infrequently angry about the sense of being neglected or abandoned by the medical profession, employers and the welfare system. The sufferer may spend much time alone, perhaps through lying down in the daytime, perhaps by being confined to the home, or perhaps because he or she is poor company for family members or friends who feel helpless and distressed in the face of the suffering. This picture is painted very vividly in the self-help book by Shone (1992). Even without pain, living like this would be a miserable existence, and one unlikely to resolve spontaneously. These problems, therefore, which arise from having continuing pain, and in part from using means of coping which work well for short-lived pains, are the main target of change in pain management.

The psychological principles of some of the techniques of pain management are clear. However, it is important to recognize them throughout, since they require changes in practice for the nurses and physiotherapists who are involved in delivering them alongside psychologists. The evidence on mood elevation by exercise in unfit and distressed people is weaker than in healthy and non-distressed people (Abele and Brehm, 1993). However, there is no doubt that learning to exercise under expert supervision, and to regain lost fitness, flexibility, strength and stamina, helps patients to develop confidence in their physical capacity, which has been severely eroded by the experience of chronic pain. Such confidence can only be developed by careful assessment of starting points and rate of progress, so that the patient has multiple and repeated success in meeting goals of increasing activity (Harding and Williams, 1995). The use of aids, such as walking sticks, orthopaedic corsets, stair lifts and railings must be questioned, since the aim is to enable the patient to be as mobile and adaptable as possible, rather than to perpetuate disability by the provision of substitutes for independent action.

Longer-term and larger-scale goals described by patients are broken down into component activities and physical requirements, and interim and short-term goals identified. Chronic pain sufferers often alternate between overactivity (in relation to their physical state), under the pressure of internal or external demands, and rest to recover from the resultant pain. Unfortunately, this is no more successful for building better physical condition and confidence in that condition than if a sportsperson were to attempt peak performance occasionally, and rest between times. The system of steady gradual specified increases in activities, using times not pain as the guide, is called pacing, and is a cornerstone of pain management.

Problems in analgesic use have been mentioned above, and one of the most important roles for the nurse in pain management is to educate patients about the rational and effective use of analgesic and psychotropic drugs, many of which are disappointing in chronic pain (McQuay, 1989; Portenoy, 1990; Brena and Sanders, 1991), and to help patients to reduce their drug intake as they learn other means of control. Patients may continue to take unhelpful drugs for a variety of reasons, including intermittent or coincident benefit. (A Schulz cartoon makes this point well. Snoopy wakes in the night with a headache, puts on his towelling dressing gown, gets some fresh air and takes an aspirin, and goes back to bed feeling better, attributing it all to the comforting dressing gown!) Other reasons include apparent expression by the doctor of belief and concern by the act of prescribing for the patient, and the temporary escape from distressing thoughts and feelings when sedated. Unfortunately, the drugs may contribute to cognitive impairment, sleep problems, and patterns of over- and underactivity. While the traditional approach has been to reduce opioids by means of a cocktail of morphine, a naturalistic comparison of cocktail with patient-controlled reduction showed the latter to be far better maintained in the longer term (Ralphs et al., 1994). Psychotropic drugs are used rather uncritically in chronic pain (Hanks, 1984), and also contribute to a range of unpleasant adverse effects including cognitive impairment (Healy, 1993).

Any process by which people develop new and more effective ways of dealing with their difficulties, extending their capacities to bring valued goals closer, and regaining lost autonomy, can clearly be construed in psychological terms. The gradual achievement of feared activities, such as many of the physical exercises and goals of mobility, approximates to graded exposure, helping to overcome fears and avoidance. While such changes were originally conceptualized purely in behavioural terms, they are now understood to involve cognitive change, as suggested by the sprinkling of terms such as 'confidence' and 'control' in the paragraphs describing the treatment components. Part of the cognitive teaching in pain management programmes makes this explicit, and helps patients to articulate the principles of good problem-solving, and of habit change and maintenance of those changes.

Some pain-management programmes choose to restrict their cognitive interventions to counselling (for which there is no track record of efficacy in pain management, where patients usually require new knowledge and skills), and/or to teaching the cognitive attention-based strategies described above. While this may be suitable for populations mildly disabled by the pain, it is a disservice to distressed patients, who have rarely had access to psychological help (distinct from pharmacotherapy or psychiatric diagnostics) for anxiety and depression of varying severity, but related to their pain. Cognitive therapy methods are well described in Williams (1992) and in

Blackburn and Davidson (1990), in Moorey and Greer (1989) for cancer patients, and in relation to pain, in Philips (1988) and Williams and Erskine (1994). Their main focus is to bring to awareness and to subject to scrutiny the content of the patients' beliefs and the connections between those beliefs and the patients' behaviour and feelings, insofar as these are problematic. This makes it possible to change those beliefs and the associated behaviour and feelings. For instance, the patient who believes (often from childhood) that he or she should strive to achieve as high a standard (in quantity or quality) as possible in any task, and that to opt to do less is morally reprehensible, will tend to push him or herself beyond the limits of fitness and tolerance. The result is often that the patient collapses, takes prolonged rest to recover, experiences increased anxiety and is bitterly disappointed at the high cost of the achievement. All of these will contribute to increased problems in managing the pain. In addition, such behaviour confuses those who know the patient, and who see him or her mowing the lawn or washing the windows one day, and unable even to stand for a few moments the next.

Of course there is no suggestion that cognitive therapy skills can be acquired from a book and practised on patients. It requires careful discussion to help patients to identify internal and external influences on their pain, to distinguish pain from other forms of distress, and to question some of their assumptions in the light of new information. Self-help books by Shone (1992) and by Broome and Jellicoe (1987) are recommended, and their use can be facilitated by a sympathetic partner, friend or health professional. Friends and family members play a complex part in the development of the patient's coping strategies, both helpful and unhelpful. While a very anxious and solicitous spouse may encourage the patient's disability and dependence, such patients tend to be more satisfied with life in general and with their marriages than those whose spouses are more detached. However, it is no doubt helpful to engage important people in the patient's life, whether family members, neighbours, workmates, or the general practitioner, in encouraging the changes the patient makes in pain management.

There is good evidence for the efficacy of pain management overall (Flor et al., 1992), although few controlled studies. Following pain management, patients were on average better than before treatment, and than untreated controls on a range of outcome measures covering activity, return to work, drug use and psychological measures. Improvements were also greater from pain management programmes than from treatment by single elements of the programme, such as physical therapy. While comparison with control groups is desirable, it is important to note that chronic pain patients have had little benefit from previous treatments, and therefore will have generally low expectations of future treatments (Peck and Coleman, 1992). Results of programmes in the UK have been published of an in-patient programme

(Ralphs, 1993) by Williams et al. (1993), and of out-patient programmes by Skinner et al. (1990) and Luscombe et al. (1995). All showed improvements in function and activity, psychological health, and drug and other health-care use, generally lasting to follow-up periods of up to one year.

# ■ CONCLUSION

It is hard to summarize the many ways in which psychological variables are part of the experience of pain, and therefore to suggest the variety of treatments which may be of help to the pain sufferer. The repeated finding that psychological variables account for far more of the differences in disability, daily function and health-care use than do medical and disease variables, or personal variables such as age, sex or education (Jensen and Karoly, 1992; Jensen et al. 1994), or of personality (Gamsa, 1994a, b) still eludes many researchers, who therefore do not measure these variables, and many clinicians, who make assumptions based on outdated models and stereotypes. I hope that this chapter challenges some of those models, implicit and explicit, and offers suggestions for more productive and more satisfying interactions with people in pain.

# ■ REFERENCES

**Abele, A. & Brehm, W.** (1993) Mood effects of exercise versus sports games: findings and implications for wellbeing and health. In: Maes, S., Leventhal, H. & Johnston, M. (eds) *International Review of Health Psychology*, Vol. 2. John Wiley & Sons, Chichester, pp. 53–80.

**Blackburn, I.-M. & Davidson, K.** (1990) *Cognitive Therapy for Depression and Anxiety.* Blackwell Scientific Publications, Oxford.

**Brena, S.F. & Sanders, S.H.** (1991) Opioids in nonmalignant pain: questions in search of answers. *Clinical Journal of Pain* **7**, 342–345.

**Broome, A. & Jellicoe, H.** (1987) *Living with Your Pain.* British Psychological Society, Leicester, in association with Methuen, London.

**Dolce, J.J., Doleys, D.M., Raczynski, J.M., Lossie, J., Poole, L. & Smith, M.** (1986) The role of self-efficacy expectancies in the prediction of pain tolerance. *Pain* **27**, 261–272.

**Fernandez, E. & Turk, D.C.** (1989) The utility of cognitive coping strategies for altering pain perception: a meta-analysis. *Pain* **38**, 123–135.

**Flor, H., Fydrich T. & Turk, D.C.** (1992) Efficacy of multidisciplinary pain treatment centers: a meta-analytic review. *Pain* **49**, 221–230.

**Flor, H., Haag, G. & Turk D.C.** (1986) Long-term efficacy of EMG biofeedback for chronic rheumatic back pain. *Pain* **27**, 195–202.

**Flor, H., Turk, D.C. & Birbaumer, N.** (1985) Assessment of stress-related psychophysiological reaction in chronic back pain patients. *Journal of Consultative Clinical Psychology* **53**, 354–364.

**Fordyce, W.E.** (1976) *Behavioural Methods for Chronic Pain and Illness.* CV Mosby, St Louis.

**Frank, J.D. & Frank, J.B.** (1991) *Persuasion and Healing*, 3rd edn. Johns Hopkins University Press, Baltimore.

**Gamsa, A.** (1994a) The role of psychological factors in chronic pain. I. A half century of study. *Pain* **57**, 5–15.

**Gamsa, A.** (1994b) The role of psychological factors in chronic pain. II. A critical appraisal. *Pain* **57**, 17–29.

**Gracely, R.H.** (1992) Evaluation of multi-dimensional pain scales. *Pain* **48**, 297–300.

**Hanks, G.W.** (1984) Psychotropic drugs. *Postgraduate Medical Journal* **60**, 881.

**Harding, V.H. & Williams, A.C. deC.** (1995) Extending physiotherapy skills using a psychological approach: cognitive behavioural management of chronic pain. *Physiotherapy* **81**, 681–688.

**Healy, D.** (1993) *Psychiatric Drugs Explained.* Mosby, Guildford.

**Jensen, M.P. & Karoly, P.** (1992) Pain-specific beliefs, perceived symptom severity, and adjustment to chronic pain. *Clinical Journal of Pain* **8**, 123–130.

**Jensen, M.P., Turner, J.A., Romano, J.M. & Lawler, B.K.** (1994) Relationship of pain-specific beliefs to chronic pain adjustment. *Pain* **57**, 301–309.

**Jessup, B.A. & Gallegos, X.** (1994) Relaxation and biofeedback. In: Wall, P.D. & Melzack, R. (eds) *Textbook of Pain*, 3rd edn. Churchill Livingstone, Edinburgh, pp. 1321–1336.

**Linden, W.** (1990) *Autogenic Training: A Clinical Guide.* Guildford Press, New York.

**Luscombe, F.E., Wallace, L., Williams J. & Griffiths, D.P.G.** (1995) A District General Hospital pain management programme. *Anaesthesia* **50**, 114–117.

**McQuay, H.J.** (1989) Opioids in chronic pain. *British Journal of Anaesthesia* **63**, 213–226.

**Meichenbaum, D.** (1993) Changing conceptions of cognitive behavior modification: retrospect and prospect. *Journal of Consulting and Clinical Psychology* **61**, 202–204.

**Melamed, B.G.** (1977) Psychological preparation for hospitalization. In: Rachman, S. (ed.) *Contributions to Medical Psychology*, Vol. 1. Pergamon Press, Oxford, pp. 43–74.

**Melzack, R. & Wall, P.D.** (1965) Pain mechanisms: a new theory. *Science* **150**, 971.

**Moorey, S. & Greer, S.** (1989) *Psychological Therapy for Patients with Cancer.* Heinemann Medical Books, Oxford.

**Morgan, J.P.** (1989) American opiophobia: customary underutilization of opioid anagesics. In: Hill, C.S. & Fields, W.S. (eds) *Advances in Pain Research and Therapy*, Vol. 11. Raven Press, New York, pp. 181–189.

**Peck, C. & Coleman, G.** (1991) Implications of placebo theory for clinical research and practice in pain management. *Theoretical Medicine* **12**, 247–270.

**Philips, H.C.** (1988) *The Psychological Management of Chronic Pain: A Treatment Manual.* Springer, New York.

**Portenoy, R.K.** (1990) Chronic opioid therapy in nonmalignant pain. *Journal of Pain and Symptom Management* **5**, S46–S62.

**Portenoy, R.K. & Payne, R.** (1992) Acute and chronic pain. In: Lowinson, J.H., Ruiz, P. & Millman, R.B. (eds) *Comprehensive Textbook of Substance Abuse*. Williams and Wilkins, Baltimore, pp. 691–721.

**Ralphs, J.** (1993) The cognitive behavioural treatment of chronic pain. In: Carroll, D. & Bowsher, D. (eds.) *Pain Management and Nursing Care*. Butterworth-Heinemann, Oxford, pp. 59–67.

**Ralphs, J.A., Williams, A.C.deC., Richardson, P.H., Pither, C.E. & Nicholas, M.K.** (1994) Opiate reduction in chronic pain patients: a comparison of patient-controlled reduction and staff controlled cocktail methods. *Pain* **56**, 279–288.

**Richardson, P.H.** (1994) Placebo effects in pain management. *Pain Reviews* **1**, 15–32.

**Richardson, P.H.** (1995) Placebos: their effectiveness and modes of action. In: Broome A. & Llewelyn, S. (eds) *Health Psychology: Processes and Applications*, 2nd edn. Chapman & Hall, London, pp. 35–51.

**Rodin, J.** (1986) Aging and health: effects of the sense of control. *Science* **233**, 1271–1276.

**Royal College of Surgeons of England & The College of Anaesthetists** (1990) *Commission on the Provision of Surgical Services. Report of the Working Party: Pain after Surgery*. Royal College of Surgeons, London.

**Rybstein-Blinchik, E.** (1979) Effects of different cognitive strategies on chronic pain experience. *Journal of Behavioral Medicine* **2**, 93–101.

**Rybstein-Blinchik, E. & Grzesiak, R.C.** (1979) Reinterpretative cognitive strategies in chronic pain management. *Archives of Physical Medicine and Rehabilitation* **60**, 609–612.

**Shone, N.** (1992) *Coping Successfully with Pain*. Sheldon Press, London.

**Skevington, S.M.** (1990) A standardised scale to measure beliefs about controlling pain: a preliminary study. *Psychology and Health* **4**, 221–232.

**Skinner, J.B., Erskine, A., Pearce, S. Rubenstein, I., Taylor, M. & Foster, C.** (1990) The evaluation of a cognitive behavioural treatment programme in outpatients with chronic pain. *Journal of Psychosomatic Research* **34**, 13–19.

**Spanos, N.P., Carmanico, S.J. & Ellis, J.A.** (1994) Hypnotic analgesia. In: Wall, P.D. & Melzack, R. (eds) *Textbook of Pain*, 3rd edn. Churchill Livingstone, Edinburgh, pp. 1349–1366.

**Thompson, S.C.** (1981) Will it hurt less if I can control it? A complex answer to a simple question. *Psychological Bulletin* **90**, 89–101.

**Turk, D.C., Meichenbaum, D.H. & Berman, W.H.** (1979) Application of biofeedback for the regulation of pain: a critical review. *Psychological Bulletin* **86**, 1322–1338.

**Turk, D.C., Meichenbaum, D. & Genest, M.** (1983) *Pain and Behavioral Medicine*. Guilford Press, New York.

**Turner, J.A. & Chapman, C.R.** (1982a) Psychological interventions for chronic pain: a critical review. I. Relaxation training and biofeedback. *Pain* **12**, 1–21.

**Turner, J.A. & Chapman, C.R.** (1982b) Psychological interventions for chronic pain: a critical review. II. Operant conditioning, hypnosis, and cognitive-behavioral therapy. *Pain* **12**, 23–46.

**Vandereycken, W. & Meermann, R.** (1988) Chronic illness behavior and noncompliance with treatment: pathways to an interactional approach. *Psychotherapy and Psychosomatics* **50**, 182–191.

**Waddell, G.** (1991) Low back disability: a syndrome of Western civilization. *Neurosurgery Clinics of North America* **2**, 719–738.

**Weisenberg, M.** (1987) Psychological intervention for the control of pain. *Behaviour Research and Therapy* **25**, 401.

**Weissman, D.E. & Haddox, J.D.** (1989) Opioid pseudoaddiction – an iatrogenic syndrome. *Pain* **36**, 363–366.

**Williams A.C.deC. & Erskine, A.** (1994) Chronic pain. In: Broome, A. & Llewelyn, S. (eds) *Health Psychology*, 2nd edn. Chapman & Hall, London, pp. 353–376.

**Williams, A.C.deC., Nicholas, M.K., Richardson, P.H., Pither, C.E., Justins, D.M., Chamberlain, J.H., Harding, J.R., Ralphs, J.A., Jones, S.C., Dieudonne, I., Featherstone, J.D., Hodgson, D.R., Ridout, K.L. & Shannon, E.M.** (1993) Evaluation of a cognitive behavioural programme for rehabilitating patients with chronic pain. *British Journal of General Practice* **43**, 513–518.

**Williams, J.M.G.** (1992) *The Psychological Treatment of Depression: A Guide to the Theory and Practice of Cognitive Behaviour Therapy*, 2nd edn. Routledge, London.

# Patient teaching: A pain management strategy

## ■ INTRODUCTION

Several assumptions underpin this title: first and foremost the claim that 'teaching' has a role in pain management, but secondly that staff can have a teaching role or have something to teach those who are suffering from pain. Linked to these assertions is also the belief that pain can be managed and that conveying knowledge or skills helps patients in pain.

These issues will be reviewed in the context of pain care in this chapter. However, in order to assess the efficacy and appropriateness of some of the approaches to patient teaching, certain complexities, definitions and interventions should be examined initially. As most of the studies on benefits of patient teaching have studied 'short-term' or acute pain situations, the second section is devoted to redressing the balance and focuses on techniques which may be of use to those with chronic illness. Further research directions are suggested throughout this chapter and the theoretical foundations of more current work are explored as a way of addressing practice issues. The final section discusses which approaches may be deemed valuable and feasible for nurses to master and integrate into their care plans, and what educational and management strategies might be necessary to encourage widespread acceptance.

## ■ COMPLEXITIES OF PATIENT 'TEACHING' FOR NURSES

Features which differentiate information-giving from patient teaching are important to address as they highlight the complexities of helping patients cope with illness problems such as pain. Information-giving is essential for the process of reducing anxiety and preparing people for new events. Coupled with this is the constant feedback from patients and their families that they do not receive adequate information. This may well demonstrate their great need for information rather than the lack of attention given to this aspect of care. However, it may also indicate the fact that the type of information given is not relevant to their needs or that it is not in a form which is sufficiently accessible.

Provision of information has conventionally been seen as a predominantly one-way passage rather than an exchange. Therein lies the problem. If nursing staff control the process, this may reflect their own priorities rather than those of the people they aim to help. Despite the powerful evidence from research studies which demonstrate that patients who receive extra standardized information prior to surgery recover more rapidly, suffer less pain and receive less analgesia (Johnson and Wallace, 1993), standardized packages of information may be less effective than a more individualized or tailored approach. Given that nurses wish to optimize their care, they should take guidance from most of these researchers and employ more inter-active individualized approaches.

Once informative interventions become individualized, the process starts to resemble 'patient teaching' in which information is supplied after a careful assessment of need (Wilson-Barnett, 1988). However, in these current cash-limited days of compromise, nurses must not abandon either a standardized plan for supplying information whenever possible or the deeper more individualized approach. Open communication and accurate assessment will hopefully guide practitioners to supply information in a way which will be relevant (McCaffery and Beebe, 1989). There is a role for both written and spoken information-giving and, as long as staff attempt to support this with a deeper and more complete process of understanding, it remains extremely important.

Patient teaching is therefore seen as a process of providing information to enhance knowledge and skills. In Chapter 7, Williams discusses a range of psychological techniques for managing pain which rely very heavily on education and the provision of information for the sole purpose of empowering patients and enhancing skills. For those in pain this is an ambitious goal with many facets which complicate the task. The extent to which the term 'teaching' is appropriate in many situations should also be questioned. There may be many aspects of knowledge that are seen as relevant by staff which may also help patients or their relatives to understand their condition and treatment. For many, however, this is a short-lived process, and there is still an enduring need for support and problem-solving. Unfortunately, the connotations and previous work in this area tend to imply that professionals should provide the teaching and the patient becomes the pupil. For some brief encounters, this may be necessary but for long-term relationships a far more egalitarian approach to management is required.

So many of the previous studies evaluating patient teaching interactions aimed to increase compliance and knowledge (Redman, 1992), and the far more meaningful goals of better health status or improved coping were rarely assessed. Not only does this demonstrate a lack of understanding or focus on the client's welfare, it probably also reflects the difficulties involved in supporting adjustment and measuring improvement over time.

## ■ NURSING INTERVENTIONS FOR THOSE WITH CHRONIC PAIN PROBLEMS

Given the positive advantages which have ensued from intense or acute interventions of additional information-giving or teaching, it is now possibly time to build on these studies and see whether interventions of a similar type could benefit patients with longer-term pain problems. Although the ideal outcome would be a pain-free patient, as seen in Chapter 7, a more realistic goal for so many would be adjustment and an active life despite the pain. There seems to be consensus that careful assessment and an understanding of the patient's beliefs and situation is a prerequisite to any therapeutic intervention. For instance, this interactive approach is promoted by Infante and Mooney (1987) when writing about orthopaedic pain. Likewise Slack and Faut-Callahan (1991) talk about active involvement of the patients with thorough assessments of their coping styles and appraisals. It follows that this requires substantial and knowledgeable assessment, often undertaken through several interviews. As part of this process and in guidelines for caring for those in pain, these authors assume that nurses will believe the patient's report of pain, understand the total significance of the pain to patients and tailor interventions to an individual's ability to participate in pain-control measures.

Once more the labels attached to interventions seem imprecise. Patient teaching discussed in the context of chronic pain management in many papers resembles a counselling approach, with the ultimate goal that the patient identifies his or her own problems and with support attempts to develop strategies to improve his or her situation. The extent to which suggestions are made by the therapist or nurse may depend on several factors. If the patient asks for specific information, if they are seeking advice or alternative strategies or if they are testing the knowledge of the practitioner, the interactions may appear more like 'patient teaching'. Mixed modes of counselling may be most helpful, but the skill would lie in matching the needs to the style or approach, and in changing the approach accordingly to suit patients' responses.

Well-known authors discuss counselling needs for those with chronic pain (e.g. Stewart, 1987). High incidence of emotional morbidity has been detailed and the goal of alleviating depression associated with pain is relevant for those who are attempting to cope and prevent depressive reactions to pain. If over half those recognized to suffer from chronic pain are also clinically depressed, this has clear implications for the psychological approaches required. They may need to ventilate and explain their feelings and would probably not be able to engage in more practical conversations on how to alleviate symptoms or on which alternative strategy to employ. Those fighting to master their pain, in contrast, would be searching for this type of advice and eager to try out new therapies.

Successful teaching-counselling studies in several specialities have provided many indicators for pain management, one of the most poignant issues being the inclusion of spouses or relatives during interventions (see Wilson-Barnett, 1988). This may seem obvious when current philosophies of client participations, family centred care and partnership in decision-making are encouraged. However, studies evaluating teaching frequently focus this on the patient alone. Alleviating the concerns of both partners should be seen as important, to avoid transfer of anxiety and promote full rehabilitation. Relatives may require different information or support, yet the benefits of either counselling couples or arranging support groups for longer-term adjustment are invaluable as shown by a multicentre nurse-led study in the USA (Dracup et al., 1984).

For those in pain, alleviation of stress through the provision of a supportive 'significant other' should help and, as studies in the acute situation have shown, pain is reduced if anxiety is lowered (Hayward, 1975). Nursing staff are probably quite familiar with the effect of parental influence on children's pain behaviour, yet all too often family members are not encouraged or helped to provide this valuable support to adults. Providing a massage or engaging in relaxation together may also be intrinsically important, easily taught by a nurse and a useful life skill for the future.

Monitoring patients' informational needs is therefore crucial to providing relevant input. This in itself, studied systematically, would be invaluable evidence. Success of such research would, of course, be dependent on devising methods to record patients' needs during periods of intense and moderate pain over the short and longer term. Comparative studies of various models of interventions are also required for those with chronic pain. Advice-giving and/or active explorations/counselling should be assessed for their relevance and effectiveness when correlated with different patients' personality and coping styles. For as Rimer et al. (1992) conclude:

*'Few systematically developed and carefully evaluated pain control patient education programmes have been reported.' (p. 171)*

## ■ THEORETICAL ISSUES

More sophisticated understanding of the mechanisms by which interventions and thereby principles for practice to alleviate symptoms or assist coping is required. Several problems have been identified while evaluating teaching input and there are now many ideas on which patient factors influence successful outcomes for these interventions.

Ley (1988) discusses the milieu, clarity of information, priorities and structuring of input. Although he tends to envisage a physician-led process, he also discusses the relevance for a readiness of the recipient. Well-known dangers of information overload, technical language, and insufficient time for reflection and evaluation are also documented. He includes work which demonstrates that individuals tend to believe and adhere to advice when it is received from an authoritative figure. However, in 'pain situations' most people are very motivated to try anything which is recommended, the main barrier to successful adherence often being intense anxiety about the cause and duration of their suffering.

Factors that affect the success of psychological interactions, such as teaching or counselling, also relate to moods and attitudes of the recipient. If someone does not believe in or have faith in the therapist, or fails to participate fully in discussions, interventions are unlikely to work. Although more evidence on these interactions is required, the theoretical explanations of Bandura's (1977) selfefficacy have been well received and seem extremely pertinent to those with pain problems.

The essence of Bandura's theory lies in recognizing self-perception as a vital component of motivation in changing behaviour. Belief in one's capabilities to master a specific challenge is seen as essential. Therapy should therefore be directed to enhancing self-image and confidence. Goals should be staged and realistic so that mastery is possible and experience of achievement builds upon a sense of self-efficacy. Thus expectations of success are seen to control attempts to succeed. Although this model has mostly been applied to health education situations, where so-called healthy people have altered 'risk' behaviours, there are lessons for pain control. When considering the implications of this model for research and practice in the context of pain control, it is important to recognize that an individual's attempts to achieve a goal are governed by expectations. Although each situation must be seen as quite specific, an individual will have certain expectations, that is 'efficacy expectations', when faced with a challenge. This expectation will primarily depend on that person's own previous experience or performance accomplishments seen as the most potent source of efficacy expectation. Secondly, vicarious experience may influence expectations through witnessing others either succeeding or failing to achieve similar goals. Third, expectations may be influenced through verbal persuasion and encouragement. Lastly, the physiological state also influences feelings of self-efficacy.

After the initial appraisal of what has to be faced has been 'placed' in the context of one's own perceived capabilities, expectations of outcome are considered. The whole consideration is dependent on which coping strategies are available, how successful they are likely to be and whether one can apply these coping strategies.

Fundamental to the application of this model in therapy is the understanding that a level of difficulty should be estimated by the individual. In order to employ the notion of developing a greater sense of self-efficacy, a nurse would work with a client to establish a list of tasks necessary to cope with a situation. Each should be quite specific, context related and seen as necessary to achieving an over arching goal. To put this in the realm of pain management, a negotiated plan for a patient and partner might be devised with a nurse. Starting with less difficult challenges such as not mentioning pain for an hour, or performing a physical activity without groaning may be relevant. When ascending the hierarchy one might find a specified relaxation session to be performed daily or an activity directed towards the benefit of others. Ultimately component tasks may build on success or regular achievement and, with a strong sense of self-efficacy, the individual may set him/herself extremely challenging tasks such as engaging in a sport or participation in a social event without thinking about his/her pain.

Another facet of relevance to overall success in self pain management and to concepts of self-efficacy is 'control'. Notions of controlling one's environment and reactions are seen as essential to well-being in the psychological literature. Wallston's (1989) discussion of control and assessment of perceptions, and desire for control indicates the complexity of this concept. However, it is sufficiently robust to have promoted research and, although few consistent findings are available, it seems that by enhancing feelings of self-control, through information-giving or providing some additional responsibilities, patients feel better. Those in pain may benefit from feeling they have control over elements in their environment to compensate for the many unpredictable events which seem to face them through illness (Victor et al., 1986)

Whether nurses are attempting to strengthen feelings of personal efficacy or environmental control, particular types of intervention may be useful. Given that patient teaching has been interpreted so widely and is so closely related to counselling, it is important to realize that the way the individual thinks about his/her pain and him/herself may determine the outcome of any intervention. Fisherman (1992) has stressed that cognitive-behavioural therapy is valuable for some who have enduring pain. By distinguishing pain from 'suffering behaviour' a nurse can encourage an individual to think differently about his/her sensations and ways of coping. Pain needs to be 'isolated' and not integrated into a person's whole existence. Mixed strategies of cognitive therapy, which combine controlling negative thoughts with more physical therapies such as exercise or relaxation, are considered invaluable options when treating individuals who all seem to react so differently to pain-related problems.

Thus various techniques might be employed during these sessions to help mastery of pain. Imagery, relaxation and yoga can be useful in an attempt to conquer the invalidity and yoga may also be taught in an attempt to reduce the unsocial behaviour associated with chronic pain.

Future studies might continue to evaluate such interventions. To date experimental evaluations of relaxation therapy have mainly involved those with cardiovascular or respiratory disorders. Positive pain mediators such as lowered blood pressure and more perceived support might be maximized in a study assessing relaxation teaching sessions to couples where pain is a problem. One such study, looking at the effects of relaxation on chronic non-malignant pain, was undertaken by Seers (1993) (see Chapter 13). This sort of intervention might be compared with or augmented by a more open counselling approach by nurse researchers and health psychologists.

Encouraging data from a Delphi survey (Mobily et al., 1993) undertaken in the USA demonstrates that a sizeable proportion of specialist nurses are undertaking various forms of cognitive-behavioural techniques. The research team aimed to provide a consensus on the most efficacious forms of therapy. Relaxation, distraction and guided imagery were included in the survey in order to provide a list of activities or a protocol for each. Nurses provided information and preferences on methods deemed most successful. Standardization of approach was sought for clinical purposes and also to facilitate future evaluative research. Clearly this study demonstrates that specialists are applying these strategies widely, albeit with a variety of approaches. Thus accounts of well-run nurse clinics and knowledgeable practitioners helping people through expert strategies and support can be found.

In summary, principles of teaching adults should be uppermost in the mind of any nurse. Working in partnership and with spouses, rather than imposing any approach to pain management is essential. Clearly it is the patient who manages his/her pain and there are opportunities for the nurse to assist. Yet complex adverse influences such as poor motivation or negative emotions, discouragement from others, or lack of commitment, or incompetence from staff may hinder success.

## ■ POLICY AND PRACTICE IMPLICATIONS

Theoretically there can be little dispute that several approaches to pain management are encompassed under the umbrella term of 'teaching' and are beneficial. Whether it is the support offered or the specific strategies which alleviate suffering, a need for such intervention is generally expressed by patients. Few studies evaluate specific interventions and there is virtually no experimental evidence on the benefits of specific interventions for those suffering from chronic pain. However, there are many reasons for this; perhaps the most powerful being the gravity of resourcing problems facing nurses, the long-term nature of such illness and the complexity of numerous factors affecting pain and behaviour (Ferrell et al., 1991). More research evidence would be helpful in advising those who wish to improve practice. In future, for instance, case description, and systematic recording and analysis should be possible in centres engaged in such care. However, matching personal characteristics with optimal interventions needs carefully controlled experimental studies and more sophisticated measurement of interventions, coping and efficacy.

From this account it should be apparent that a sophisticated and progressive professional approach for informing and supporting patients and their partners is required. Guidelines for practice are required but, of necessity, would need to be flexible, taking account of the complexities of this field and recognizing the gaps in research evidence. However, the great need for advancement in this area of care must be evident from this book. Nurses need to take up the challenge of pain care by becoming more involved in research development of practice. In order to do this, however, far more resources need to be devoted to educational preparation and to coordination of service provision.

The pre- and post-registration level nursing studies of pain assessment and intervention need to be augmented by more integration and supervision within practice placements. Several opportunities in acute care settings are afforded by the numerous surgical and medical conditions presenting with severe pain. Despite analgesics being so effective when administered appropriately, evidence of poor assessment and treatment abounds. This could be corrected by a careful nursing plan, working through with patients the best approach and giving them more control of these acute situations. Nurses have a direct responsibility for this and should work closely with doctors, psychologists and pharmacists ensuring both good coordination of care and their own constant updating of pain medications.

At the more specialist level, evidence of improved outcome from nurses 'teaching' and pain management is growing (see Wilson-Barnett and Beech, 1994). However, invaluable work, demonstrating the power of sensitive and focused care/counselling is still required, although impossible unless more of these posts are implemented. 'Pain clinics' exploit most of the interventions discussed here and nurses are centrally involved. Perhaps more integration of these staff with ward and community teams is required to support patients and develop nursing expertise more widely.

Increasingly the developing consumerism and involvement of patients in choices will promote the 'low-tech' nurse-intense treatments, such as 'teaching' or psychological interventions. They are appreciated by those with pain problems, reduce negative emotions associated with pain and enhance perceived control. Given that outcome-driven services are required, this provides the ideal formula for tailoring nursing care to patient need. Such a priority should be recognized by management and promoted through strengthening the skills and practice of nursing staff in this area.

## ■ REFERENCES

**Bandura, A.** (1977) *Social Learning Theory.* Prentice Hall, Englewood Cliffs, NJ.

**Dracup, K., Meleis, A. & Edlefsen, P.** (1984) Family focused cardiac rehabilitation: a role supplementation programme for cardiac patients and spouses. *Nursing Clinics of North America* **19**, 113–124.

**Ferrell, B.R., McCaffery, M. & Grant, M.** (1991) Clinical decision-making and pain. *Cancer Nursing* **14**, 289–297.

**Fishman, B.** (1992) The cognitive behaviour perspective on pain management in terminal illness. Cognitive behavioural therapy. *Hospice Journal: Physical, Psychosocial and Pastoral Care of the Dying* **8**, 73–88.

**Hayward, J. C.** (1975) *Information – A Prescription Against Pain.* RCN Study of Nursing Care Series. Royal College of Nursing, London.

**Infante, M.C. & Mooney, N. E.** (1987) Interactive aspects of pain assessment. *Orthopaedic Nursing* **6**, 31–34.

**Johnson, J. & Vogele, C.** (1993) Benefits of psychological preparations for surgery: an analysis. *Annals of Behavioural Medicine* **15**, 4 Sept.

**Ley, P.** (1988) *Communicating with Patients.* Chapman & Hall, London.

**McCaffery, M. & Beebe, A.** (1989) *Pain. Clinical Manual for Nursing Practice.* CV Mosby, St Louis.

**Mobily, P.R., Herr, K.A. & Kelly, L.S.** (1993) Cognitive-behavioural techniques to reduce pain: a validation study. *International Journal of Nursing Studies* **30**, 537–548.

**Redman, B.K.** (1992) *The Process of Patient Education*, 7th edn. CV Mosby, St. Louis.

**Rimer, B.K., Kedziera, P. & Levy, M.H.** (1992) The role of patient education in cancer pain control. *Hospice Journal: Physical, Psychosocial and Pastoral Care of the Dying* **8**, 171–191.

**Seers, K.** (1993) Maintaining people with chronic non-malignant pain in the community: teaching relaxation as a coping skill. Report submitted to the Department of Health on completion of a post-Doctoral Nursing Research Fellowship.

**Slack, J. & Faut-Callahan, M.** (1991) Pain management. *Nursing Clinics of North America* **26**, 463–476.

**Stewart, W.** (1987) Counselling and pain relief. *British Journal of Guidance and Counselling* **15**, 140–149.

**Victor, J.S., McEnvoy, B., Becker, M. H. & Rosenstock, I. M.** (1986) Self-efficacy. *Health Education Quarterly* **13**, 73–91.

**Wallston, K.A.** (1989) Assessment of control in health-care settings. In: Steptoe, A. & Appels, A. (eds) *Stress Personal Control and Health*. John Wiley & Sons, Chichester, pp. 85–103.

**Wilson-Barnett, J.** (1988) Patient teaching or patient counselling. *Journal of Advanced Nursing* **13**, 215–222.

**Wilson-Barnett, J. & Beech, S.** (1994) Evaluating the clinical nurse specialist: a review. *International Journal of Nursing Studies* **31**, 561–572.

# The management of children's pain

For most children pain is an integral part of life (Helman, 1990), and may include the cut or bruise from a tumble in the playground, a painful throat as a result of tonsillitis or the pain of an injection following routine childhood immunizations. Some painful childhood situations are difficult to avoid and indeed may provide a valuable learning experience for the child and his/her family. However, there can be little doubt that in many cases children experience pain which could be alleviated. This chapter will explore the problem of pain in children, some of the factors which have contributed to its undertreatment and the ways in which more effective pain management can be achieved.

## ■ THE EPIDEMIOLOGY OF PAIN IN CHILDREN

Little is known about the epidemiology of pain in children (Anand and Hickey, 1987; Eland, 1988). It is suggested that as paediatric pain has relatively little social impact, unlike adult pain, the costs of which can be calculated in terms of lost work days and benefits claimed, there is not the same incentive to investigate the extent of the problem (Goodman and McGrath, 1991). However, if one accepts that admission to hospital is almost certainly associated with some degree of pain (Zajac, 1992), be it as the result of a disease process, injury, or as a result of the investigations and treatment of illness, the number of children involved has increased steadily since 1974. In 1991 the actual numbers were estimated to be in the region of 800 children per 10,000 population (Audit Commission, 1993). The physical and psychological suffering of the children involved and of their families is worthy of further consideration. Effective pain management may result in earlier discharge from hospital (US Department of Health and Human Services, 1992) and the 'well-analgesed' child may experience fewer complications, particularly after surgery. Greipp (1992) described the effect of pain on the sufferer as 'devastating and dehumanizing', and as nurses we have an ethical obligation to address the needs of children. Similarly, we should attempt to identify and address factors which may compromise effective pain management.

## ■ BARRIERS TO EFFECTIVE PAEDIATRIC PAIN MANAGEMENT

Several authors have identified factors, or as they should more accurately be called 'myths', which can contribute toward children receiving suboptimal pain management (McCaffery and Beebe, 1989; Watt-Watson and Donovan, 1992; Burr, 1993).

### ▪ Pain perception and the developing nervous system

It has been suggested that there is a fundamental difference in the nervous system of an infant, when compared to an adult (Swafford and Allen, 1968), which precludes the infant feeling pain. An infant does not have a fully myelinated nervous system, but in adults a large number of nerve fibres which transmit pain impulses are also unmyelinated. Myelination serves to insulate nerve fibres, thereby speeding up the transmission of impulses, but does not affect the quality of the impulses. However, as pain is a subjective learned experience, it is theoretically more accurate to refer to an infant's aversive response to a noxious stimulus as nociception rather than pain.

## ▪ Children's ability and willingness to communicate about their pain

The myth that children are more tolerant of pain than adults has arisen from a variety of factors. Children may not have the verbal skills to convey their experience to others, or perhaps it is more accurate to suggest that health care professionals need to become more conversant with the language that children use. Jerrett and Evans (1986) identified several unusual pain descriptors used by children aged 5–9½ years. These included 'yucky', 'dizzy', 'snow' and 'sausage'. Verbally competent children may choose not to reveal they have pain if they find the resultant pain management intervention unacceptable.

## ▪ The professionals know best?

It has been suggested that children may not realize that there is an alternative to experiencing pain, or that the health care professionals know when they have pain and therefore intervene when it is appropriate. Lack of intervention on the part of the health care professionals may be taken by the child as an indication that everything that can be done is being done. This last point is particularly important when one considers that the majority of prescriptions for paediatric pain relief are for prn (*pro re nata*), or when required medication. Alex and Ritchie (1992) suggest that children in pain rely on nursing staff to administer medication rather than initiating the process themselves. LaMontagne et al. (1991) also identified discrepancies in pain ratings between children, nursing staff and medical staff. The children rated their pain higher than the nurses or medical staff, and this inevitably led to inadequate pain management.

## ▪ Playing, sleeping and pain

There is a suggestion that children who are able to engage in play or other activities, or who are able to sleep do not have much pain. Children tend to be very adept at using distraction mechanisms. Play, books, television and music enable the child to focus on something pleasant and to shift pain away from the centre of their awareness to the periphery. The pain does not go away, but for as long as the distraction lasts, the child's awareness of pain is diminished. Distraction therapy can be a very effective and beneficial intervention when used appropriately, but children should not be allowed to cope with unremitting pain by the use of this technique alone. Children who have been left to rely on distraction therapy will often sleep as a result of exhaustion.

## ▪ Addiction

Concerns have been expressed about the use of opiates for pain management in children, that their use may result in the child becoming addicted or that they are more likely to experience respiratory depression. There can be little doubt that the use of opiate analgesia is potentially dangerous, since children and adults alike may experience oversedation and respiratory depression (Gourlay and Boas, 1992; Farmer and Harper, 1992), if they do not receive appropriate nursing care, and when the pharmacokinetics of the drugs used are not fully understood. However, this should not preclude their use in the paediatric population but rather it suggests that the health care professionals involved in the care of these children should be more vigilant. The incidence of opiate addiction resulting from the therapeutic use of this group of drugs in the adult population is generally overestimated by nursing staff (McCaffery and Ferrell, 1990) and, since there is no evidence to suggest that addiction occurs more frequently in the paediatric population, the risk is likely to be exaggerated in this patient group as well.

## ■ CHILDREN'S PERCEPTION OF PAIN

Children's perception of their pain is influenced by many factors and, although they can be considered individually, a child's pain perception is more than the sum of these individual influences. From birth children have complete neural pathways which can transmit painful impulses. However, a child's ability to locate pain is limited by his/her previous experiences and also by his/her knowledge of the body. For nurses working within the hospital environment, it is important to recognize that children of 2 and 3 years of age have poorly defined body boundaries. A child may, for example, become highly distressed at the prospect of an injection into an existing intravenous line, because he/she cannot distinguish where his/her body ends and the intravenous line begins, therefore an injection into the line will cause him/her pain. Children's pain perception is influenced by their own emotions, which are largely influenced by the emotions of their parents or primary carer. This concept of emotional contagion is crucially important in the care of hospitalized children. Frightened, anxious parents create fear and anxiety in their child, which in turn reinforces the parents' concerns (Glasper and Thompson, 1993). Children undergoing painful procedures identified the presence of a parent as the most important factor to help them cope with the situation (Gadish et al., 1988), but if the parents are unable to support their child psychologically because of their own anxieties, the child's level of stress will be increased and therefore pain perception will be heightened.

A Piagetian model of cognitive development can be applied to a child's understanding of pain (McCready et al., 1991; Hurley and Whelan, 1988). The sensory-motor period is between birth and 2 years of age, and at approximately 6 months children develop a pain memory and manifest anticipatory distress prior to a previously experienced painful procedure. Between the ages of 2 and 7 years (pre-operational phase) children believe that others can see or understand their pain in the way that they do (egocentrism), and that it can also be caused by others, particularly as a punishment for bad behaviour. Pain is perceived as 'my own' and exists in the present only. They cannot relate pain to future or positive outcomes and therefore are unable to rationalize the potential benefits of an analgesic injection for pain relief. Older children (7–12 years of age, the concrete operational phase) begin to have some concept of mental pain, are beginning to formulate their own ideas of death and loss, and may also relate current pain experiences to previous occurrences. Sociocultural factors also begin to affect their perceptions of pain. Children of 12 years and above (the formal-operational phase) largely function as adults, although their ability to understand and process a situation may be initially curtailed by their limited experiences. Adolescents are also very aware of the social expectations imposed upon them, and may be concerned that experiencing pain will prevent them conforming to the 'norm'. At this stage they are able to make clear distinctions between physical, mental and emotional pain. An awareness of how a child is processing his/her pain experience, may provide valuable information when selecting pain-management interventions.

## ■ PAEDIATRIC PAIN MANAGEMENT AND THE MULTIDISCIPLINARY TEAM

Pain-management interventions which adopt a purely biomedical approach fail to acknowledge the complexity of the pain experience and are therefore unlikely to be successful. The contributions of the multidisciplinary team may radically influence the way in which paediatric pain is managed. Individuals may have a direct impact on the child's pain management, for example, the psychologist and play therapist may work together to instruct children and their families on non-pharmacological pain management interventions. Physiotherapists may have experience using transcutaneous electrical nerve stimulate (TENS) machines, or heat and cool pads, and may also provide education for the nursing staff on exercise regimens. They may also advise on splinting and other aids which may reduce pain. Educational input from the teacher provides distraction, but also helps to maintain structure and ensures that the child's basic needs are met. Medical staff are responsible for prescribing appropriate analgesic medication. However, the nurse as the child's advocate has a vital role in ensuring that the medical staff are given accurate, up-to-date information which is supported by appropriate physiological observations and by the use of pain assessment tools to enable the medical staff to prescribe suitable analgesia, which reflects the needs of the child. Pharmacists and medical engineering departments may have an indirect beneficial effect on the child's pain management by ensuring that appropriate drugs doses have been prescribed and that the necessary equipment is available.

The nurse's role, as part of this multidisciplinary team, encompasses many different aspects. Akinsanya (1985) suggests that pain and nursing are inextricably linked, and as such the nurse has a crucial role to play in the management of pain. The nursing process, using a conceptual or theoretical model, enables the nurse and her client to adopt a problem-solving approach to the client's situation. In paediatric nursing, models which focus on the child and family provide the framework for the four stages of the nursing process: assessment, planning, implementation and evaluation. Although these stages are frequently considered to be a linear progression, it is more appropriate to conceptualize the process as a cyclical model. The emphasis of this approach is to consider pain as a biopsychosocial experience, which affects the child and also the family unit. As such, each of the stages of the nursing process must adopt a holistic approach, involving the child (whenever possible) and the parents (or primary carers). Assessment should consider not only the source or potential source of the pain, but also individualized factors, which may influence the child's pain perception. Chapter 5 has a detailed discussion of pain assessment tools for use in the paediatric setting, but assessment should involve more than the use of tools for measuring or assessing pain. Planning and implementing the use of pain interventions should include the use of pharmacological and non-pharmacological methods, and of course should reflect the child's developmental level. Evaluating the pain management strategies used can be by direct means using self-report pain measurement tools or by indirect methods, for example, by observing how the child is managing activities or by monitoring vital signs. It is important when negotiating the goal or desired outcome of pain management strategies with the child and family that realistic and achievable goals are set (see later), which demonstrate a connection between the problem and the proposed intervention. For example, the goal 'David will not complain of postoperative pain' may be achieved by several methods, many of which do not include the amelioration of pain (Walker and Campbell, 1989).

## ■ PAIN MANAGEMENT INTERVENTIONS

Before considering the analgesic interventions available for the paediatric patient, it is relevant to consider the goal of pain management. In the USA, Burokas (1985) asked nurses caring for postoperative paediatric patients to state their goal of pain relief, and 12% gave the response of complete pain relief, 61.2% stated that their aim was to relieve as much pain as possible, and almost 28% said that their aim was to relieve enough pain for the patient to function or merely to enable the child to tolerate their pain.

The expected goal of pain relief should be negotiated with the child whenever possible and with his/her family. In this situation the nurse's role is as an educator, to enable the child and family to obtain adequate information so that they may make an informed decision. The informed decision should consider not only the beneficial effects of the available analgesic interventions but also their potential side-effects and complications. The child's need for comforting and coping interventions, such as parental presence, transitional objects, and games and toys, as an integral part of the pain-management strategy should also be discussed. The negotiation of goal setting is particularly important when addressing the needs of the child with chronic pain or the child with a painful terminal disease. The child and family must feel comfortable with the goal of pain management and the strategy which will be employed to achieve this goal. They must also realize that all pain management should be dynamic and responsive to the changing needs of the individuals involved.

## ■ PROCEDURAL PAIN

Even so-called 'minor' invasive procedures, such as finger pricks for blood sampling, venepuncture and insertion of intravenous cannulae can be a source of considerable distress to the child and his/her family. Such procedures can occur routinely within a health care environment and the professionals involved may become inured to the effect that these activities have on the child and family. Wherever possible, painful invasive procedures should be 'clustered' together and the child and family should be adequately prepared both physically and psychologically for the proposed procedure. 'Clustering' the procedures will be of benefit to the child because he/she will then have periods of 'pain-free' time, barring emergencies. If at all possible, painful procedures should not be performed in the child's 'own space', because the hospitalized child requires an area of sanctuary where unpleasant things do not happen. If the child's bed or room is invaded because an unpleasant procedure has been performed there, the safe area is removed. Similarly, painful procedures should not be carried out in the play area. Care should be taken to note that the room where the procedure is to be undertaken is at an appropriate temperature, to remove 'frightening things' and to ensure that books, toys or even music cassettes are available to distract the child during the procedure. The mother or father should be physically in a position to support their child.

### ■ The pharmacological management of procedural pain

Procedural pain management can be achieved by the use of analgesic, anaesthetic or sedative agents, or a combination of these three. The action of analgesic agents will be explored later in this chapter.

## Sedative agents

These produce sedation and hypnosis, skeletal muscle relaxation and reduce anxiety. They do not provide analgesia and are therefore sometimes used in combination with opiate analgesia, thereby increasing the risk of respiratory depression. Commonly used drugs include diazepam, temazepam, triclofos sodium and trimeprazine tartrate.

## Anaesthetic agents

Ketamine hydrochloride can be given via the intravenous or intramuscular route, and has good analgesic properties when used in a subanaesthetic dose. The state of unconsciousness produced is known as 'dissociative anaesthesia', where children may appear only mildly sedated and maintain their body tone. The incidence of respiratory depression is rare, but it is estimated that ketamine hydrochloride may produce post-emergence delirium, manifested by dreams and hallucinations in one third of patients (Zelter et al., 1989). It should therefore be used with caution in children and under strict supervision.

Inhaled nitrous oxide (Entonox) may be of value for some children, as a potent analgesic which has minimal cardiovascular and respiratory effects. The 'demand delivery' system of administration restricts its suitability to children who are willing and able to cooperate; the mask or mouthpiece delivery system will preclude its use for some children.

Local anaesthetic infiltration of the proposed procedural area, for example, prior to suturing of a small laceration, has often been avoided in children, because the local anaesthetic solution can cause pain and discomfort which is more distressing to the child than the suturing procedure. Davidson and Boom (1992) established that warming the lignocaine solution to a temperature of 37°C reduces the pain associated with subcutaneous injection.

Local anaesthetic creams can be used to anaesthetize the skin, prior to local infiltration with lignocaine, venepuncture or intravenous cannulation. EMLA (eutectic mixture of local anaesthetics) applied under an occlusive dressing approximately one hour before the proposed procedure generally results in decreased pain. Local changes as a result of the use of EMLA cream include redness or blanching as a result of vasoconstriction, which can be problematic if the patch has been applied prior to intravenous cannulation. EMLA should be used with caution in infants owing to reports of methaemoglobinaemia (reduced oxygen-carrying capacity) occurring as a result of its use (Frayling et al., 1990).

Ametop gel (4% amethocaine gel) again applied under an occlusive dressing, generally produces anaesthesia in approximately 30 minutes and the duration of anaesthesia lasts for up to six hours (Lawson et al., 1995). Amethocaine also has a known vasodilatory action, and this may result in small veins becoming more prominent, thereby facilitating cannulation. This more rapid onset and prolonged duration of action may have some advantages in busy paediatric units where, owing to other circumstances, it is often difficult to adhere to strict timing for the application of topical local anaesthetics.

## ■ PHARMACOLOGICAL PAEDIATRIC PAIN MANAGEMENT

The use of prn (*pro re nata*) analgesia has frequently led to children receiving inadequate pain relief. Evidence suggests that nurses, when confronted with an upper and lower limit on the amount of analgesia they can administer, will give the child the lower amount, and will administer the analgesia as infrequently as possible (Gonzalez et al., 1993). A deeper understanding of the pharmacological agents involved may lead to enhanced pain relief for the paediatric patient (see also Chapter 6).

### ▮ Opiate analgesia

Effective pain management relies on the selection of the most appropriate drug administered via a route which is acceptable and appropriate for the individual child, and which will maintain a constant, therapeutic plasma level of the chosen analgesic.

Morphine sulphate is the gold standard against which all other opioid analgesics are compared and can be administered by several different routes. When an intermittent dosing regimen is prescribed, better quality pain relief will be achieved if the medication is given regularly and around the clock in the acute phase of the pain. Selecting an appropriate route of administration can have considerable impact on the compliance of the child, because many children may deny having pain if they are aware that analgesia will be administered via the intramuscular route. Children may also find the use of rectal suppositories distressing. The intravenous route is most acceptable to children, but thought must be given to the placement of the intravenous cannula. This method of administration is certainly one of the most effective in maintaining a steady plasma level of the drug.

However, with many analgesic regimens, children become the passive recipients of care, but their psychological needs may be better addressed if they are enabled to become active participants in their pain management regimen. Patient-controlled analgesia (PCA), a method of empowering the patient to manage their own pain, can be used successfully with children as young as 4 or 5 years of age. Morphine sulphate is generally considered the drug of choice for paediatric PCA (Rauen and Ho, 1989; Bender et al., 1990; Gureno and Reisinger, 1991). Identifying children who may be suitable for PCA therapy is based not only on their chronological age, but also on their cognitive ability, their physical ability to use a handset or demand device and their willingness to participate in PCA. In general, a more flexible approach to programming the PCA device is used with children, which reflects their different needs. Education, reinforcement, continuous monitoring and evaluation of the technique are vital to ensure success.

The greater solubility of diamorphine, which allows effective doses to be administered in smaller volumes, may be of value in the care of the terminally ill child, particularly when the subcutaneous route is being used. There is also a suggestion that diamorphine may have an enhanced euphoric effect, which may also be of benefit for the terminally ill child.

Sublingual buprenorphine may be of value for children who do not require or are not suitable for parenteral opiates, but for whom the oral route is not available. Younger children may require considerable instruction on the sublingual route and it may be helpful to make a 'game' out of administration and guess how long the child can hold the tablet under the tongue before it disappears. The use of a hand-held mirror will help to reinforce how the tablet disappears. The nurse caring for the child must rigorously monitor the child for signs of nausea and vomiting which can accompany the administration of sublingual buprenorphine. If children experience this side-effect, they may be very reluctant to take the medicine on a subsequent occasion if this side-effect is not managed effectively.

Although papaveretum was once used fairly extensively for paediatric pain management, recently its use has diminished. Papaveretum BPC is a mixture of opium alkaloids (morphine 50%, codeine 3.8%, noscapine 19% and papaverine 5%, approximately), and as a result of the reported genotoxicity of noscapine it should be used with extreme caution in females of child-bearing potential (Gatehouse et al., 1991). A noscapine-free preparation is obtainable, but other analgesics which are more readily available may provide equally satisfactory pain relief, without the complications of obtaining a particular preparation or inadvertently administering the wrong formulation.

Codeine phosphate can be used for children with mild to moderate pain and may be particularly useful for children following cranial surgery. It should not be used to provide long-term analgesia because of the high incidence of constipation which can result. The use of paracetamol and codeine phosphate synergistically can provide enhanced pain relief.

## ▪ Non-opiate analgesia

Until recently one of the most common criticisms about the analgesics available for children was the lack of a suitable intermediary between opiate analgesia and paracetamol. The use of non-steroidal anti-inflammatory drugs (NSAIDs), particularly diclofenac sodium, has largely addressed this problem. Balanced analgesia, a method of blocking or modifying pain pathways at several different points has been widely advocated as a means of achieving more effective pain management (Morton, 1993) and the NSAIDs have been used increasingly to achieve balanced analgesia. Diclofenac sodium can be given orally, rectally or intramuscularly, although the latter route is rarely used because it can be extremely painful. The dispersible preparation enables the drug to be given in small amounts which increases its suitability for children. These drugs also have an anti-pyretic effect. The side-effects which may be encountered are mainly indigestion-like symptoms after prolonged usage. The NSAIDs are generally contraindicated in children with bleeding disorders, and they should be used with caution in children who have a history of asthma as they can precipitate wheeziness. Although their use has been associated with acute renal failure in adults owing to the effect of prostaglandins on renal function, the incidence of renal toxicity in normal, healthy children is low. Their use in children with pre-existing renal disease is generally contraindicated.

Paracetamol can be extremely effective against mild to moderate pain, particularly when it is associated with a fever. Failure of paracetamol as an analgesic is often the result of erratic administration which fails to maintain a therapeutic plasma level. Many preparations are available and children may become extremely loyal to the preparation they are used to receiving, thereby improving compliance.

The use of aspirin for paediatric pain management is largely prohibited because of the association between aspirin ingestion and the occurrence of Reye syndrome, toxic encephalopathy. It may be used with caution in children over the age of 12 years, but it is generally considered preferable to use diclofenac sodium. However, children with juvenile chronic arthritis may find aspirin particularly useful (Foale, 1995).

## ■ NON-PHARMACOLOGICAL PAIN MANAGEMENT

As pain is a multidimensional experience, nursing interventions to care for the child in pain must reflect this approach, because adopting a purely biomedical pain management strategy fails to recognize the impact of the individual's thoughts, feeling and concerns on their pain perception. There can be little doubt that in many situations nurses need to actively employ non-pharmacological pain management strategies to enable her/him to effectively care for her/his patients. Non-pharmacological interventions can be broadly divided into two categories: cognitive-behavioural interventions or physical agents.

### ▮ Physical non-pharmacological agents

The simple action of 'stroking a child's hurt to make it better' is a technique which parents frequently employ. The action of stroking or massaging increases A beta nerve fibre activity and thereby closes the 'gate', reducing the transmission of pain impulses and therefore alleviating pain. The application of heat pads or cool pads has a similar effect and may also reduce muscle spasm, which is frequently associated with pain. In some circumstances rest and immobilizing the painful area may also be necessary. The use of TENS in children is not well documented, but may be considered for particular cases. Lander and Fowler-Kerry (1993) suggest that the use of TENS may be of value in reducing the pain associated with venepuncture. Care must be taken when preparing a child for the use of TENS because children may find the sensation distressing. For example, it may be helpful to demonstrate its use on a parent before approaching the child. When the parents have described to their child how TENS 'feels' it may be preferable to demonstrate its use firstly on a non-painful area before applying the electrodes in the appropriate area. Electrode placement can be something of a trial and error experience; inappropriate electrode placement may result in ineffective therapy or actually cause pain. There is also a suggestion that, as the child controls the TENS, there is also a degree of 'placebo response' (Eland, 1993). Notwithstanding this it may prove valuable in specific cases and certainly its use is worthy of further exploration in current paediatric pain management.

### ∎ Cognitive-behavioural interventions

Cognitive-behavioural interventions can make a valuable contribution to the care of the child in pain and the reader is referred to Chapter 7 for a more comprehensive discussion of this technique.

As with all aspects of pain management, the role of the nurse is to negotiate with the child and his/her family about the types of non-pharmacological pain management interventions they have used previously or which they think would be of value to them, and to educate and empower them in their use. It is, however, imperative that the nurse acknowledges her/his own limitations in this area, and that support and help from the department of psychological medicine is available and readily sought.

### ∎ A holistic approach to painful dressing changes – a case study

Kate, aged 12 years, required twice-weekly dressing changes to deep, ulcerated lesions on her left arm, left knee, the inner aspect of her left calf and the outer aspect of her right thigh. Dressing changes were potentially painful and Kate was extremely anxious. Previously the procedure had been carried out under general anaesthesia; however, as the wounds were healing, it was felt to be appropriate to explore undertaking the procedure without anaesthesia. Kate had two main concerns, firstly that the dressing changes would hurt and secondly that the wounds were not healing. A plan of care for the dressing changes was drawn up by Kate, her mother and the nursing staff, which included both pharmacological and non-pharmacological interventions.

Explanations were given to Kate and her mother about the use of nitrous oxide (Entonox) for painful procedures. The idea of being in control of her own analgesia appealed to Kate, the equipment was shown to her and she 'practised' using the mouthpiece delivery system.

Kate and her psychologist worked out a series of statements that she would use during the dressing change. Her favourite statements were: 'This is okay. I'm doing really well' and 'Relax, there's nothing to worry about'. She also explored the use of imagery, and decided to focus on her home as she had been hospitalized for some time. Kate also practised deep breathing exercises. The nurses encouraged her to breathe deeply, hold the breath and then let it out slowly. This rhythmic breathing also facilitated Kate's use of the Entonox.

When Kate felt prepared, the decision was made by her and her mother, and the nursing and medical staff to undertake the dressing changes without anaesthesia. Information, preparation and control were vital to her ability to cope with the procedure. The nursing staff planned with her in what order the dressings would be removed, and for much of the initial removal of bandages and padding she was an active participant. Seeing her wounds for the first time understandably provoked a great deal of anxiety, and the nurses and her mother encouraged her to breathe deeply and to use the Entonox. She was also encouraged to use her positive statements and to 'imagine' herself at home. Kate found it helpful to 'name' the larger wounds and this gave her and her mother a focus to monitor their healing.

Although Kate stated that the first dressing change without anaesthesia was not painful, when her wounds were redressed she became very tearful and distressed. It is important to recognize that this type of procedure can be a very emotional experience for the child. Kate was made comfortable and her favourite music was played, her mother stroked her hair, and she was given positive reinforcement by the nursing staff about how well she had managed and also how well her wounds were healing. On subsequent dressing changes there was no further display of distressed emotion when the procedure was completed, the Entonox was available, but was not used and Kate was very firmly in charge of the procedure.

## ■ SPECIAL CONSIDERATIONS

### ▮ Pain management in infants and neonates

Despite all the evidence to suggest that neonates and infants can and do experience pain, many anxieties remain about the use of analgesic agents in these age groups. As with all pain patients, it is important to adopt a multidimensional approach to pain management, and to recognize the valuable contribution that the delivery of high-quality nursing care can make to their well-being (Sparshott, 1989). However, the neonate and infant also require analgesic interventions, which are tailored to their individual needs. It is important to recognize that the metabolism of morphine is significantly altered in this age group. The elimination half-life is prolonged and there is decreased clearance of morphine, therefore infants may attain higher serum concentrations of morphine with a continuous infusion, which will decline more slowly after the infusion has been discontinued (Goldman and Lloyd-Thomas, 1991). It is also suggested that they may be more sensitive to the respiratory depressant effects of morphine, and therefore require assiduous monitoring and appropriate intervention should this occur (Lloyd-Thomas et al., 1995). Prescribing regimens vary but should generally be started at the lower end of the therapeutic range for the child's weight. Paracetamol may be prescribed for this group of patients, with normal liver function, for use in the short term without concern for hepatotoxicity (Lloyd-Thomas, 1990).

## ■ The child undergoing surgery

Surgical procedures can be a major source of pain for many children. Although many of the pharmacological interventions previously mentioned can be used to provide postoperative pain relief, effective surgical pain management is a broad subject and therefore requires further consideration.

Surgical pain can be managed at three stages during the procedure: before surgery by the use of premedications, immediately before or during the surgical procedure, and after the surgery has been completed. The use of premedications is a fairly contentious issue. Intramuscular preparations have a low level of acceptability for the child, family and often the nursing staff, whilst oral preparations are often unpalatable, and the child may require a great deal of persuasion before he/she will take the mixture. Indeed many institutions are now advocating that children undergoing surgery should not be premedicated. However, there can be little doubt that, for some procedures, such as major throat surgery and cardiac surgery, and for some children who are particularly anxious, the use of a preoperative premedication is desirable, if not essential. The general goal of a premedication is to provide perioperative analgesia and also some sedation, reduce secretions, maximize haemodynamic stability during induction and to make the entire induction process more tolerable for all concerned (McIlvaine, 1989). These goals can be successfully achieved by the use of oral premedicants and, whenever possible, intramuscular premedications should be avoided.

In addition to general anaesthesia, several analgesic techniques can be used immediately prior to surgery or during the operative procedure. These

include the use of intravenous fentanyl, an opiate which when used intravenously has a rapid rate of onset and a relatively short duration of action,
and local anaesthetic techniques, including the use of peripheral nerve blocks,
such as penile blocks prior to circumcision, ring blocks of digits prior to
toenail surgery or suturing lacerations, and of course inguinal blocks prior
to herniotomy or orchidopexy. Central nerve blocks, particularly via the
caudal route, are also frequently used in children (Lloyd-Thomas, 1990).
Caudal blocks can provide adequate analgesia both during and after surgery
involving lower limbs, anoperitoneal, genitourinary and abdominal surgery
below the level of the umbilicus. The addition of diamorphine to the local
anaesthetic solution may potentiate the analgesic action but this technique
is not suitable for children undergoing day-care surgery because of the risk
of respiratory depression. Lumbar and thoracic extradural blocks may be
used to provide analgesia during surgical procedures and also when maintained as a continuous infusion during the postoperative period to provide
postoperative analgesia. Again a combination of local anaesthetic and opiate
analgesia is generally used.

The nursing staff caring for children receiving continuous extradural infusions must be aware of the possible side-effects and complications of the
procedure. These include the side-effects of the drugs themselves, such as
nausea and vomiting, pruritus, urinary retention, oversedation and respiratory depression as a result of the opiate and urinary retention, and sensory
changes and potentially motor blockade as a result of the local anaesthetic.
Similarly there may be technical complications such as catheter displacement
and disconnection, and accidental removal. Many parents have considerable
anxieties about the use of continuous extradural infusions in children, and
pre-operatively the technique should be fully explained to the child (where
appropriate) and his/her family. They should be encouraged to ask questions and, if they decide that they do not want their child to have analgesia
via this route, their wishes should be respected.

Even a relatively simple intervention such as wound infiltration or instilla-
tion of local anaesthetic into the wound prior to closure can provide remarkably effective analgesia following procedures such as herniotomy and
pyloromyotomy (Morton, 1993).

Although intraoperative analgesic techniques are often considered to be
beyond the scope of responsibility of the nurses caring for the child following
surgery, it is imperative that they understand what analgesic techniques
have been used, how the procedure was carried out and the likely consequences of the procedure. These should include potential side-effects, such
as sensory or motor blocks following peripheral nerve blockade, and
also the likely duration of action of analgesia. This will enable the nurse to
plan postoperative analgesic administration and thereby prevent the child

experiencing an analgesic void, when the intraoperative analgesia is no longer effective, but the postoperative intervention has not yet come into effect. As with all aspects of pain care, nurse education is vital, and in some hospitals specialist nurses are employed as members of a multidisciplinary Acute Pain Control Service, to improve patient care by educating all members of the health care team, supervising the administration of analgesia in the clinical area, auditing the quality of the service provided and undertaking research to enhance practice (Macintyre and Ready, 1996).

Postoperative analgesia should be individualized to the child and the surgical procedure he/she has undergone. Careful consideration should be given to the choice of analgesia, particularly if more than one type has been prescribed, the route of administration and the potential side-effects of the drugs chosen. At all times the nurse must act as the child's advocate and adopt a dynamic approach to the management of pain in the postoperative child.

## ∎ Juvenile rheumatoid arthritis

This inflammatory disease of an unknown inciting agent gives rise to joint stiffness and pain, night pain, limitation of mobility and interference with the activities of daily living (Whaley and Wong, 1989). There is no specific cure for the disorder and the goals of therapy focus on preserving function, preventing physical deformities and relieving the symptoms (Seymour, 1990). Cognitive-behavioural programmes assist the children to cope with their chronic pain, by encouraging them to regulate their pain perception and to modify their pain behaviours. Physiotherapy, splinting and positioning during rest may help to prevent pain, reduce deformities and to maintain function (Beyer et al., 1992). The use of NSAIDs, such as ibuprofen or naproxen, may suppress the inflammatory process and also relieve pain.

## ∎ Sickle cell disease

It is recognized that patients in sickle cell crisis require effective analgesia immediately. The reader is referred to Chapter 11 for a discussion of some of the developmental issues involved in sickle cell disease and the ways in which these can be compromised by frequent episodes of pain. Patient-controlled analgesia has been shown to be an effective treatment strategy for adolescents and children in crisis. Pain behaviour contracts, with mutually agreed goals and professional and patient's responsibilities, enable the patient to exert some control over the hospital experience, and may provide a valuable bridge to enable the patient and health care professionals to work together to negotiate care which is acceptable to both groups (Burghardt-Fitzgerald, 1989).

# ▪ The terminally ill child

The selection of the appropriate drug and route of administration for the terminally ill child is largely determined by the stage of the disease process. General management principles are that the analgesia should be effective, that administering the analgesia should not occupy too much of the child's and family's time, and that the quality of analgesia achieved and the other effects are acceptable to the child and his/her family. In general, morphine sulphate administered orally (four hourly regularly) and titrated against the pain until relief is achieved is considered the drug and route of choice. When an effective dose has been achieved, it may be more convenient to change to a slow-release preparation, which can be given every 12 hours (Dominca and Hunt, 1993). If oral administration is no longer effective or possible, continuous subcutaneous diamorphine infusions can be administered using a syringe driver. Patient-controlled analgesia pumps can also be used to administer diamorphine subcutaneously and may be beneficial for the older child.

# ▪ The burned child

The child who has sustained a burn injury confronts the nurse caring for him/her with a multiplicity of pain dilemmas. The major difficulty for the nurse is the need to reconcile his/her caring role whilst potentially contributing to the child's pain when carrying out complex and lengthy treatments. Other obstacles are the myths which continue to abound about the nature of burn pain. Kelly (1994) states that a child who has sustained full-thickness burns does not feel pain, whereas Carr et al. (1993) state that a child who has sustained overwhelming injury will have destroyed nociceptors and indeed the nerves themselves but, around the viable margin of the wound, damaged nerve endings remain which may be hypersensitive. Knighton and Palozzi (1992) suggest that full-thickness burns may also give rise to deep somatic pain as a result of inflammation and ischaemia.

The initial or emergent phase of management of the burned child usually requires the administration of intravenous opiates, in small incremental doses. This route of administration may prove problematic if the child has sustained fluid loss as a result of the injury. However, the apparently more accessible intramuscular route may give rise to unreliable absorption of the drug. For children who are willing and able to cooperate, the use of Entonox may be considered. The acute phase follows the emergent phase and lasts until partial thickness wounds are healed, or full-thickness wounds have been grafted. During this phase, background pain may be low to moderate. However, during procedures such as dressing changes and physiotherapy, the pain may become severe to excruciating. Slow-release morphine preparations via the oral or rectal route with supplemental morphine prior to painful procedures may be helpful in this situation. Carr et al. (1993) warn against the routine use of fentanyl as tolerance can rapidly develop, with the child requiring ever-increasing doses to control his/her pain. The rehabilitative phase follows the acute phase and lasts until the wound(s) has completed matured. The return of nerve function may be associated with pain, and neuronal tissue can also be trapped in the scar, causing pain in a wound which is completely healed. As the scar tissue matures, itching and pain during exercise can occur. Itching can be particularly distressing. During this phase, simple analgesics, NSAIDs and antidepressants, such as low-dose amitriptyline, may be of value. Throughout the care of the child with burns, the nurse must address the child's pain needs using both pharmacological interventions and non-pharmacological methods of pain relief. Other members of the health care team, such as psychologists, physiotherapists, play therapists and counsellors, may be a valuable resource, not only contributing to the recovery of the child and his/her family, but also assisting the nursing staff in coming to terms with their role in the child's management.

## ■ CONCLUSION

Although there can be little doubt that interest in paediatric pain management has increased substantially over the past few years and that this has resulted in considerable changes in clinical practice (Howard, 1993), there is still a pressing need to improve the care of the child in pain or potential pain and that of his/her family. Indeed, pain relief has been identified as one of the ten indicators for measuring the quality of paediatric care in hospitals (Audit Commission, 1993). Nurses have a central role in the management of the child in pain, and it is vital that they are empowered to develop the necessary skills, knowledge and awareness to fully embrace this role, and that pain-management strategies are developed which reflect the changing environment of health care provision, and the individual needs of children and their families.

## ■ REFERENCES

**Akinsanya, C.Y.** (1985) The use of knowledge in the management of pain: the nurse's role. *Nurse Education Today* 5, 41–46.

**Alex, M.R. & Ritchie, J.A.** (1992) School-aged children's interpretation of their experience with acute surgical pain. *Journal of Pediatric Nursing* 7, 171–180.

**Anand, K.J.S. & Hickey, P.R.** (1987) Pain and its effects in the human neonate and fetus. *New England Journal of Medicine* 317, 1321–1329.

**Audit Commission** (1993) *Children First: A Study of Hospital Services.* HMSO, London.

**Bender, L.H., Weaver, K. & Edwards, K.** (1990) Postoperative patient-controlled analgesia in children. *Pediatric Nursing* 16, 549–554.

**Beyer, J.E., Clegg, S.A., Foster, R.L. & Hester, N.O.** (1992) Clinical judgement in managing the crisis of children's pain. In: Watt-Watson, J.H. & Donovan, M.I. (eds) *Pain Management Nursing Perspective*. Mosby Year Book, St Louis.

**Burghardt-Fitzgerald, D.C.** (1989) Pain-behavior contracts: effective management of the adolescent in sickle-cell crisis. *Journal of Pediatric Nursing* **4**, 320–325.

**Burokas, L.** (1985) Factors affecting nurses' decisions to medicate pediatric patients after surgery. *Heart and Lung* **14**, 373–378.

**Burr, S.** (1993) Myths in practice. *Nursing Standard* **7**, 4.

**Carr, D.B., Osgood, P.F. & Szyfelbein, S.K.** (1993) Treatment of pain in acutely burned children. In: Schechter, N.L. Berde, C.B. & Yaster, M. (eds) *Pain in Infants, Children and Adolescents*. Williams & Wilkins, Baltimore.

**Davidson, J.A.H. & Boom, S.J.** (1992) Warming lignocaine to reduce pain associated with injection. *British Medical Journal* **305**, 617–618.

**Dominca, F. & Hunt, A.** (1993) Children's hospices. In: Glasper, E.A. & Tucker, A. (eds) *Advances in Child Health Nursing*. Scutari Press, Harrow.

**Eland, J.M.** (1988) Persistence in pediatric pain research: one nurse researcher's efforts. *Recent Advances in Nursing* **21**, 43–62.

**Eland, J.** (1993) The use of TENS with children. In: Schechter, N.L., Berde, C.B. & Yaster, M. (eds) *Pain in Infants. Children and Adolescents*. Williams & Wilkins, Baltimore.

**Farmer, M. & Harper, N.J.N.** (1992) Unexpected problems with patient controlled analgesia. *British Medical Journal* **304**, 574.

**Foale, H.** (1995) The child with musculoskeletal or articular dysfunction. In: Campbell, S. & Glasper, E.A. (eds) *Whaley And Wong's Children's Nursing*. Times Mirror International Publishers, Barcelona.

**Frayling, I.M., Addison, G.M., Chattergee, K. & Meakin, G.** (1990) Methaemoglobinaemia in children treated with prilocaine-lignocaine cream. *British Medical Journal* **301**, 153–154.

**Gadish, H.S., Gonzalez, J.L. & Hayes, J.S.** (1988) Factors affecting nurses' decisions to administer pediatric pain medication postoperatively. *Journal of Pediatric Nursing* **3**, 383–390.

**Gatehouse, D.G., Stemp, G., Pascoe, S., Wilcox, P., Hawker, J. & Tweats, D.J.** (1991) Investigations into the induction of aneuploidy and polyploidy in mammalian cells by the anti-tussive agent noscapine hydrochloride. *Mutagenesis* **6**, 279–283.

**Glasper, E.A. & Thompson, M**. (1993) Preparing children for hospital admission. In: Glasper, E.A. & Tucker, A. (eds) *Advances in Child Health Nursing*. Scutari Press, Harrow.

**Goldman, A. & Lloyd-Thomas, A.R.** (1991) Pain management in children. *British Medical Bulletin* **47**, 676–689.

**Gonzalez, J.C., Routh, D.K. & Armstrong, F.D.** (1993) Differential medication of child versus adult postoperative patients: the effect of nurses' assumptions. *Children's Health Care* **22**, 47–59.

**Goodman, J.E. & McGrath, P.J.** (1991) The epidemiology of pain in children and adolescents: a review. *Pain* **46**, 247–264.

**Gourlay, G.K. & Boas, R.A.** (1992) Fatal outcome with the use of rectal morphine for postoperative pain control in an infant. *British Medical Journal* **304**, 766–767.

**Greipp, M.E.** (1992) Undermedication for pain: an ethical model. *Advances in Nursing Science* **15**, 44–53.

**Gureno, M.A. & Reisinger, C.L.** (1991) Patient controlled analgesia for the young pediatric patient. *Pediatric Nursing* **17**, 251–254.

**Helman, C.G.** (1990) *Culture, Health and Illness*, 2nd edn. Wright, London.

**Howard, R.** (1993) Preoperative and postoperative pain control. *Archives of Disease in Childhood* **69**, 699–703.

**Hurley, A. & Whelan, E.G.** (1988) Cognitive development and children's perception of pain. *Pediatric Nursing* **14**, 21–24.

**Jerrett, M. & Evans, K.** (1986) Children's pain vocabulary. *Journal of Advanced Nursing* **11**, 403–408.

**Kelly, H.** (1994) Initial nursing assessment and management of burn-injured children. *British Journal of Nursing* **3**, 54–59.

**Knighton, J.A. & Palozzi, L.** (1992) Relief of burn pain in adults and children. In: Watt-Watson, J.H. & Donovan, M.I. (eds) *Pain Management Nursing Perspective*. Mosby Year Book, St Louis.

**LaMontagne, L.L., Johnson, B.D. & Hepworth, J.T.** (1991) Children's ratings of postoperative pain compared to ratings by nurses and physicians. *Issues in Comprehensive Pediatric Nursing* **14**, 241–247.

**Lander, J. & Fowler-Kerry, S.** (1993) TENS for children's procedural pain. *Pain* **52**, 209–216.

**Lawson, R.A., Smart, N.G., Gudgeon, A.C. & Morton, N.S.** (1995) Evaluation of an amethocaine gel preparation for percutaneous analgesia before venous cannulation in children. *British Journal of Anaesthesia* **75**, 282–285.

**Lloyd-Thomas, A.R.** (1990) Pain management in paediatric patients. *British Journal of Anaesthesia* **64**, 85–104.

**Lloyd-Thomas, A.R., Howard, R.F. & Llewellyn, N.E.** (1995) The management of acute and post-operative pain in infancy and childhood. In: Aynsley-Green, A., Ward-Platt, M.P. & Lloyd-Thomas, A.R. (eds) *Stress and Pain in Infancy and Childhood*. Bailliere Tindall, London.

**Macintyre, P.E. & Ready, L.B.** (1996) *Acute Pain Management A Practical Guide.* W.B. Saunders, London.

**McCaffery, M. & Beebe, A.** (1989) *Pain Clinical Manual for Nursing Practice.* C.V. Mosby, St Louis.

**McCaffery, M. & Ferrell, B.** (1990) Do you know a narcotic when you see one? *Nursing* **20**, 62–63.

**McCready, M., MacDavitt, K. & O'Sullivan, K.K.** (1991) Children and pain: easing the hurt. *Orthopaedic Nursing* **10**, 33–42.

**McIlvaine, W.B.** (1989) Perioperative pain management in children: a review. *Journal of Pain and Symptom Management* **4**, 215–229.

**Morton, N.** (1993) Balanced analgesia for children. *Nursing Standard* **7**, 8–10.

**Rauen, K.K. & Ho, M.** (1989) Children's use of patient-controlled analgesia after spine surgery. *Pediatric Nursing* **15**, 589–593.

Seymour, J. (1990) The hidden pain. *Nursing Times* **86**, 16–17.

Sparshott, M. (1989) Pain and the special care baby unit. *Nursing Times* **85**, 61–64.

Swafford, L. & Allen, D. (1968) Pain relief in the pediatric patient. *Medical Clinics of North America* **52**, 31.

US Department of Health and Human Services (1992) *Acute Pain Management: Operative or Medical Procedures and Trauma.* Agency for Health Care Policy and Research, Rockville.

Walker, J.M. & Campbell, S.M. (1989) Pain assessment, nursing models and the nursing process. *Recent Advances in Nursing* **24**, 47–61.

Watt-Watson, J.H. & Donovan, M.I. (1992) *Pain Management Nursing Perspective.* Mosby Year Book, St Louis.

Whaley, L.F. & Wong, D.L. (1989) *Essentials of Pediatric Nursing.* Mosby Year Book, St Louis.

Zajac, J. (1992) Pediatric pain management. *Critical Care Nursing Quarterly* **15**, 35–51.

Zelter, L.K., Jay, S.M. & Fisher, D.M. (1989) The management of pain associated with pediatric procedures. *Pediatric Clinics of North America* **36**, 941–961.

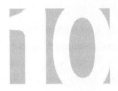

# Managing postoperative pain: problems and solutions

## ■ INTRODUCTION

This chapter adopts a problem-solving approach to the management of postoperative pain. It does this firstly by assessing the nature of acute pain and the incidence and prevalence of the problem in the surgical population. Contributing factors such as attitudes and beliefs regarding pain, knowledge and assessment of pain are explored. Strategies to improve pain management are discussed with particular emphasis on the assessment of pain for the surgical patient; and finally, organizational factors, the role of the multidisciplinary team and the development of Acute Pain Services (APS). Although analgesia is not the only way to manage postoperative pain and nurses are ideally in a position to teach patients other strategies (Spencer, 1989), this chapter does not focus on therapeutic interventions *per se* as these are explored in other chapters. Nonetheless, their role in the overall management of pain is extremely important, and it is assumed that the nurse will be familiar with such strategies and their use.

The nurse obviously has a unique role in the management of the patient's pain, in that she/he is the one who spends most of her/his time with the patient. However, the role is complex as the nurse, patient, doctor and organizational variables all contribute to create a unique situation. A reflective practitioner is required not only to be aware of these but also to be able to do something about them.

## ■ THE NATURE OF ACUTE PAIN

The International Association for the Study of Pain (IASP, 1986) define pain as:

> *'An unpleasant sensory and emotional experience associated with actual or potential tissue damage, or described in terms of such damage.'*

The definition offered by McCaffery (1972), however, reflects the subjective and personal nature of the pain:

> *'Pain is whatever the patient says it is and exists whenever he says it does.'*

Acute pain is generally characterized by being associated with a specific event including: (a) trauma, such as a sports injury, burn or accident; (b) a disease, such as migraine, headache, gout and sickle cell crisis, cancer or myocardial infarction; or (c) therapy, such as surgery, dental work or diagnostic procedures (Donovan, 1990). Acute pain usually has a sudden onset and foreseeable end. When it lasts more than 6 months, it is termed chronic pain.

## ■ THE EFFECTS OF UNCONTROLLED PAIN

In the postoperative period, pain needs to be managed effectively so that chronic pain does not develop. The reasons cited for the sound management of pain often focus on the ethical nature of allowing uncontrolled pain (see Chapter 4 for further discussion). Whilst it is unethical to allow a patient to suffer, it is also extremely detrimental to their postoperative recovery. When pain is acute and uncontrolled the patient is unlikely to move, preferring to lie as still as possible to avoid inducing excruciating pain. This has several unwanted side-effects. Respiratory function may be compromised, and coughing and deep breathing may be avoided, thus predisposing them to chest infections (Craig, 1981). The physiotherapist obviously has a crucial role in the postoperative period, but to gain maximum cooperation from the patient he/she needs to be pain free.

Phillips and Cousins (1986, p. 24) describe how skeletal muscle immobilization, venous stasis and platelet aggregation can predispose to the formation of deep vein thrombosis (DVT) in the surgical patient. Increasing venous return by leg exercises and early ambulation can reduce the likelihood of DVT formation, but a patient in pain is usually unwilling to move about the bed or get up hourly for a short walk.

Other unwanted side-effects of uncontrolled pain can include lack of trust between the nursing staff and the patient. They may feel that no one believes their pain or that there is nothing they can do about it, which can then result in the patient feeling increased anxiety. The relationship between pain, anxiety, perceived helplessness or powerlessness, and patients undergoing surgery is discussed by Walding (1991) and Williams in Chapter 7 of this book. There is a suggestion that, by decreasing the perception of powerlessness, the intensity of the pain experience may also decrease.

## ■ INCIDENCE AND PREVALENCE OF POSTOPERATIVE PAIN

Despite the dramatic advances in pain control over the past 10 years, many patients in both hospital and the community continue to suffer unrelieved pain (Bonica, 1980; Mather and Mackie, 1983; Ketovuori, 1987; Royal College of Surgeons, 1990) and up to three-quarters of patients experience moderate to severe pain whilst in hospital (Marks and Sachar, 1973; Cohen, 1980; Weiss et al., 1983).

Donovan et al. (1987) conducted a study to determine the incidence and characteristics of pain in a random population of 353 patients in a large mid-western hospital in America. Data were collected using portions of the McGill Pain Questionnaire (MPQ). The use of this tool is important as several studies (Melzack, 1975; Dubisson and Melzack 1976; Turk et al., 1985) have been conducted that reveal the MPQ to be a reliable and valid multi-dimensional measure of pain that can be used with a large variety of patient groups with different types of pain (see Chapter 5 for a fuller discussion on methods of pain assessment). Their findings revealed that 58% of patients experienced *excruciating* pain, and fewer than half of these patients had a member of the health care team ask about their pain or note the pain on the patient record.

One of the main mitigating factors for this sad state of affairs was that the dose of analgesia administered over a 24-hour period was less than a quarter of the amount ordered. These findings were similar to the previous study by Marks and Sachar (1973), who concluded that physicians under-prescribed analgesics and nurses gave even less than was prescribed.

Owen et al. (1990) conducted a survey of 259 elective surgical patients, concerning their expectations of pain and their pain relief. The findings indicated that pain relief was ineffective with 39% of patients experiencing moderate pain at 72 hours and 21% severe pain.

These findings are also consistent with some of the findings from Seers (1987) in the UK. She found in her sample of 80 surgical patients that over 21% of patients had between 'very bad' or 'agonizing' pain on the first post-operative day and, when pain was made worse by coughing or moving, nearly 70% of patients reported very bad pain. Interestingly, she also found that some patients continued to experience pain after the fourth day of surgery. Melzack et al. (1987) similarly found that patients with pain that persisted beyond the fourth day following surgery comprise a substantial portion of the patients in a surgical ward (31%). They are often older and tend to use more words to describe their pain and are helped less by their prescribed analgesic medications.

## ■ FACTORS CONTRIBUTING TO THE POOR MANAGEMENT OF POSTOPERATIVE PAIN

To participate fully and to be effective in the management of postoperative patients' pain, the nurse needs to understand the factors that contribute to ineffective pain relief. To ignore this body of literature is to be ignorant of some of the most powerful influences that have clearly limited our ability to provide optimum pain relief in the surgical setting. Nurses' attitudes and beliefs, assessment of postoperative pain and and nurses' knowledge of pain will be considered in more depth, to illuminate some of the inadequacies, but also to offer solutions.

As already discussed (in Chapter 2), the classic studies by Davitz and Davitz (1981) exploring nurses' ratings of suffering demonstrated that social and cultural background clearly influenced the nurses' assessment of the degree of pain a patient was suffering. Those nurses who had experienced pain themselves were more empathetic to patients' pain and suffering but, through the course of the nurses' education, their reactions to patients' physical pain tended to decrease. A similar finding was supported by Ketovuori (1987) who asked 22 patients after gynaecological surgery to describe their wound pain using the Finnish Pain Questionnaire. The questionnaire was also presented to a total of 62 surgical nurses (29 who had previously experienced wound pain and 33 who had not) for them to describe patients' pain at its highest intensity on the third day. Findings revealed that those nurses who had experienced wound pain scored higher values for the patients' pain and those nurses who had not experienced previous pain more accurately described the patients' pain.

Bendelow (1993) has taken the research in a new direction by exploring the relationship between perceptions of pain and the social characteristics of the individual, with an emphasis on the role of gender in the process. Using a multimethod approach, the findings reveal socio-cultural explanations of why women are thought to 'cope better with pain', as both male and female respondents expressed the opinion that men would take longer to admit they were experiencing pain or seek treatment. These findings clearly have implications for the assessment of pain in the clinical setting. The evidence for a relationship between culture and inferences of pain or suffering has often been inconclusive owing to small numbers in their samples or conflicting findings with previous studies (Dudley and Holm, 1984; Reizian and Melies, 1986; Holm et al., 1989). There does, however, seem to be agreement that nurses' inferences of suffering are directly or indirectly related to their own psychological characteristics and acquired beliefs about suffering and pain. We cannot always change these characteristics but, by being aware that we may have them, we can strive to avoid influential judgements on others' pain that may result in incorrect assessment of the information available to us.

How to address beliefs and attitudes is a difficult problem. The use of vignettes to simulate 'real life' is valuable but, under normal clinical conditions, the nurse has access to subtle cues from the patients' voice and facial expression, which are difficult to do justice to in a written description. The nurse is also able to select the cues to which she/he attends (von Baeyer, 1984). Having said this, one study found that half of the pain information available from patients was not noted and, in over a third of the cases, the information recorded did not agree with that provided by the patient (Camp, 1988).

Sofaer (1992, p. 82) advocates using role play to help nurses understand the feelings of the patients who experience pain and to understand their own feelings in relation to providing pain relief. This role play utilizes two scenarios. In the first, one person portrays the patient who is in severe pain and the other is a busy disbelieving nurse. During the second scenario, one person plays the role of a patient in severe pain and the other portrays a nurse who believes the patient. The observations of the group and the feelings of each of the participants is then noted. The exercise is one which clearly explores the real nature of the nurse–patient relationship, and facilitates understanding of beliefs, attitudes and feelings in relation to pain.

## ■ NURSES' ASSESSMENT OF POSTOPERATIVE PAIN

From studies in this area it would seem reasonable to conclude that nurses have been shown to infer less pain than the patient is actually experiencing (Camp, 1988; Choiniere et al., 1990). Seers (1987) took a sample of 80 patients admitted for elective surgery, and interviewed them before surgery and twice a day after surgery for 7 days. They and the nurses were asked to rate their pain on a pain relief and verbal rating scale. A questionnaire that explored various aspects of postoperative pain relief was completed by 28 staff. Interestingly the findings revealed that nurses consistently underestimated the intensity of the patients' pain. For 77% of the time, nurses and patients did not agree about the intensity of the pain: 54% of nurses rated the patients' pain at a lower level than the patients did, and 13% rated it at a higher level. Her findings also indicated that pain assessment was not a high priority in nursing care. Further research suggests that nurses tend to categorize patients according to overt pain behaviours and may not believe them even when they signal that pain is becoming a distressing symptom (Wakefield, 1995).

Another study comparing patients' ratings of their pain and nurses' was conducted on 47 patients admitted to a coronary care unit (Bondestam et al., 1987). A numerical pain-rating scale was used (graded 0–10) to measure pain. Although a positive correlation was found between the patients' and nurses' pain assessments ($r = 0.76$; $p=<0.001$), 23% of nurses underestimated the patients' pain and 20% overestimated their pain.

Documentation of pain assessment formularizes the pain assessment process and is essential to the provision of individualized care from both the legal and professional perspectives. Relatively few studies have considered the documentation of pain assessments (Camp and O'Sullivan, 1987; Graffam, 1990), yet the findings have indicated that a minimal amount of data is recorded. In one survey (Donovan et al., 1987), over half of the patients could not remember being asked by a nurse about their pain and in only half of the medical charts was there any note of pain progress.

Similarly Camp and O'Sullivan (1987) found that, despite the fact that patients described their pain in areas that should be included and documented in pain assessment, documentation of this information was conspicuously lacking. Nurses documented less than 50% of what the patients reported. Albrecht et al. (1992) similarly found that nurses perceived themselves as documenting patient response to analgesic medication much more frequently than they actually did. There would appear to be a discrepancy in the decision-making process and it was suggested that education had not addressed the importance of documenting patient response to analgesia.

Failure to document a patient's response to analgesia or a nursing intervention negates all attempts to manage pain effectively, as there is no basis on which to guide practice further. Documenting such evaluation facilitates sound assessment for future pain-relief strategies, continuity of care and accountability.

# ■ NURSES' KNOWLEDGE OF PAIN

As previously discussed, a lack of knowledge has often been cited for the inability of nurses to assess pain systematically and document their findings. Studies on nurses have generally used survey techniques to explore their knowledge and attitudes regarding a variety of issues, such as knowledge of narcotics, beliefs about addiction and respiratory depression, and non-pharmacological treatment modalities.

Watt-Watson (1987) examined the knowledge base related to pain assessment and narcotic administration of 106 graduate nurses and 101 baccalaureate nursing students. Data were collected using a questionnaire. The findings revealed that a lack of knowledge about pain assessment and narcotic administration was evident. This is seemingly typical of many of the surveys that have been conducted to determine nurses' knowledge regarding such issues (Charap, 1978; Rankin and Snider, 1984; Camp and O'Sullivan, 1987).

McCaffery and colleagues (1990) conducted a survey of the current nursing knowledge about pharmacological management of among 2459 nurses attending a pain workshop in the United States. Their findings demonstrated a significant lack of knowledge regarding the definition of narcotic and opioid drug classification. They found that less than 25% correctly identified the incidence of addiction following the use of opioids for pain relief as less than 1%.

Similarly in the UK, Bourbonnais and Wilson-Barnett (1992) identified and compared the knowledge of nurses working in intensive therapy and hospice settings. Their findings indicated that, although hospice nurses were more knowledgeable, both groups demonstrated a lack of knowledge in specific content areas.

Concern about narcotic addiction and respiratory depression are commonly expressed by nurses as a reason for withholding narcotic administration. Morgan (1985) has written about 'American opiophobia', the customary underutilization of opioid analgesics, and claims that physicians undertreat severe pain owing to their irrational and undocumented fear that appropriate use of opioids will lead to addiction. The literature supports the suggestion that it would be safe to assume nurses also suffer from this fear (Marks and Sachar, 1973; Charap, 1978; Cohen, 1980; McCaffery et al., 1990; Lavies et al., 1992). Table 10.1 summarizes the correct definitions of terms that frequently are incorrectly defined, relating to narcotic administration.

Respiratory depression has been known to occur in less than 1% of the population receiving narcotic analgesia (Marks and Sachar, 1973; Porter and Jick, 1980), and yet surveys continue to identify this as a significant concern of doctors and nurses. In one study, nurses incorrectly attributed analgesia

*Table 10.1* Correct definitions of addiction, tolerance and physical dependence

| Descriptor | Fact |
| --- | --- |
| Addiction | This is a behavioural pattern characterized by compulsive drug-seeking behaviours. It leads to an overwhelming desire for the acquisition and use of the drug, for purposes other than pain relief. |
| Tolerance | This is manifest by a clinical requirement for a higher dose of the drug in order to achieve the original analgesic effect. |
| Physical dependence | Physical dependence is manifest when withdrawal symptoms occur following abrupt cessation of the chronic use of opioids. |

to be the cause of respiratory changes during the days after surgery rather than uncontrolled pain as the cause (Cohen, 1980).

Of those studies exploring nurses' knowledge, the final paragraph usually makes reference to the need for further education (Hosking, 1985; Camp and O'Sullivan, 1987; Watt-Watson, 1987), yet there are relatively few studies that have evaluated the outcomes of introducing an educational programme. Sofaer (1983) conducted a study to assess the practicability and effectiveness of a clinically based educational programme for all levels of ward nurses on pain management. Although the outcome of the study revealed such an approach was beneficial in terms of patient outcomes, it still did not manage to include all staff (those working nights did not participate) and long-term evaluation did not occur.

The development of a pain assessment tool and an ongoing educational programme was incorporated using an action research approach by Davis (1988). The focused educational programme (inclusion of trained staff only; educational needs of untrained staff was not mentioned) used lectures, video material (unspecified), discussion and journals. Nurses' attitudes to pain management were ascertained prior to the start of the programme and after the trial period of one month. He found that staff demonstrated a positive change in attitude after the programme. Although a knowledge questionnaire was given to staff, no mention of the findings occur in the paper.

Knowledge and attitudes must be addressed within educational curricula but linked to this must be a reappraisal of the nature of the organizational situation (the context) in which these decisions are made. Since the seminal work of Fagerhaugh and Strauss (1977), it would seem that little research has addressed the issues that might be more influential than all the research elicited on nurses' knowledge, attitudes and beliefs. This is the day-to-day reality of assessing the patient in pain and the nature of the environment in which this takes place. Research in this area has sadly been neglected, yet the working environment and clinical work in hospital since registration have been perceived to be the most influential experiences in learning about pain and its management (Bourbonnais and Wilson-Barnett, 1992). It also appears that the level of clinical expertise has important implications for pain management and this is discussed by King in Chapter 15. The role of the organization and the multidisciplinary team are discussed further in this chapter.

## ■ PAIN ASSESSMENT AND THE SURGICAL PATIENT

Pain assessment tools can be invaluable in aiding accurate pain assessment (Thompson, 1989) as the subjective nature of pain is difficult to communicate effectively. Only patients can measure their pain accurately and nurses should provide them with assessment tools to help them communicate their pain accurately (for further discussion of pain assessment tools, refer to Chapter 5). In the surgical patient there are a number of factors, related to the patient, that can affect the reliability of any assessment tool. It is the purpose of this section to explore these influences in more detail.

That patients' postoperative pain experience and analgesic consumption vary following identical surgical procedure, should come as no surprise as psychological factors have been shown to modify the pain response of postoperative patients (see Chapter 2). However, pain assessment should begin in the pre-operative period, as it is essential to assess the patient's prior pain experience, coping styles related to pain, their levels of anxiety, as well as their expectations of pain.

### ■ Prior pain experience

The influence that a prior pain experience may have on the current pain cannot be ignored. Research exploring the role of prior pain experience and expectations about postoperative pain has revealed that patients' global pain ratings of past pain experiences was the single strongest partial correlate of expected pain (Walmsley et al., 1992). Obtaining information about patients' prior pain experience could assist nurses in providing them with the appropriate information about the probable level of discomfort to be expected and pain-management strategies that could be used.

### ■ Coping mechanisms

If the patient has experienced pain before, it is important to identify the strategies they used to cope with this. Often patients have a range of strategies that they find particularly helpful, such as listening to music, taking a warm bath or watching television. It is important that these are utilized as they have already been known to help. The other benefit of using prior coping strategies is that it increases the patient's feeling of self-control, which in turn can reduce anxiety and ultimately pain.

With the advent of patient-controlled analgesia (PCA), it is important to consider how the patient deals with stressful situations. It has been suggested that patients who adopt an avoidant blunting strategy would be unlikely to agree to use PCA and those who attempt to master events may benefit from the additional control PCA provides (Thomas and Rose, 1993). Nurses can be instrumental in ensuring that those patients who are likely to benefit from PCA are correctly selected; there should be assessment of their suitability. The role of PCA in pain management will be discussed further in the chapter.

## ▪ Expectations of pain

It is as important to care for the client in the pre-experience phase as it is in the post-experience one. Prior to surgery patients should be questioned about their expectations of pain. Expectations are thought to develop through observations of others, past experiences and the information that is conveyed about the pain experience. Wallace (1985) interviewed and collected data from 118 female patients undergoing laparoscopic surgery for sterilization or infertility investigation and the findings revealed that the greater the pain that was expected, the greater the pain reported at return from theatre. Also, the greater the expected pain, the greater reported postoperative fear. It was suggested that as pain expectancy was positively correlated with post-surgical distress, the minimization of patient fears may be the most helpful intervention. Thus, not only the provision of accurate information, but reassurance by nursing staff may significantly reduce patients' distress.

Carr (1990) showed a significant difference between patients' expectations prior to surgery and pain scores following surgery, with 76% of patients underestimating the postoperative pain they would experience. Although patients tended to expect moderate pain ('surgery is painful isn't it?'), they actually experienced moderate to severe pain. The factors contributing to these unfortunate findings are explained in the study. Similarly Lavies et al. (1992) found that patients also expected to have a significant degree of pain, usually based on previous experience of surgery. That patients have a low expectation regarding pain relief is probably one reason why there has not been public outrage.

Expectations about pain following surgery could affect a patient's motivation to attempt to find pain relief. Patients may expect severe pain, feel they have little control over the situation and thus behave accordingly.

## ▪ ORGANIZATIONAL FACTORS

Fagerhaugh and Strauss (1977) looked at the organizational setting in which pain management took place. They felt that the discrepancy between actual and potential pain relief may be due to: the work demands in the clinical area; lack of accountability surrounding pain management; and the complexity of the patient–staff relationship. They made the observation that organizations are often embedded in social worlds (hospitals in the medical world) and they can only be understood as part of the ideologies of those worlds. The ideologies of those worlds may well affect the running of given organizations. Thus, the medical model – based on empirical, quantitative approaches – may not fit the psychosocial nature of pain. It is important to consider the wider world in which pain is often managed to enable factors inhibiting pain management to be identified.

Using in-depth interviews with ward sisters/charge nurses, Evans (1992) found that 'policies and politics of pain management' emerged as a conceptual category and that the many constraints impeding effective nursing management of postoperative pain included defective policy decisions and poor interprofessional communications. James (1992) acknowledges the dominant hospital system, and suggests that these organizational problems may appear insurmountable even when staff actively seek to give 'good patient care'.

The strict policies and the sense of implicit accountability when administering controlled drugs may act to prohibit nurses administering these drugs more frequently. The time taken to find another nurse, prepare and check the drug, and administer it may also inhibit its more liberal utilization. Although it has been acknowledged that legal constraints and institutional policies can unnecessarily limit the nurse's ability to manage pain safely and effectively (Jacox et al., 1992), there is little research available that has identified the influence of such policies. Interestingly, it is the advent of PCA that has identified some of these problems and, at the same time, potentially removed some of the barriers that contribute to the ineffective management of pain.

PCA is increasingly being used to deliver opioid analgesics and its superiority to conventional methods of delivery is well proven (Bennett et al., 1982; Slattery et al., 1983; Notcutt and Morgan, 1990; Thomas et al., 1995). It has been shown to be a safe modality which allows the patient to administer small doses of analgesia, through the intravenous or epidural route, to achieve pain relief. Advantages of the method include a reduced degree of sedation, lowered patient anxiety associated with a sense of self-control and reduced demand on nursing time (Lange et al., 1988). The narrow 'therapeutic window' during which pain relief is achieved and excessive sedation is avoided, is perceived to be a further advantage (White, 1988). Patients can finely tune the effect of the analgesia and may trade off a small increase in pain against the unpleasant or unwanted side-effects of opiates, such as nausea or sedation. Another benefit of PCA has been the associated reduction in hospital stay by up to 2 days (Thomas et al., 1995).

Aitken and Kenny (1990) found that 55% of staff who worked with PCA on a postoperative cardiac surgical ward, said it reduced their workload, mainly by relieving them of the task of checking and administering controlled drugs. Thomas (1993) found that 14 out of 15 nurses completing a questionnaire about PCA said they liked it because the patient was in control and did not have to rely on nursing staff, and also because it meant that nurses did not have to check out controlled drugs constantly.

This liberal attitude has not always been present, as evident in Bast and Hayes' (1986) description of their initial experience with introducing PCA:

*'Perhaps the greatest difficulty we had to overcome – although few would admit it openly – was the fear of letting our patients have any control over their needs. We were simply afraid they'd use too much narcotic.'*

There is a need to explore the nurses' role in the administration of controlled drugs further, and in particular the influence of legal constraints and hospital policies.

## ■ THE MULTIDISCIPLINARY TEAM

Oden (1989) has attributed the problem of poor pain management to poor accountability. No one member of the medical team assumes responsibility for pain control and the assessment of analgesic interventions. Nurses believe that the anaesthetist is the most appropriate person to manage pain relief, yet anaesthetists do not routinely visit all patients postoperatively and neither is there an incentive for them to do so (Chapman et al., 1987, cited in Winefield et al., 1990). For optimal pain relief it is essential that the team work together closely. There is a need for close liaison with therapists (such as physiotherapists and occupational therapists), so enabling the patient to partake with the maximum cooperation. Good communication and support from pharmacists is obviously an essential requisite also, since this ensures that prescriptions are correctly prescribed and dispensed. They also offer educational support.

To appreciate more fully how the multidisciplinary team could work more closely together, two strategies will be considered. Firstly, how to work more effectively with other members of the team and, secondly, the role of the acute pain team.

## ■ Achieving optimum pain relief through collaboration

Communicating with the physiotherapist concerning the timing of therapy and how the patient's pain is currently being controlled, enables the nurse to plan ahead and tailor the management of pain so that the patient can achieve maximum benefit. This ultimately will enable the patient to be actively involved in those activities which decrease the possibility of the negative effects of reduced mobility. If the patient is to achieve maximum benefit then pain must be well controlled.

Pain assessment should not take place on a drug round because the nurse is busy and the patient is not given adequate time to have their pain assessed properly. Patients may wait for the drug round before they tell the nurse that they have pain, therefore suffering between rounds. It is, therefore, much better to assess pain on a regular basis, in an unhurried manner. It need not take hours but a good assessment is a necessity for effective pain management. Sit *with* the patient and establish that you have time for them. Acknowledge that they may have pain by asking an open question such as 'how is your pain?'. This question encourages the patient to respond openly. Firstly, by acknowledging that they may have pain (i.e. you believe the patient) and, secondly, by avoiding a simple 'yes/no' response, more meaningful information is likely to be forthcoming.

Nurses often find themselves in a frustrating position when the patient still has pain despite having had analgesia. To facilitate the relief of pain, Walker and Wong (1991) outline a very effective plan of action to achieve the combination of analysis, documentation and persuasion required to change an analgesic regimen.

### Step 1: Work with the existing prescription

This entails considering that the right drug, right time, right dose and right route have all been selected. Very often a variable dose has been prescribed, so it is important to ensure the dose has been titrated against the pain (by adjusting it upwards or downwards). Time is often written as prn (*pro re nata*, meaning 'according to circumstances'), which has been shown to be ineffective for maximum pain relief as often patients do not receive the analgesia on a regular basis. If continuous relief is required, then ensure the drug is given regularly to avoid peaks and troughs. Liaise with therapists for timing to ensure that the patient has received maximum pain relief prior to activity so they are comfortable enough to give the maximum cooperation. The route of administration is commonly intramuscular, yet this has been found to be an unreliable route as peak plasma concentrations following administration have been shown to show a threefold variability in the maximum peak and up to an eightfold variability in the time of this occurrence (Austin et al., 1980). If drugs need to be given via this route, then they should be given regularly 'around the clock' to reduce plasma variability as much as possible. Postoperatively, hypotension, hypothermia and shock can all reduce the uptake of the drug that has been given intramuscularly. It is important to assess the patient for any of these conditions and have an awareness that they may contribute to ineffective analgesia.

### Step 2: Consider alternative prescriptions

Having considered all of the above variables, your patient may still be in pain. Before approaching the doctor for a change in the prescription, think of an appropriate strategy. Is it an alternative drug that is required or a change in route, dose or time? Consideration of the variety of pharmacological agents used and their onset, peak and duration is a prerequisite.

## Step 3: Talk with the doctor

In order to obtain change in the prescription, this negotiation can often be fruitful if the following are considered:

- *Consider the timing.* It is better to choose a time when the doctor is focused on the patient.
- *Be assertive.* Speak confidently and clearly, and avoid arguing or becoming defensive.
- *Establish credibility.* Support your request with precise information. Use verbal or numerical rating scales. This presents information in a manner that is difficult to challenge or avoid.
- *Anticipate questions.* If you request a change in dose or drug, then work out beforehand what that change might be. Ensure that you are up to date with the patient's vital signs as well.
- *Request a specific change.* If the doctor is unwilling to change the prescription, request a 24-hour trial of your suggestion and then a review. In that period ensure that you collect data regarding pain assessment, vital signs, sleep, appetite, etc., as this will be valuable in establishing the effectiveness of the new regimen.
- *Suggest an alternative.* If the doctor is unwilling to prescribe another drug, suggest increasing the dose or adding a non-steroidal anti-inflammatory drug to the current regimen.

## Step 4: Implement the new prescription

As soon as the new regimen commences, start to evaluate the analgesic effectiveness. Also think ahead: once pain is well controlled you may require a further alteration in the prescription, so anticipate future analgesic needs.

## ▪ Achieving optimum pain relief through an acute pain service

Experience in the USA and UK has demonstrated that a multidisciplinary approach utilizing medical, nursing, psychological and pharmacological expertise is essential to the successful provision of Acute Pain Services (APS) (Royal College of Surgeons and College of Anaesthetists, 1990). Ready et al. (1988) describes most elegantly the inception of an APS whose goals in developing and implementing it were:

1. To improve postoperative analgesia.
2. To train anaesthesiology residents in methods of postoperative pain management.
3. To apply and advance new analgesic methods.
4. To carry out clinical research in the area of postoperative pain management.

Nurses have an important role to play if the advent of the APS are to be successful, and support for the development of such teams is endorsed in the recommendations of the report by the Royal College of Surgeons and College of Anaesthetists (1990). Although the initiatives include advanced techniques, there is strong emphasis on educational initiatives for all staff involved in pain management. A more recent paper by Notcutt and Austin (1995) suggests that each hospital should have a broader 'Pain Management Service', which should empower nurses and doctors to relieve pain successfully as well as providing expertise in handling different problems, for example, through education. Education is a powerful strategy to challenge current practices and improve pain management.

The development of newer methods of analgesia administration, such as patient control of opioid administration, continuous intravenous infusion and intraspinal administration of opiates or local anaesthetics, has provided the opportunity for greater pain relief and avoided some of the problems associated with traditional intramuscular narcotic administration (Hord and Kokenes, 1989). The APS can enable such developments to be used, allowing patients to be nursed on a general ward rather than in intensive care and high dependency areas, where good pain control may be dependent on the number of beds available.

Evidence has suggested that the introduction of the APS may lead to a change in the attitude of all groups of staff in the management of post-operative pain.

The reduced morbidity, faster convalescence and improved satisfaction in patients who receive adequate postoperative pain relief provide economic justification for the introduction of PCA (Justins, 1992; Thomas and Rose, 1993). In the UK some hospitals have already commenced an APS and Dening (1993) briefly discusses some of these services.

## ■ CONCLUSION

A problem-solving approach is necessary if the effective management of postoperative pain is to be a reality. This chapter has considered some of the factors that have been elicited through research that contribute to ineffective pain management. Solutions to problems have been offered and recent developments in this area explored. If pain is to be effectively managed in the postoperative period and the advantages of new methods of analgesia delivery are to be exploited to their full potential, then nurses and doctors need to have the appropriate education to enable them to function effectively within the multidisciplinary team. Other key players in the team, such as physiotherapists and occupational therapists, should receive similar educational input and, where possible, strategies such as shared learning and role play should be utilized to facilitate real-life situations and encourage multidisciplinary collaboration. There is an urgent need to redress the current educational strategies, both from the amount and content (in pre-registration nursing/medicine and continuing education curricula) but also the methods used to deliver them. These strategies will facilitate the development of pain teams and encourage multidisciplinary collaboration, as well as disbanding some of the current factors that are known to inhibit effective pain management, in particular, ineffective communication between patient, nurse and doctor.

The 1980s and early 1990s have seen rapid changes in the nature of surgery resulting in more acutely ill patients being nursed in general wards, shorter in-patient stay and increased day surgery. Effective pain management must be seen as central to the delivery of quality patient care for the surgical patient. We must not continue to make the same mistakes, but grasp the changes and nurse proactively, ensuring that the oversights of the past are not repeated in the future.

# ■ REFERENCES

**Aitken, H.A. & Kenny, G.** (1990) Use of patient controlled analgesia in postoperative cardiac surgical patients – a survey of ward staff attitudes. *Intensive Care Nursing* **6**, 74–78.

**Albrecht, M., Cook J., Riley, M. & Andreoni, V.** (1992) Factors influencing staff nurses' decisions for non-documentation of patient response to analgesic administration. *Journal of Clinical Nursing* **1**, 243–251.

**Austin, K.L., Stapleton, J.V. & Mather, L.E.** (1980) Multiple intramuscular injections: a major source of variability in analgesic response to meperidine. *Pain* **8**, 47.

**Bast, C. & Heyes, P.** (1986) PCA: a new way to spell pain relief. *Registered Nurse* August, 18–20.

**Bendelow, G.** (1993) Pain perceptions, emotions and gender. *Sociology of Health and Illness* **15**, 273–294.

**Bennett, R.L., Batenhorst, R.L. & Bivens, B.A.** (1982) Patient-controlled analgesia: a new concept of postoperative pain relief. *Annals of Surgery* **195**, 700–705.

**Bondestam, E., Hovgren, F., Johanson, G., Jern, J., Herlitz, J. & Holmberg, S.** (1987) Pain assessment by patients and nurses in the early phase of acute myocardial infarction. *Journal of Advanced Nursing* **12**, 677–682.

**Bonica, J.J.** (1980) Pain research and therapy: past and current status and future needs. In: Ng, L.K.Y. & Bonica, J.J. (eds) *Pain Discomfort, and Humanitarian Care.* Elsevier, Amsterdam, pp. 1–46.

**Bourbonnais, F. & Wilson-Barnett, J.** (1992) A comparative study of intensive therapy unit hospice nurses' knowledge on pain management. *Journal of Advanced Nursing* **17**, 362–372.

**Camp, D.** (1988) A comparison of nurses' recorded assessment of pain with perceptions of pain as described by cancer patients. *Cancer Nursing* **11**, 237–243.

**Camp, D.L. & O'Sullivan, P.** (1987) Comparison of surgical and oncology patients' descriptions of pain and nurses' documentation of pain assessments. *Journal of Advanced Nursing* **12**, 593–598.

**Carr, E.C.J.** (1990) Postoperative pain – patients' expectations and experiences. *Journal of Advanced Nursing* **15**, 89–100.

**Chapman, P.J., Ganendran, A., Scott, R.J. & Basford, K.E.** (1987) Attitudes and knowledge of nursing staff in relation to management of postoperative pain. *Australia and New Zealand Journal of Surgery* **57**, 447–450.

**Charap, A.D.** (1978) The knowledge, attitudes, and experience of medical personnel treating pain in the terminally ill. *The Mount Sinai Journal of Medicine* **45**, 561–580.

**Choiniere, M., Melzack, R., Girard, N., Rondeau, J. & Paguin, M.** (1990) Comparison between patients' and nurses' assessment of pain and medication efficacy in severe burn injuries. *Pain* **40**, 143–152.

**Cohen, F.** (1980) Post-surgical pain relief: patient's status and nurses' medication choice. *Pain* **9**, 265–274.

**Craig, D.B.** (1981) Postoperative recovery of pulmonary function. *Anaesthesia and Analgesia* **60**, 46.

**Davis, P.** (1988) Changing nursing practice for more effective control of postoperative pain through a staff initiated educational programme. *Nurse Education Today* **8**, 325–331.

**Davitz, J.R. & Davitz, L.L.** (1981) *Inferences of Patients' Pain and Psychological Distress*. Springer, New York.

**Dening, F.** (1993) Patient-controlled analgesia. *British Journal of Nursing* **2**, 274–277.

**Donovan M.I.** (1990) Acute pain relief. *Nursing Clinics of North America* **25**, 851–861.

**Donovan M., Dillon, P. & McGuire, L.** (1987) Incidence and characteristics of pain in a sample of medical–surgical inpatients. *Pain* **30**, 69–78.

**Dubuisson, D. & Melzack, R.** (1976) Classification of clinical pain descriptions by multiple group discriminant analysis. *Experimental Neurology* **51**, 480.

**Dudley, S.R. & Holm, K.** (1984) Assessment of the pain experience in relation to selected nurse charcteristics. *Pain* **18**, 179–186.

**Evans, J.** (1992) The nursing management of postoperative pain: policies, politics and strategies. *Journal of Clinical Nursing* **1**, 226.

**Fagerhaugh, S.Y. & Strauss, A.** (1977) *Politics of Pain Management: Staff–Patient Interaction*. Addison-Wesley, London.

**Graffam, S.** (1990) Pain content in the curriculum – a survey. *Nurse Educator* **15**, 20–23.

**Holm, K., Cohen, F., Dudas, S. et al** (1989) Effects of personal pain experience on pain assessment. *IMAGE: Journal of Nursing Scholarship* **21**, 72–75.

**Hord, A.H. & Kokenes, C.** (1989) Postoperative pain: a review of management methods. *Hospital Formulary* **24**, January, 28–40.

**Hosking, J.** (1985) Knowledge and practice. *Nursing Mirror* **160**, ii–vi.

**International Association for the Study of Pain** (1986) Pain terms: a current list with definitions and notes on usage. *Pain* (Suppl). **3**, S216.

**Jacox, A., Ferrell, B. & Heidrich, G.** (1992) Managing acute pain: a guideline for the nation. *American Journal of Nursing* May, 49–55.

**James, N.** (1992) Care = organisation + physical labour + emotional labour. *Sociology of Health and Illness* **14**, 488–509.

**Justins, D.M.** (1992) Acute pain. In: *Pathophysiological Mechanisms of Pain; Past and Future Therapy, Proceedings of an International Conference.* IBC Tec Services, London.

**Ketovuori, H.** (1987) Nurses' and patients' conceptions of wound pain and the administration of analgesia. *Journal of Pain and Symptom Management* **2**, 213–219.

**Lange, M.P., Dahn, M.S. & Jacobs, L.A.** (1988) Patient-controlled analgesia versus intermittent analgesia dosing. *Heart and Lung* **17**, 495–498.

**Lavies, N., Hart, L., Rounsefell, & Runciman, W.** (1992) Identification of patient, medical and nursing staff attitudes to postoperative opioid analgesia; stage 1 of a longitudinal study of postoperative analgesia. *Pain* **48**, 313–319.

**Marks, R. & Sachar, E.** (1973) The undertreatment of medical inpatients with narcotic analgesia. *Annals of Internal Medicine* **78**, 173–181.

**Mather, L. & Mackie, J.** (1983) The incidence of postoperative pain in children. *Pain* **15**, 271–282.

**McCaffery, M.** (1972) *Nursing Management of the Patient with Pain.* J.B. Lippincott, Philadelphia.

**McCaffery, M., Ferrel, B. & Page, E.** (1990) Nurses' knowledge of opioid analgesic drugs and psychological dependence. *Cancer Nursing* **13**, 21–27.

**McGuire, D.** (1992) Measuring pain. In: Frank-Stromborg, R. (ed.) *Instruments for Clinical Research.* Oncology Nursing Society, Boston.

**Melzack, R.** (1975) The McGill Pain Questionnaire: major properties and scoring methods. *Pain* **1**, 277.

**Melzack, R., Abbot, F., Zackon, W., Mulder, D.S. & Davis, W.** (1987) Pain on a surgical ward: a survey of duration and intensity of pain and the effectiveness of medication. *Pain* **29**, 67–72.

**Morgan, J.** (1985) American opiophobia: customary underutilisation of opioid analgesics. *Advances in Alcohol Substance Abuse* **5**, 163–173.

**Notcutt, W.G. & Austin, J.** (1995) The acute pain team or the pain management service? *The Pain Clinic* **8** (2), 167–174.

**Notcutt, W. & Morgan, R.J.** (1990) Introducing patient controlled analgesia into a District General Hospital. *Anaesthesia* **45**, 401–406.

**Oden, R.V.** (1989) Acute postoperative pain: incidence, severity, and the etiology of inadequate treatment. *Anaesthesia Clinics of North America* **7**, 1–15.

**Owen, H., McMillan, V. & Rogowski, D.** (1990) Postoperative pain therapy: a survey of patients' expectations and their experiences. *Pain* **41**, 303–307.

**Phillips, G.D. & Cousins, M.J.** (1986) Neurological mechanisms of pain and the relationship of pain, anxiety and sleep. In: Cousins, M.J. & Phillips, G.D. (eds) *Acute Pain Management.* Churchill Livingstone, Edinburgh.

**Porter, J. & Jick, H.** (1980) Addiction rare in patients treated with narcotics. *New England Journal of Medicine* **302**, 123.

**Rankin, M. & Snider, B.** (1984) Nurses' perceptions of cancer patients' pain. *Cancer Nursing* **1**, 149–155.

**Ready, L.B. Oden, R., Chadwick, H.S., Beneditti, C., Rooke, G.A. & Wild, L.M.** (1988) The development of an anaesthesiology-based postoperative pain management service. *Anaesthesiology* **68**, 100–106.

**Reizian, A. & Meleis, A.I.** (1986) Arab-Americans' perceptions of and responses to pain. *Critical Care Nurse* **6**, 30–37.

**Royal College of Surgeons and College of Anaesthetists** (1990) *Commission on the Provision of Surgical Services. Report of the Working Party on Pain after Surgery.* RCS and RCAnaes, London.

**Seers, K.** (1987) Perceptions of pain. *Nursing Times* **83** (48), 37–39.

**Slattery, P.J., Harmer, M., Rosen, M. & Vickers, M.D.** (1983) An open comparison between routine and self-administered postoperative pain relief. *Annals of the Royal College of Surgeons of England* **65**, 18–19.

**Sofaer, B.** (1983) Pain relief – the core of practice. *Nursing Times* **79** (47), 38–42.

**Sofaer, B.** (1992) *Pain: A Handbook for Nurses.* Chapman & Hall, London.

**Spencer, K.** (1989) Postoperative pain: the alternative to analgesia. *The Professional Nurse* July, 479–480.

**Thomas, V.J** (1993) Patient and staff perceptions of PCA. *Nursing Standard* **7** (28), 37–39.

**Thomas, V.J. & Rose, F.D.** (1993) Patient-controlled analgesia: a new method for old. *Journal of Advanced Nursing* **18**, 1719–1726.

**Thomas, V.J., Heath, M., Rose, D. & Flory, P.** (1995) Psychological characteristics and the effectiveness of patient-controlled analgesia. *British Journal of Anaesthesia* **74**, 271–276.

**Thompson, C.** (1989) The nursing assessment of the patient with cardiac pain on the coronary care unit. *Intensive Care Nursing* **5**, 147–154.

**Turk, D.C., Rudy, T.E. & Salovey, P.** (1985) The McGill Pain Questionnaire reconsidered: confirming the factor structure and examining appropriate uses. *Pain* **21**, 385.

**von Baeyer** (1984) Consequences of nonverbal expression of pain: patient distress and observer concerns. *Social Science and Medicine* **19**, 1319–1324.

**Wakefield, A.B.** (1995) Pain: an account of nurses' talk. *Journal of Advanced Nursing* **21**, 905–910.

**Walding, M.F.** (1991) Pain, anxiety and powerlessness. *Journal of Advanced Nursing* **16**, 388–397.

**Walker, M. & Wong, D.L.** (1991) A battle plan for patients in pain. *American Journal of Nursing* June, 32–36.

**Wallace, L.M.** (1985) Surgical patients' expectations of pain and discomfort: does accuracy of expectations minimise post-surgical pain and distress? *Pain* **22**, 363–373.

**Walmsley, P.N.H., Brockopp, D.Y. & Brockopp, G.W.** (1992) The role of prior pain experience and expectations on postoperative pain. *Journal of Pain and Symptom Management* **7**, 34–37.

**Watt-Watson, J.** (1987) Nurses' knowledge of pain issues: a survey. *Journal of Pain and Symptom Management* **2**, 207–211.

**Weiss, D., Sriwatanakul, K., Alloza, J., Weintraub, M. & Lasagna, L.** (1983) Attitudes of patients, housestaff and nurses towards postoperative analgesic care. *Anaesthesia and Analgesia* **62**, 70–74.

**White, P.F.** (1988) Use of patient-controlled analgesia for management of acute pain. *JAMA* **259**, 243–247.

**Winefield, H.R., Katsikitis, M., Hart, L.M. & Rounsefell, B.F.** (1990) Postoperative pain experiences: relevant patient and staff attitudes. *Journal of Psychosomatic Research* **34**, 543–552.

# 11

## Sickle cell disease pain

Sickle cell disease (SCD) is the most prevalent haemoglobinopathy in northern Europe (WHO Advisory Group on Hereditary Disease, 1985) and primarily affects the Caribbean and African population and also small numbers of people from the Mediterranean and the Middle East (National Association of Health Authorities, 1991). Data on estimated annual births of infants with a major haemoglobin disorder in the UK reveal that around 129 babies are born with the disease every year (Modell and Anionwu, 1996). This figure is based on the 1991 census data and is therefore a very conservative estimate.

## ■ PATHOPHYSIOLOGY

SCD is a group of genetic blood disorders including sickle cell anaemia (SS), sickle haemoglobin C disease (SC), sickle cell β thalassaemia (Sβ Thal) (Konotey-Ahulu, 1991; Midence et al., 1993). SCD occurs as a result of a mutation in the haemoglobin synthesis (see Serjeant, 1992, for further reading).

The sickle mutation is found in large geographic areas, which include Africa, the Middle East, the Mediterranean region and Asia. Its frequency is increased in areas where malaria is prevalent because the sickle cell gene offers protection against this parasite. The sickle cell gene is, therefore, most common in people who have descended from these regions. In Britain it occurs predominantly in African–Caribbeans and West Africans, and currently there are estimated to be 9000 people affected by the disorder in Greater London (Streetly et al., 1997).

The highest rate of mortality occurs during the first 5 years of life as a result of infection, and another peak occurs in the 20–24-year age range (Serjeant, 1992). Although recent improvements in medical care have raised life expectancy (Brozovic and Davies, 1987), survival beyond the age of 40 is unusual and recent research conducted in the USA revealed that the median age of death is 42 for males and 48 for females (Platt et al., 1994).

SCD is characterized by the production of a predominance of haemoglobin S (HbS) causing a structural change in red blood cells producing a 'sickle' shape, which leads to a number of life-threatening problems for the SCD sufferer. Clinically, episodes of significant 'sickling' often take place suddenly and without warning, and are so characteristic of the disease that they have earned the name 'sickle cell crises'. Acute splenic sequestration is common in young children (under the age of 6 years) and is one of the most common causes of very early death. It is poorly understood, but it occurs when there is a sudden pooling of red cells into the spleen causing splenic enlargement, severe abdominal pain, acute anaemia, peripheral circulatory failure, shock and sometimes death (Midence and Elander, 1994).

Other complications are delayed growth and a delay in the onset of puberty, priapism, avascular necrosis, strokes and enuresis. Pregnancy is a hazard, because there is an increased incidence of painful crises, and miscarriages and stillbirths are likely. An increase in knowledge and improvement in medical care, particularly the prophylactic use of penicillin, has brought about a reduction in the numbers of childhood deaths.

## ■ ACUTE EPISODES OF PAINFUL SICKLING CRISIS

The most frequent and intractable physical problem experienced by individuals with SCD is painful crises, which require admission into hospital. The most frequent sites of pain are lumbar spine, femur and abdomen. These painful (bony) vaso-occlusive crises account for 91% of hospital admissions in this patient population. These pains often last a week or two, sometimes persisting for weeks and appear to be related to an increased susceptibility to bloodstream infection. In central London, painful crises account for the second greatest number of admissions, with an average length of stay of 7 days (Yardumian, 1993).

In another study involving nine sickle cell patients, Waters and Thomas (1995) found that the average time spent in hospital over a 12-month period was 33.3 days. This inevitably causes severe disruption to the educational and social aspects of life, which, in turn, has consequences for achievement capabilities and psychosocial adjustment.

Individuals vary in the number of painful crises experienced, but most SCD patients experience one or two severe episodes per year requiring hospital admission (Varni and Walco, 1988). This suggests that a significant proportion of the painful crises requiring medical and nursing care occurs in only a small percentage of the SCD population. Shapiro (1989) and Brozovic et al. (1987) have shown that the proportion in need of frequent medical intervention is approximately one-fifth of the SCD population. In the study involving nine hospitalized SCD patients, Waters and Thomas (1995) found that five patients had more than 4 weeks sick leave per year owing to painful crises.

### ■ Precipitating factors

Painful crises are often precipitated by dehydration, exertion, infection, stress, fatigue, cold (including air conditioning) and swimming in cool water (Shapiro, 1991). However, the majority of painful episodes occur without any identifiable trigger. Serjeant et al. (1994) also found that exposure to cold (e.g. being caught in the rain or swimming), physical exertion and the emotional stress of college exams or arguments precipitated crises among the SCD patients in Jamaica.

Dehydration can lead to a reduction in plasma volume and an increase in the blood viscosity, which in turn interferes with the normal blood flow. Exertion and stress can reduce the level of oxygen in the blood, which makes the red cells susceptible to sickling (Midence and Elander, 1994).

## ■ TREATMENT AND MANAGEMENT

Minor crises are managed at home with oral analgesics but hospitalization becomes necessary when the pain is so severe that oral analgesics are ineffective. On admission to hospital, the three essential components of treatment are analgesia, hydration and the identification and treatment of underlying infections (Midence and Elander, 1994). Pharmacological therapy is therefore the mainstay of treatment and opioids are usually required. Most hospitals use either continuous subcutaneous or intramuscular morphine or pethidine (Davies and Brozovic, 1989).

Patient-controlled analgesia (PCA) has been found to be a very successful analgesic method among children and adolescents in the USA (Schecter et al., 1988). The PCA system consists of a syringe pump and a timing device. The patient activates the system by pressing a button, causing a small dose of analgesic to be delivered into the venous system. Simultaneously a lockout device is activated ensuring that another dose cannot be delivered until the first dose has had time to exert its full effect. PCA use among the SCD population in the UK has been much more limited.

## ■ PROBLEMATIC PAIN MANAGEMENT

The management of pain in this group of patients appears to be problematic (Vichinsky et al., 1982). Both patients' expectations about pain relief and attitudes of staff concerning the provision of that relief contribute to the inadequacy of the situation (Weisman et al., 1992). Ingrisano (1986) suggests that when a patient enters the hospital in a painful crisis, he or she must assume a sick role, whilst at the same time gain adequate analgesia. The first is a dependent/passive role and the latter necessarily involves assertive behaviour/active role.

The patients' perception of their lack of control whilst occupying the sick/dependent role elicits pain behaviour, which is frequently disproportionate to the disease process (Ingrisano, 1986; Waters, 1992) in an attempt to gain pain relief. Emotional reactions to sickle cell pain becomes exaggerated by the problems of inadequate recognition and treatment of pain by health care professionals (Gil, 1989). Many doctors and nurses who have limited experience of managing SCD may become excessively concerned about narcotic use, and confused and frustrated when attempting to manage painful episodes (Waters, 1992; Weisman et al., 1992).

On the other hand, some health care professionals who see only a few patients with SCD may misinterpret a patient's pain behaviour as 'faking' or drug seeking. Evidence that nurses misinterpret pain behaviour as 'faking' or 'drug seeking' comes from a recent study by Alleyne and Thomas (1994). In this study, not only did the majority of patients discern that the nurses doubted their pain status, they also provided evidence of nurses appearing to deliberately prolong the process.

Fears about opiate dependence shown by health care professionals is a major obstacle to effective pain control in SCD. Vichinsky (1982) reported that out of 600 sickle cell patients there was no incidence of drug addiction.

However, Brozovic et al. (1986) noted that, among 101 SCD patients in Great Britain, 13 were addicted and seven were drug dependent.

Such conflicting evidence regarding drug dependency and drug addiction only serves to muddy the water even more. Nevertheless, Midence and Elander (1994) remind us that even the few drug-addicted or drug-dependent patients are entitled to treatment when they are in pain. According to Shapiro (1991) the undertreatment of sickle cell pain is attributed to the combined effects of a general lack of education about pharmacological treatment of pain and an antagonistic relationship between patients and staff. This impairs compassionate and competent intervention.

The assessment of pain in the SCD patient appears to be non-existent, since it is generally the patients who have to draw the nurses' attention to their pain (Alleyene and Thomas, 1994; Waters and Thomas, 1995). Nursing enquiries about pain are usually confined to drug rounds suggesting that nurses place a low priority on providing pain relief. As with postoperative pain (see Chapter 10), other researchers believe that inappropriate prioritization of pain relief by nurses may be influenced by their fear about addiction (Murray and May, 1988; Schecter et al., 1988) and overdosing (Payne, 1989) with narcotic analgesia in those in sickle cell crisis.

However, the withholding of analgesia may itself lead to preoccupation with pain relief and sick-role behaviours, where patients must legitimate their pain (Ballas, 1990). Patients whom nurses had observed laughing, talking or watching television prior to a request for analgesic were considered not to be experiencing genuine pain (Waters and Thomas, 1995). As Waters and Thomas have argued, this highlights a lack of understanding concerning individual differences in the capacity to cope with pain. It may well be that patients were engaging in distraction when they were displaying these behaviours, but these were interpreted by the nursing staff to be incompatible with genuine pain experience. It seems that they have to be 'rolling around in agony' before they receive any attention (Alleyne and Thomas, 1994).

The frequent reporting of these and other examples of poor practice, stimulated The Working Party of The Standing Medical Advisory Committee on Sickle Cell, Thalassaemia (SMAC, 1994) and other haemoglobinopathies, to recommend prompt administration of effective analgesics, which should be monitored by trained staff. It also recommends that a pain management protocol should be available in hospitals that treat SCD patients and that this should be a mandatory requirement in specialist haemoglobinopathy units.

## ■ COMMUNICATION PROBLEMS

Pain can be seen as a communication problem, since responses to relieve pain and alleviate suffering require the presence of pain to be communicated to another person who can act to relieve it (Somerville, 1993). Those who cannot verbalize and communicate their pain are often regarded as not being in pain; Somerville (1993) suggests that failure to treat children's pain is a manifestation of this phenomenon. She further argues that it is easy to detach from those with whom we cannot communicate, or those with whose status or position we do not identify. With respect to sickle cell pain management, we must also add colour and culture to this list, and these disparities adversely affect the communication process (Shapiro, 1991).

In failing to identify with people we also depersonalize them (Somerville, 1993) and sometimes we deliberately avoid communication with others in order to take advantage of this reaction. In the study concerned with 'The management of sickle cell crisis as experienced by patients and their carers' by Alleyne and Thomas (1994), patients with SCD reported that they had to employ attention-seeking strategies for any interaction with the nursing staff, or else they were otherwise largely left alone. Nurses themselves did not demonstrate any interaction that they had initiated with the patients, other than the administration of analgesic medication.

Sickle cell patients who took part in a pilot study (using a cognitive-behavioural approach to manage sickle cell pain) (Thomas et al. 1996) as well as those that I have counselled, have stated that they are not treated as individuals by health care professionals, but rather like 'animals' and without respect. Nurses seem to believe that individualizing care for sickle cell patients is an impossible and unrealistic task, and this is exemplified in the following statement of a nurse taking part in Alleyne and Thomas' study:

> 'You're meant to treat them as individuals, but when you go in a bay and there are four of them in, you can't say, do you want pethidine as well?'

This statement suggests that nurses not only have major difficulties in seeing sickle cell patients as individuals in their own right but it also demonstrates a lack of systematic assessment of sickle cell pain.

Whereas an inability to communicate about pain can be depersonalizing because there is no basis for understanding, the communication of pain may also be blocked because of the way people choose to express the pain. Severe pain possesses an individual to the point where he/she becomes 'the pain' (Somerville, 1993). As discussed in Chapter 2, there are ethnic differences in the expression of pain which can strengthen the depersonalizing effect. Somerville goes on to say that other people may then act to de-identify from the pain that is seen as the person rather than to identify with the person who is in pain. If a person cannot identify with someone, then it becomes difficult to be empathetic. Certainly the majority of patients in Waters and Thomas' study (1995) estimated nurses' sympathy for their pain to be very low indeed. Furthermore, patients found that nurses never offered comfort measures or verbal support as means of providing relief. If they did offer such support, it was done on such rare occasions, that patients felt in need of more emotional support. Prashar et al. (1985) and Anionwu (1992) have argued that improving professional awareness through education is a necessary step towards improving poor practice. There are a number of haemoglobinopathy courses which have been implemented with this purpose in mind.

## ■ POSSIBLE SOLUTIONS

One explanation for nurses' reliance on pharmacological intervention as a substitute for offering verbal support or complementary methods of relief is due to a general lack of knowledge about the sickle cell crises and the disease process (France-Dawson, 1990) and the specific psychological challenges that SCD present to individual sufferers. Although this chapter is concerned with pain management in SCD, a brief overview of psychological issues will be presented.

I believe that an appreciation of the psychological issues is likely to facilitate better understanding of the type of coping strategies utilized during painful crises and the ways in which these can influence the interaction with health care professionals. It is also very pertinent, since it appears from the literature that it is the poorly adjusted SCD patients who are more likely to be admitted to hospital and therefore with whom nurses are likely to interact.

SCD has been with us for a considerable number of years, yet there is a dearth of UK-based research that addresses the psychological reactions of people with SCD. Our current understanding of the psychological reactions and the experience of psychosocial problems has, therefore, been gained largely from research undertaken almost exclusively in the USA. I would like to emphasize at this stage that the majority of SCD sufferers cope extremely well and consequently do not manifest psychological difficulties. Indeed, as Barbarin (1994) has argued, it is remarkable how psychologically unscathed many children with SCD are when we consider the degree of poverty, physical handicap and family instability that they have to face. For this reason, Barbarin believes that children with SCD are resilient.

In considering the adjustment of the adult population, most people with SCD are in a relatively healthy psychological state and research suggests that, although psychosocial factors influence the frequency of painful crises, it is only a small percentage of the total sickle cell population that accounts for the majority of hospitalizations. For example, over a period of 6 years, Williams et al. (1983) conducted a survey of 300 patients, and found that only 5% had ten or more admissions, 30% had 3–9 admissions, 36% up to two and 29% had none.

Research carried out by Gil et al. (1992) has also demonstrated that significant numbers of adult sickle cell sufferers work, are active socially and recreationally, and are psychologically well adjusted. There are, however, many sufferers for whom the reverse is also true and, while disease severity can explain some of the variability, the bulk of the research evidence strongly suggests that psychological factors are more crucial in determining adjustment (Vinchinsky, 1982; Gil et al., 1989, 1992; Hurtig et al., 1989; Midence et al., 1993). The evidence suggests that patients who cope poorly, lead limited lives and are poorly adjusted psychologically are also more likely to be heavily dependent on hospital services for pain management.

## ■ PSYCHOLOGICAL CONSIDERATION OF SICKLE CELL DISEASE

In keeping with other chronic disorders, adverse psychological reactions and consequences in SCD occur as a result of the interpretation of individuals and families affected by the disease (Williams et al., 1983). The individual's reactions to chronic illness are dependent on a number of variables, but family and parental reactions are major determinants of psychological adjustment (Whitten and Fischoff, 1974).

It is not uncommon for parents to feel guilty about having passed on the disease to the child and consequently they may compensate by being overprotective or by overindulging the child. For example, Williams et al. (1983) has found that American mothers may overfeed their baby with SCD in an attempt to correct the anaemia or, in their desperation, they may use home remedies that friends or relatives have prepared, in an attempt to improve their child's symptoms. Alternatively, they may constantly seek the advice of health care professionals and become dependent on a few select members of this group in an attempt to relieve their anxieties.

Since SCD is an inherited disorder, psychosocial adjustment begins in infancy and therefore explanations of psychological concerns are best understood within a developmental perspective. In infancy, painful episodes interrupt the child's development by interfering with parent–infant bonding. Hospitalization can engender feelings of abandonment and helplessness in the child, which are further compounded by the unpleasant and painful procedures inherent in medical care (Whitten and Fischoff, 1974). The child with SCD is likely to experience constant fear of the unknown, particularly when no effort is made to reassure the child.

Peer acceptance is an important issue for the school age child but frequent absence from school owing to sickle-related illness interrupts peer relationships. In addition, the inability to participate in strenuous activity further reduces the opportunities for peer acceptance and can cause isolation. Research carried out by Williams et al. (1983) identified a number of anxiety-provoking events which influenced the onset of crisis in children. For example, anxiety about a teacher's reaction, illness of the mother and being disappointed by the father were identified as factors precipitating the onset of a crisis. In general, it appears that an increase in physical symptoms can be anticipated when the patient is undergoing life-event changes. The child who has been brought up in a family environment where understanding and support have been provided constantly throughout the illness will develop a good self-concept and adaptive coping skills.

Adolescence is characteristically known to be a period that requires significant adaptation (Coleman and Hendry, 1990) and, as such, it is not surprising that its onset heralds a particularly difficult time for significant numbers of SCD sufferers (Hurtig and White, 1986a, 1986b). According to Erickson (1963), the adolescent's chief developmental task is identity formation and peer relationships are crucial to this activity.

An adolescent with SCD may have delayed onset of puberty and physical growth, which can cause him/her to appear much younger and therefore unacceptable by his/her non-affected peers. Yellow eyes caused by jaundice, physical disability and dental deformities are some of the side-effects of the disease that cause embarrassment and problems with self-esteem.

The adolescent with SCD may develop reactive depression or alternatively she/he may not want to be limited by the disease and deliberately participate in stressful activities in an attempt to prove to her/his peers that she/he is 'normal'. Therefore he/she may exacerbate the illness for short periods of time (Whitten and Fischoff, 1974). Social isolation, absenteeism and reduced peer group activity were identified by Vichinsky et al. (1982) as social indicators of poorly compensated adolescent patients and these problems seem to be particularly related to hospitalization. Psychological morbidity was evident in the increased incidence of depression, anxiety and neurosis.

The extent to which the adult with SCD adjusts is dependent on positive adaptation in childhood and adolescence. Therefore, an adult who has not resolved the major issues during childhood and adolescence will have many of the same concerns of a maladjusted adolescent (Whitten and Fischoff, 1974; Williams et al., 1983; Hurtig and White, 1986a, 1986b). Thoughts of marriage and career aspirations, and the ability to maintain lasting intimate relationships may preoccupy the young adult. For some, this period marks the return of painful symptoms after a relative 'honeymoon period' (Holbrook and Phillips, 1994) and, therefore, requires a degree of readjustment.

This is a period in which a number of end-organ problems becomes manifest. These include: recurring episodes of acute chest syndrome, necrosis of the end of long bones and recurring episodes of renal symptoms. Mortality from end-organ failure becomes a real possibility (Serjeant, 1992; Holbrook and Phillips, 1994) and, as a consequence, the young adult perceives a constant threat, which is intensified with each crisis that requires hospitalization (Thomas et al., 1994). This and the occurrence of death among friends of the same age and among other siblings with SCD renders some young adult SCD patients acutely aware of a shortened life span (Holbrook and Phillips, 1994).

Regarding psychosocial problems, Nadel and Portadin (1977) found a positive relationship between depression and the frequency of painful crises. Gil et al. (1989) found that negative thinking such as catastrophizing and passive adherence to medical treatment were related to frequency and severity of painful crises. For a more detailed account of the relevant developmental issues, the reader is referred to Whitten and Fischoff (1974), Williams et al. (1983) and Thomas et al. (1994).

During the past decade, the research with diverse pain populations has convincingly shown that the assessment of psychological, social and behavioural factors adds enormously to our understanding of pain problem and patient adjustment (Gil, 1989). If nurses and other health care professionals can fully recognize that psychosocial factors are important determinants of overall psychological adjustment to SCD, then this knowledge should facilitate a more holistic approach to management strategies.

## ■ THE IMPORTANCE OF PATIENT-CONTROLLED ANALGESIA IN THE MANAGEMENT OF SICKLE CELL PAIN

As we saw in Chapter 2, loss or lack of control is aversive and related to poor outcome. Sickle cell patients frequently experience feelings of helplessness and depression, which in turn exacerbates pain (Pallister, 1992). It has been demonstrated within the context of acute surgical pain that increasing the patients' sense of control is beneficial in bringing about a decrease in the pain experience (Thomas et al., 1995). Therefore, methods such as PCA that increase personal control are very important.

There are several reasons for believing that the use of PCA in the treatment of sickle cell pain might prove valuable. Firstly, although it has been demonstrated that PCA provides safe effective postoperative pain control in all age groups, including children as young as 7 years old, to date only limited information is available concerning the use of PCA in the management of sickle cell crisis pain despite its significant theoretical advantage (Schecter et al., 1988; Holbrook, 1990). Secondly, PCA allows self-administration of analgesics removing dependence on hospital staff and therefore reducing the potential for conflict. This is vital since this group of patients consider their pain to be consistently underestimated by carers (Franklin, 1990; Alleyne and Thomas, 1994).

A third aspect in which sickle cell treatment may benefit from PCA concerns the extent to which the patient is in control of his or her situation. As with all chronic illness, loss of control resulting in helplessness is a major feature of sickle cell disease (Weisman and Schecter, 1992). Enabling the sickle patient to become an active participant in the control of his or her pain would go some way towards reducing the helplessness and therefore improve the quality of care. Another way in which PCA will be of value to the sickle cell sufferer is that it offers instant treatment of pain compared to an average of 30 minutes to provide analgesia via the intramuscular method, therefore it significantly reduces the amount of time that the individual is in pain.

In terms of a fifth measure, PCA may also be more beneficial for the sickle cell patient than a conventional intramuscular analgesic regimen. For example, a number of studies (Clark et al., 1989; Thomas, 1991; Thomas et al., 1995) have shown that surgical patients treated with PCA are discharged on average 2 days earlier than those treated with intramuscular injections. This suggests that as well as achieving effective pain relief, PCA provides an increased sense of control, which promotes a sense of well-being and speeds recovery. Since repeated hospitalizations lead to disruption of education and career prospects, reduced self-esteem and poorer social adjustment (Hurtig and White, 1986a, 1986b), any facility that is likely to return the young sickle cell patient back to the community is a positive asset that should be utilized. In addition, research has shown that SCD patients would like to become more involved in their pain management (Waters and Thomas, 1995). PCA affords this involvement.

## ■ MULTIDIMENSIONAL APPROACHES TO THE MANAGEMENT OF SICKLE CELL DISEASE-RELATED PAIN

It is now well established that the treatment of pain can be enhanced by approaches that incorporate psychological, social and behavioural components (Keefe et al., 1986). However, the management of sickle cell pain in many British hospitals focuses exclusively on the physical aspects of pain, ignoring the psychological and sociocultural dimensions.

Evidence from the USA suggests that the use of psychological techniques to complement medical treatment already provided will be of long-term benefit. Thomas et al. (1984) found that a variety of self-management skills involving progressive relaxation, thermal biofeedback, self-hypnosis and cognitive strategies brought about a 50% reduction in casualty visits, hospital admissions and analgesic intake.

Vichinsky et al. (1982) demonstrated the benefits of a multidisciplinary approach in managing the pain associated with SCD. By providing adequate analgesic therapy and extensive counselling they were able to reduce morbidity and hospitalization. Most striking was a 58% decrease in casualty visits, and a 44% decrease in admissions.

In the UK, a pilot study which utilizes cognitive therapy (CT) to pain management was carried out between November 1994 and April 1995 by the present author and colleagues (Thomas, Wilson-Barnett, Goodhart and Pelle). The main objective of a CT programme is to reduce helplessness and enhance personal control by motivating individuals to assume more responsibility and involvement towards their condition. The purpose of this pilot study was to determine the feasibility of implementing a community-based pain management on the well-being of adolescents and young adults with SCD living in London. This intervention, therefore, represents a departure from the usual approach by seeking to provide pain management strategies for SCD pain that also takes account of the psychological and social consequences of this condition.

The study involved 30 patients with sickle cell disease (SS genotype) whose age ranged from 15 to 35 years of age. Patients were randomly allocated to one of the following groups.

## ■ Group 1: Cognitive therapy for the management of chronic pain

This involved weekly one-hour sessions, for 6 months, with a qualified cognitive therapist who taught the following: cognitive therapy, relaxation training and health education information.

## ■ Group 2: The placebo-attention group

This is included because it is possible that being with the cognitive therapist may alone result in improvement. This group also had weekly one-hour 'non-directive' sessions for 6 months with the same qualified therapist. These sessions were patient-led and patients allocated to this group used the sessions for discussing the types of problems they encountered in hospital and to explore the feelings associated with these problems.

The CT and attention-placebo sessions were held in a community hall.

## ■ Group 3: Waiting list control

Patients in this group received conventional medical treatment only.

The following were used in all patients after randomization, before the intervention and at 6 months' follow-up in all groups:

- General Health Questionnaire 30 (GHQ 30) (Goldberg and Williams, 1988) – to assess anxiety and depression.
- State-trait Anxiety Scale (Spielberger, 1983) – to assess state anxiety and trait.
- Coping Strategies Questionnaire (Rosenthial and Keefe, 1989) – to assess coping strategies.
- Pain Self-efficacy Questionnaire (Nicholas, 1988) – to assess patients' perception of their ability to cope with pain.

### ▪ Results

Preliminary analyses failed to reveal any significant difference between the groups on any of the psychological outcome measures. This is not surprising since we were dealing with small numbers of patients. However, as a feasibility initiative, this study has provided some useful insights concerning patient compliance, attrition rates and the appropriateness of the psychological measures. Levels of psychological morbidity were high enough to warrant psychological intervention. For example, the average GHQ score was 11, much higher than the recommended 3–4 cut-off threshold for psychiatric disorder. Even allowing for inflation by somatic symptoms, this score is high. The mean state anxiety score was 50, well above the age-related norms of 36.5 (Spielberger, 1983).

Positive correlations were achieved between GHQ ($r = 0.44$; $p < 0.001$), state anxiety ($r = 0.47$; $p < 0.0001$), trait anxiety ($r = 0.55$; $p < 0.0001$) and pain experience. These correlations imply that high psychological distress scores were related to severe pain. Since it is well established that anxiety (Thomas et al., 1995) and depression (Tyrer et al., 1989) can intensify pain, it is not at all surprising that the physical approach employed for managing sickle cell crisis pain in British hospitals has been largely inadequate.

There were no significant differences found between the groups in terms of pre- and post-intervention outcome measures, but there was a most encouraging observation of a trend in the reduction of psychological distress (average GHQ scores = 7), and an increase in pain self-efficacy scores (scores improved from 22 to 32) after CT intervention.

Preliminary analyses of the effects on admission rates have revealed no significant differences in hospital admission rates, but there was a significant difference between the groups in terms of post-intervention duration of hospital stay. The mean pre-intervention duration of stay for the entire population was 10 days within the intervention groups. This was reduced to 6 days for the CT, 8 days for the attention and 11 days for the waiting list groups at post-intervention times. Analysis of variance revealed a significant difference ($F = 5.29$, df 2; $p <0.001$) and a *post hoc* Scheffe test revealed that the longest duration occurred within the waiting list control. Because of the small numbers of patients in each group it is not possible to make any definitive claims. However, as a feasibility initiative, this study has provided some useful insights.

In addition, patients were generally very positive about this approach and claim that they are using the strategies they have learnt to manage the pain and its associated stress on a regular basis. Many commented that they really valued having someone to 'really listen' to them and some felt that it was the first time that health care professionals had shown any interest. This pilot study has laid the foundation for a larger study which began in April 1996.

# ■ CONCLUSIONS AND RECOMMENDATIONS

Patients with SCD have severe, recurrent and unpredictable pain which is exacerbated by psychosocial problems. Pain management is rendered extremely problematic by the negative attitudes and poor understanding of staff as well as the maladaptive coping behaviour of some of the patients. Some of the research evidence presented highlights some examples of very poor practice and it is my belief that this inferior care arises because nurses (and doctors) lack awareness of the psychological challenges with which patients have to contend. The physical toll that is exacted by this disease also goes largely unnoticed. Education on the physical and psychosocial aspects of SCD is therefore crucial.

The use of a formal, documented pain assessment is important to the provision of effective pain control and the evaluation of pain medications. Assessment should also involve the identification and encouragement of continued use of pre-existing positive coping strategies (Gil et al., 1989). Although some research has been undertaken to assess the coping strategies of SCD patients in the USA (Gil et al., 1989, 1992; Thompson et al., 1992) very little research of this nature has been conducted in the UK. The evidence suggests that the systematic assessment of coping strategies in pain patients can be reliably assessed and is predictive of pain and adjustment (Gross-Rosenthiel, 1986; Gil et al., 1992). Chapter 10 also provides useful strategies for assessing and managing pain.

In the UK, Anionwu (1977) has argued for a considerable time that it is important to harness the wide-ranging resources that SCD patients possess. Research in this area is, therefore, needed as a necessary first step in order to provide effective multidisciplinary pain management interventions for this population.

The use of pain behaviour contracts is another solution, and reports from the USA have demonstrated that this a particularly effective way of managing the adolescent in a painful crisis (Burghardt-Fitzgerald, 1989). This is a very useful strategy which fosters the development of confidence and personal control in the adolescent. The development of the pain behaviour contract should occur in partnership with the patient if it is to be successful. Contracts include a variety of levels which differ according to dosage, frequency of medication and the degree of independent activity. The type of activities involved in the contract include out of bed activity, activities of daily living, deep breathing exercises and the use of relaxation. After 24 hours on any given analgesic dosage and activity regimen, readiness to progress to the next level is assessed and, if the adolescent is not ready to progress to the next level, the current level should remain.

In the UK, pain behaviour contracts for individual patients have been introduced by a few haematologists with some success. Trust is a crucial component to this and all pain management initiatives. However, as Waters and Thomas (1995) have argued, in order for trust to develop between nurses and these patients, the patients need to feel that their pain is consistently recognized and believed. The involvement of a clinical or health psychologist is essential if the multidimensional nature of pain is to be fully addressed (Thomas et al., 1994; Kesse, 1995).

## ■ ACKNOWLEDGEMENT

I would like to thank Eric Kesse and Sandra Beech who helped in putting together some of the material for this chapter.

## ■ REFERENCES

**Alleyne, J. & Thomas, V.J.** (1994) The management of sickle cell crisis as experienced by patients and their carers. *Journal of Advanced Nursing* **19**, 725–732.
**Anionwu, E.** (1977) Self-help in sickle cell anaemia. *World Medicine* **12**, 89–91.
**Anionwu, E.** (1992) Sickle cell disorders and the school child. *Health Visitor* **65**, 120–122.
**Ballas, S.K.** (1990) Treatment of pain in adults with sickle cell disease. *American Journal of Haematology* **34**, 49–54.
**Barbarin, O.A.** (1994) Risk resilience in adjustment to sickle cell disease: integrating focus groups, case reviews and quantitative methods. In: Nash, K.B. (ed.) *Psychosocial Aspects of Sickle Cell Disease*. The Haworth Press, New York, pp. 97–121.
**Brozovic, M. & Davies, S.C.** (1987) Management of sickle cell disease. *Post Graduate Medical Journal* **63**, 605–609.
**Brozovic, M., Davies, S.C., Yardumian, A., Bellingham, A., Marsh, G. & Stephens, A.D.** (1986) Pain relief in sickle cell crises. *Lancet* (September 13th) 624–625.
**Brozovic, M., Davies, S.C. & Brownell, A.I.** (1987) Acute admissions of patients with sickle cell disease who live in Britain. *British Medical Journal* **294**, 1206–1208.
**Burghardt-Fitzgerald D.C.** (1989) Pain-behaviour contracts: effective management of the adolescent in sickle cell crisis. *Paediatric Nursing* **4**, 320–324.
**Clark, E., Hodsman, N. & Kenny, G.** (1989) Improved post-operative recovery with patient controlled analgesia. *Nursing Times* **85** (9), 54–55.
**Coleman, J.C. & Hendry, L.** (1990) *The Nature of Adolescence*. Routledge, London.
**Davies, S.C. & Brozovic, M.** (1989) The presentation, management and prophylaxis of sickle cell disease. *Blood Reviews* **3**, 30–44.
**Erickson, C.** (1991) Hypno-analgesia in sickle cell anaemia. *Paediatric Research* E **29** (9a), Abstract.
**Erikson, E.H.** (1963) *Childhood and Society*, 2nd edn. Free Press, New York.
**France-Dawson, M.** (1990) Sickle cell conditions and health knowledge. *Nursing Standard* **4**, 30–34.
**Franklin, I.** (1990) *Sickle Cell Disease: A Guide for Patients, Carers and Health Workers*. Faber and Faber, London.

**Gil, K.M.** (1989) Coping with sickle cell disease pain. *Annals of Behavioural Medicine* **11**, 48–57.

**Gil, K.M., Abrams, M., Phillips, G. & Keefe, F.** (1989) Sickle cell disease pain: relations of coping strategies to adjustment. *Journal of Consulting and Clinical Psychology* **57**, 725–731.

**Gil, K.M., Abrams, M., Phillips, G. & Williams, D.A.** (1992) Sickle cell disease pain: 2. Predicting health care use and activity level at 9 months follow-up. *Journal of Consulting and Clinical Psychology* **60**, 267–273.

**Goldberg, D. & Williams, P.** (1988) *Users' Guide to the General Health Questionnaire.* NFER Nelson, Basingstoke Press, Basingstoke, Hampshire.

**Gross-Rosenthiel, A.** (1986) The effects of coping strategies on the relief of pain following surgical interventions for lower back pain. *Psychosomatic Medicine* **48**, 229–241.

**Holbrook, T.** (1990) Patient controlled analgesia pain management for children with sickle cell disease. *Journal of the Association for Academic Minority Physicians* **1**, 93–96.

**Holbrook, C.T. & Phillips, G.** (1994) The natural history of sickle cell disease and the effects on biopsychosocial development. In: Nash, K.B. (ed.) *Psychosocial Aspects of Sickle Cell Disease.* The Haworth Press, New York, pp. 7–18.

**Hurtig, A.L. & White, L.S.** (1986a) Children and adolescents: the unexpected terrain of emotion and development. In: Hurtig, A. & Viera, T. (eds) *Sickle Cell Disease: Psychological and Psychosocial Issues.* University of Illinois Press, Chicago, pp. 24–39.

**Hurtig, A.L. & White, L.S.** (1986b) Psychosocial adjustment in children and adolescents with sickle cell disease. *Journal of Paediatric Psychology* **11**, 411–427.

**Hurtig, A.L., Koepke, D. & Park, K.B.** (1989) Relation between severity of chronic illness and adjustment in children and adolescents with sickle cell disease. *Journal of Paediatric Psychology* **14**, 117–132.

**Ingrisano, C.** (1986) Planning patient care for the adolescent. In: Hurtig, A.L. (ed.) *Sickle Cell Disease: Psychological and Psychosocial Issues.* University of Illinois Press, Chicago, pp. 84–149.

**Keefe, F.J., Gil, K.M. & Rose, S.C.** (1986) Behavioural approaches in multidisciplinary management of chronic pain: programs and issues. *Clinical Psychology Review* **6**, 87–113.

**Kesse, E.** (1995) Psychology meets haematology: a role for psychologists in the management of sickle cell disease. *Clinical Psychology Forum* **83**, 29–32.

**Konotey-Ahulu, F.I.D.** (1991) *The Sickle Cell Disease Patient: Natural History from a Clinico-epidemiological Study of the first 1550 Patients of Korle Bu Hospital Sickle Cell Clinic.* Macmillan, London.

**Midence, K. & Elander, J.** (1994) *Sickle Cell Disease: A Psychosocial Approach.* Radcliffe Medical Press, Oxford.

**Midence, K., Fuggle, P. & Davies, S.C.** (1993) Psychosocial aspects of sickle cell disease in childhood and adolescence. *British Journal of Clinical Psychology* **32**, 271–280.

**Modell, B. & Anionwu, E.** (1996) Guidelines for screening haemaglobin disorders: service specifications for low and high prevalance. In: *Ethnicity and Health: Reviews of Literature and Guidance for Purchasers in the Areas of Cardiovascular Disease, Mental Health and Haemoglobinopathies, CRD Report 5.* University of York, NHS Centre, York.

**Murrey, N. & May, A.** (1988) Painful crisis in sickle cell disease: patients' perspective. *British Medical Journal* **297**, 452–454.

**Nadel, C. & Portadin, G.** (1977) Sickle cell crises: psychological factors associated with onset. *New York Journal of Medicine* **77**, 1075–1078.

**National Association of Health Authorities** (1991) Haemaglobinopathies: review of services for black and minority ethnic people. *Words about Action Bulletin* no. 4, January.

**Nicholas M.K.** (1988) Paper presented at the British Psychological Society Conference, St Andrews University.

**Pallister, C.J.** (1992) A crisis that can be overcome: management of sickle cell disease. *Professional Nurse* 509–513.

**Payne, R.** (1989) Pain management in sickle cell disease: rationale and techniques. *Annals of the New York Academy of Sciences* **565**, 189–206.

**Platt, O.S., Brambilla, D.J., Rosse, W.F., Milner, P.F., Castro, O., Steinberg, M.H. & Klug, P.P.** (1994) Mortality in sickle cell disease: life expectancy and risk factors for early death. *New England Journal of Medicine* **330**, 1639–1644.

**Prashar, U., Anionwu, E. & Brozovic, M.** (1985) *Sickle Cell Anaemia – Who Cares?* Runnymede Trust, London.

**Rosenthiel, A.K. & Keefe, F.J.** (1983) The use of coping strategies in chronic low back pain patients: relationship to patient characteristics and current adjustment. *Pain* 1733–1744.

**Schecter, N.L., Berrin, F.B. & Katz, S.M.** (1988) The use of patient controlled analgesia in adolescents with sickle cell pain crisis. *Journal of Pain and Symptom Management* **3**, 1–5.

**Serjeant, G.R.** (1992) *Sickle Cell Disease*, 2nd edn. Oxford Medical Publications, Oxford.

**Serjeant, G.R., Ceulaer, C.D., Lethbridge, R., Morris, J., Singhal, A. & Thomas, P.** (1994) Painful crises in sickle cell disease. *British Journal of Haematology* **87**, 586–591.

**Shapiro, B.S.** (1989) The management of pain in SCD. *Paediatric Clinics of North America* **36**, 1029–1043.

**Shapiro, B.S.** (1991) Sickle cell disease related pain. *International Association for the Study of Pain Newsletter* January/February, 2–4.

**Somerville, M.A.** (1993) Death of pain. In: Gebhart, G.F., Hammond, D.L. & Jensen, T.S. (eds) *Proceedings of the 7th World Congress on Pain: Progress in Pain, Research & Management*, Vol. 2. IASP Publications, Seattle, pp.41–58.

**Spielberger, C.D.** (1983) *Manual for the State-Trait Anxiety Inventory: STAI (Form Y) Self Evaluation Questionnaire.* Consulting Psychologists Press, Palo Alto, CA.

**Standing Medical Advisory Committee on Sickle Cell, Thalassaemia and Other Haemoglobinopathies** (1994) Report. Department of Health. HMSO London.

**Streetly, A., Maxwell, K. & Mejia, A.** (1997) *The Fair Shares for London Report; Sickle Cell Disorders in Greater London: A Needs Assessment of Screening and Care Services*. Marks and Spencer Publications, London.

**Thomas, J.E., Koshy, M., Peterson, L., Dorn, L. & Thomas, K.** (1984) Management of pain in SCD using biofeedback therapy: preliminary study. *Biofeedback and Self-regulation* **9**, 413–420.

**Thomas, V.J.** (1991) Personality Characteristics and the Effectiveness of Patient Controlled Analgesia. Unpublished PhD dissertation, Goldsmiths' College, London University.

**Thomas, V.** (1996) A community-based cognitive behavioural pain management programme for patients with sickle cell disease: A pilot study. Abstracts of the Llandudno meeting. *Journal of the Pain Society* **12**, 63.

**Thomas, V., Kesse, E. & Pelle, J.** (1994) Sickle cell disease and psychosocial problems: are health psychologists playing their part? *Health Psychology Update* **18**, 17–22.

**Thomas, V.J., Heath, M.L., Rose, F.O. & Flory, P.** (1995) Psychological characteristics and the effectiveness of patient controlled analgesia. *British Journal of Analgesia* **74**, 271–276.

**Thompson, R.J., Jr, Gil, K.M., Abrams, M.R. & Philips, G.** (1992) Stress, coping and psychological adjustment of adults with sickle cell disease. *Journal of Consulting and Clinical Psychology* **60**, 433–440.

**Tyrer, S.P., Capon, M., Peterson, D.M. et al** (1989) The detection of psychiatric illness and psychological handicaps in British pain clinic population. *Pain* **36**, 63–74.

**Varni, J.W. & Walco, G.A.** (1988) Chronic and recurrent pain associated with paediatric diseases. *Issues in Comprehensive Paediatric Nursing* **11**, 145–158.

**Vichinsky, E.P., Johnson, R. & Lubin, B.H.** (1982) Multi-disciplinary approach to pain management in sickle cell disease. *American Journal of Paediatric Haematology/Oncology* **4**, 328–332.

**Waters, J.** (1992) The Nurse's Role in the Management of Sickle Cell Crisis Pain. BSc undergraduate dissertation, King's College, University of London.

**Waters, J. & Thomas, V.J.** (1995) Pain from sickle cell crisis. *Nursing Times* **91**(16), 29–31.

**Weisman, S.J. & Schecter, N.L.** (1992) Acute pain: mechanisms and management. In: Hord, A.H., Ginsberg, B. & Preble, L.M. (eds) *Sickle Cell Anaemia Pain Management*. Mosby Year Book, St Louis.

**Whitten, C.F. & Fischoff, J.** (1974) Psychological effects of sickle cell disease. *Archives of Internal Medicine* **133**, 681–689.

**Williams, I., Earles, A.N. & Pack, B.** (1983) Psychological considerations in sickle cell disease. *Nursing Clinics of North America* **18**, 215–229.

**World Health Organisation Advisory Group on Hereditary Diseases** (1985) *Community Approaches to the Control of Hereditary Diseases*. Unpublished WHO document HMG/WG/85.10. (Obtainable free from the Hereditary Disease Programme, WHO, Geneva, Switzerland.)

**Yardumian, A.** (1993) Setting the scene on sickle cell care. Paper presented at the *London Sickle Cell Conference*, October.

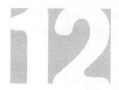

# Cancer pain and its management

## ■ INTRODUCTION AND BACKGROUND

There is a powerful association between pain and cancer in the mind of the public, which tends to be regarded as an inevitable fearful aspect of the disease. This unfortunate perception usually stems from an experience of having known, or heard about, someone who has suffered excruciating pain in the course of terminal cancer. In truth, there is no need for most patients to suffer from pain. If properly applied, the current state of knowledge of the causes of pain and methods of controlling it allow successful palliation in 95–99% of the patients with pain related to cancer (Bonica, 1979). Adequate and appropriate pain management are important nursing responsibilities, especially when caring for the person with cancer pain (Spross et al., 1990).

Cancer-related pain is a multidimensional experience consisting of the following components (Ahles et al., 1983; McGuire, 1987):

- Physiological (organic causes of pain)
- Sensory (intensity, location, quality)
- Affective (depression, anxiety)
- Cognitive (manner in which pain influences a person's thought processes, how he or she views the meaning of pain)
- Behavioural (pain-related behaviours)
- Sociocultural components (demographic, social and cultural factors that are related to the experience of pain).

The multidimensional conceptualization of pain requires an approach to assessment and management that involves multiple health care disciplines. Whether these dimensions are treated singly or together, they all contribute to the overall pain experience and all require input from different health care providers. Nurses, pharmacists, physiotherapists, psychologists, occupational and social workers and the medical specialities of oncology, radiotherapy, anaesthetics, orthopaedics, neurosurgery and psychiatry are among the specific groups of professionals that have a role in the assessment and management of cancer pain. However, of all these specialists, nurses are the only group who have 24-hour contact with the patient. Their role in alleviating distress associated with pain is, therefore, paramount.

## ■ SCOPE OF THE CANCER PAIN PROBLEM

### ▪ The prevalence of pain in cancer patients

There is evidence that pain may be a problem for this group of patients. Although cancer is not usually painful at the onset or in the early stages, many patients with recurrent or metastatic disease eventually experience it. An analysis of 32 published reviews revealed that 70% of patients with progressive malignant disease had pain as a major symptom (Bonica, 1985). A series of studies using verbal reports and rating scales indicated that pain is moderate to severe in about 50% of patients with cancer, and very severe or excruciating in 30% (Daut and Cleeland, 1982). The prevalence of pain tends to increase as the disease progresses and frequently is of multiple aetiology. Certain malignancies are more often associated with cancer pain, particularly lung cancer, pancreatic cancer and primary bone cancer (Daut and Cleeland, 1982; Greenwald et al., 1987).

### ▪ Professional issues

The treatment of cancer pain is one of the most urgent issues facing health care professionals today. A number of issues have been identified which contribute to its inadequate management and some of these factors have been discussed already in Chapter 10. These can be viewed as obstacles to successful management (see Table 12.1). Some of the major reasons suggested for our failure to treat cancer pain adequately are a lack of knowledge of the mechanisms involved, a lack of teaching and insufficient application of current knowledge. McCaffery et al. (1990) have conducted three recent studies on nursing knowledge of pain. For example, a survey of 2459 nurses in the USA revealed serious deficiencies in nurses' knowledge of opioid analgesia. However, surveys have shown that nurses acknowledge educational deficiencies in relation to pain control. In a questionnaire

## *Table 12.1* *Obstacles to successful pain management*

Lack of understanding about pain

Expectation that pain should be present

Relief of pain not viewed as a goal of treatment

Inadequate or non-existent assessment

Undertreatment with analgesics

Inadequate knowledge of analgesics and other drugs

Fears of addiction, sedation and respiratory depression

Inadequate knowledge of other interventions for pain

Source: Groenwald, S., Hansen Frogge, M., Goodman, M. & Yarbro C. (eds) *Cancer Nursing Principles and Practice*, 2nd edn, p. 399. © 1992 Boston: Jones and Bartlett Publishers. Reprinted by permission.

## *Table 12.2* *Summary of a research study describing nurses' knowledge and assessment skills in the area of pain control in cancer patients (Paice et al., 1991)*

**Factors associated with adequate pain control in hospitalized post-surgical patients diagnosed with cancer**

**Aim**

To examine the pain experience of surgical oncology patients, explore the relationship between the patient's assessment of the pain, and the nurse's and doctor's assessments, and describe the pain assessment and documentation practices.

**Design**

Correlational *ex post facto* design.

**Instruments**

Structured interview collecting data from patients regarding pain experience (including intensity, location and effect of pain on functioning), pain treatment and demographic information. Nurses and doctors caring for each patient completed brief assessments of their perceptions of the patient's pain intensity.

**Sample**

A random sample of 34 cancer patients who had undergone a general surgical procedure 1–31 days previously.

**Results**

70.6% of the patients stated at the time of the interview that they were in pain, however, only 8.8% were in severe pain. 91.2% stated they had been in pain during the 24 hours prior to the interview. Approximately 40% of the patients stated that a nurse had never asked them about their pain. More than a quarter of the patients' charts did not have pain addressed in the initial postoperative nursing documentation, and less than 20% of the charts listed pain on the problem list. A review of prescription charts revealed that the amount of opioid analgesia prescribed by doctors was a larger average dose, unfortunately the amount given by the nurses was constant in comparison to results in other studies.

**Implications**

A lack of documentation leads to a lack of consistent care and an inability to evaluate the effectiveness of pain therapies. Initial assessment and ongoing documentation are vital. The education of health professionals, patients and families on the appropriate use of opioid analgesia is necessary.

study of 669 nurses from 23 countries, the majority of respondents believed that they had received little or no training in cancer pain management and an overwhelming majority thought that more emphasis should be given to management of cancer pain (Pritchard, 1988).

The persistence of myths about pain hinders progress in its management. As we have seen in the surgical setting, an unfounded concern about addiction is often expressed by nurses (McCaffery et al., 1990). They frequently overestimate the frequency with which psychological dependence on opioids occurs during pain control. For several years the World Health Organisation (WHO, 1986) has consistently reported that the likelihood of addiction occurring from the use of opioids for pain relief is very small – less than 1%.

A fundamental problem is that nurses have exhibited a deficiency in the assessment of pain (Dalton, 1989; Donovan and Dillon, 1987; Rankin and Snider, 1984). A lack of basic assessment skills, failure to acknowledge and document the existence of pain, and inaccurate documentation when the problem is known to exist prohibit patients from receiving the benefit of reasonable pain control. Evidence for the fact that nurses commonly underestimate pain and then inadequately medicate patients is demonstrated in a study by Paice et al. (1991) and summarized in Table 12.2.

## ■ MECHANISMS OF CANCER-RELATED PAIN

Pain experienced by cancer patients is, when considered strictly in terms of the underlying pathophysiological and biochemical processes, no different from the pain experienced by other people. Aetiological, clinical and psychological characteristics of both tumour- and treatment-related cancer pain, however, distinguish it from other types of pain. The basic mechanisms of pain have been considered in Chapter 1.

Malignancies can cause pain in a variety of ways. A comprehensive discussion is beyond the realms of this introductory chapter and only a few examples will be discussed. A summary of the more common causes is given in Table 12.3.

Pain and discomfort in cancer may be related to the tumour or malignancy itself, to pressure exerted by the tumour, to diagnostic testing procedures or to many of the cancer treatments that may be used. Bone destruction as a result of tumour invasion is one of the most devastating sources of pain and may be caused by primary or metastatic tumour. Primary tumours of the breast, lung, prostate and kidney are frequent causes of bone metastases and bone pain which tends to be worse on movement and on weight bearing. The quality of bone pain can range from a dull ache to a deep, oppressive, intense pain. Infiltration or compression of nerves can cause pain that is described as 'sharp' and 'burning', and there may be

*Table 12.3* Causes of pain in 100 cancer patients

| | Number of pains | | |
| --- | --- | --- | --- |
| | **Male** | **Female** | **Total** |
| **Caused by cancer (67%)** | | | |
| Bone | 30 (16) | 28 (15) | 58 (31) |
| Nerve compression | 24 (16) | 32 (15) | 56 (31) |
| Soft tissue infiltration | 21 (19) | 14 (12) | 35 (31) |
| Visceral involvement | 15 (15) | 18 (16) | 33 (31) |
| Muscle spasm | 9 (7) | 5 (4) | 14 (11) |
| Lymphoedema | — | 4 (3) | 4 (3) |
| Raised intracranial pressure | — | 2 (2) | 2 (2) |
| Myopathy | — | 2 (1) | 2 (1) |
| | 99 (42) | 105 (49) | 204 (91) |
| **Related to treatment (5%)** | | | |
| Postoperative | 1 (1) | 7 (6) | 8 (7) |
| Colostomy | 1 (1) | 1 (1) | 2 (2) |
| Nerve block | — | 2 (1) | 2 (2) |
| Postoperative adhesions | 1 (1) | — | 1 (1) |
| Post-radiation fibrosis | — | 1 (1) | 1 (1) |
| Oesophageal | — | 1 (1) | 1 (1) |
| | 3 (3) | 12 (9) | 15 (12) |
| **Associated pains (6%)** | | | |
| Constipation | 6 (6) | 5 (5) | 11 (11) |
| Capsulitis of shoulder | 1 (1) | 3 (3) | 4 (4) |
| Bedsore | — | 1 (1) | 1 (1) |
| Post-herpetic neuralgia | — | 1 (1) | 1 (1) |
| Pulmonary embolus | 1 (1) | — | 1 (1) |
| Penile spasm (catheter) | 1 (1) | — | 1 (1) |
| | 9 (9) | 10 (10) | 19 (19) |
| **Unrelated pains (22%)** | | | |
| Musculoskeletal | 19 (10) | 24 (17) | 43 (27) |
| Osteoarthritis | 2 (1) | 2 (2) | 4 (3) |
| Migraine | 1 (1) | 1 (1) | 2 (2) |
| Miscellaneous | 6 (5) | 10 (8) | 16 (13) |
| | 28 (15) | 37 (24) | 65 (39) |
| Totals | 138 | 165 | 303 (100) |

Figures in parentheses indicate number of patients in this category, as distinct from number of pains.

Reprinted with permission by McGuire, D. and Yarbro, C. Original source: Coyle, N. & Foley, K. (1987) Prevalence and profile of pain syndromes in cancer patients. In: McGuire, D. & Yarbro, C. (eds) *Cancer Pain Management*, 2nd edn. W.B. Saunders, Philadelphia, p. 25.

progressive motor and/or sensory loss. Nerve destruction (deafferentation pain, pain caused by damage to a nerve or to the spinal cord) may produce hypersensitivity, parasthesiae and lancing and/or burning pain. Vertebral metastases involving spinal nerves may occur with breast and lung cancer. Tumours causing lymphatic or venous obstruction may lead to a dull, throbbing type of pain and are often associated with a lymphoma. Ischaemic pain results when any tumour occludes arterial circulation. Visceral pain results from the involvement of abdominal, pelvic and intrathoracic organs. Pain is often a continuous dull ache but may become sharper if an organ moves or the patient changes position. Obstruction of viscera may occur with colon cancer and patients with abdominal obstruction often complain of pain that is dull and poorly localized. Finally, tumours invading the skin or mucous membranes, which are a common occurrence in patients with progressive head and neck malignancies, may cause pain associated with inflammation, ulceration, infection and tissue necrosis.

### ▮ Cancer pain syndromes

Cancer pain has been categorized according to a series of common pain disorders and their pathological mechanisms (Foley, 1979). The first and most common cause of pain in cancer patients is that caused by direct tumour involvement, for example, metastatic bone disease, nerve compression, and hollow-viscus and retroperitoneal involvement. The second group of pain syndromes, which is those associated with cancer therapy, is less frequent. These occur in the course of, or as a result of, surgery, chemotherapy or radiotherapy. The sources of pain associated with these cancer treatments are wide-ranging – from initial diagnostic procedures responsible for acute short-term pain to standard treatment modalities (surgery, radiotherapy, chemotherapy) that cause acute short-term pain and/or chronic, long-term pain. Acute pain is linked with trauma that results from surgical procedures, such as mastectomy and amputation. Potential sources of pain which may occur with particular chemotherapy agents include jaw pain, tender toes and fingers which are associated with the administration of vincristine, and stomatitis which might result following administration of the drug methotrexate. Radiotherapy can cause inflammation of the skin or irradiated organs, and radiation fibrosis of the lumbar or brachial plexus. Finally, pain can also be associated with debility for example, constipation and pressure sores. Pain may, of course, be unrelated to the cancer, such as osteoarthritis or a migraine headache. Nurses therefore have an important responsibility to assess the pain carefully as the treatment is dependent on cause.

In addition to the above method of classification, three pain syndromes of somatic, visceral and deafferentation pain have been described in patients with cancer (Potenoy, 1987). These are characterized by pain of different

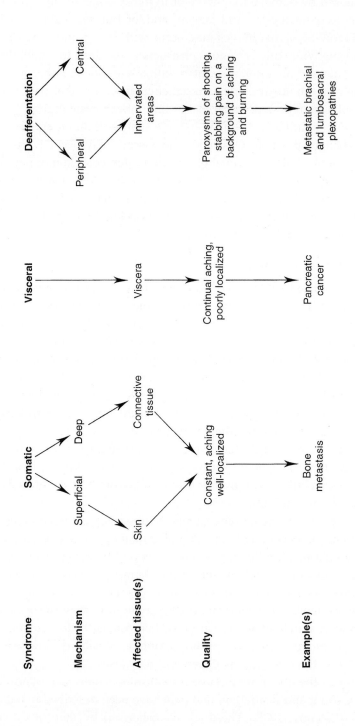

*Figure 12.1* Pain syndromes in cancer. *Reproduced with permission from McGuire and Sheidler (1992). Pain. In: Groenwald, S., Hansen Frogge, M., Goodman, M. & Yarbro, C. (eds) Cancer Nursing Principles and Practice, 2nd edn. Jones and Bartlett Publishers, Boston, p. 392.*

*Table 12.4* Multidimensional factors affecting pain threshold and pain sensitivity in individuals with cancer-related pain

| Lowered threshold/more sensitivity | | Elevated threshold/less sensitivity | |
|---|---|---|---|
| *Factor* | *Dimension* | *Factor* | *Dimension* |
| Insomnia/fatigue | Physiological | Sleep/rest | Physiological, sensory |
| Discomfort | Sensory | Relief of symptoms | |
| Anger | Affective | Reduction in anxiety/elevation of mood | Affective |
| Anxiety | | Diversional activities | Cognitive behavioural |
| Depression | | | |
| Fear | | | |
| Sadness | | | |
| Boredom | Cognitive behavioural | Medications (analgesics, anxiolytics, antidepressants) | Physiological, affective, behavioural |
| Mental isolation | | | |
| Social abandonment | Sociocultural | Companionship/ sympathy/ understanding | Sociocultural |

Reprinted with permission by McGuire, D. and Yarbro, C. Original source: McGuire, D. (1987) The multidimensional phenomenon of cancer pain. In: McGuire, D. & Yarbro, C. (eds) *Cancer Pain Management,* 2nd edn. W.B. Saunders, Philadelphia, p. 8.

qualities, located in different anatomic parts of the body, and caused by different mechanisms (see Fig. 12.1). It is important to note that many cancer patients with pain will have one or more of these three syndromes simultaneously, and that each response varies with different therapeutic approaches.

The discussion above relates to the physiological dimension of cancer pain. However, the multidimensional model of cancer-related pain (see Table 12.4) can inform our understanding of the multiple factors that may affect an individual's perception and interpretation of pain. Factors that decrease the pain threshold should be assessed: insomnia, fatigue, boredom, sadness, anger, anxiety, financial concerns, social isolation, and fear of death or of worsening pain. Tolerance is enhanced by adequate rest and sleep, diversion, mood elevation, empathy, antidepressants, antianxiety agents and analgesics. The nurse can use this information constructively by attempting to fulfil the needs which raise the pain threshold and by preventing the problems occurring which lower the pain threshold and therefore exert a significant impact on the pain experienced by a patient.

# ■ ASSESSMENT AND MANAGEMENT

Foley (1985) has outlined what she believes to be the initial principles upon which effective nursing assessment and management of cancer pain rests. These include complete assessment of the history of pain, use of appropriate diagnostic procedures to determine its nature, early treatment with analgesics and continual reassessment of the patient's response to prescribed therapy.

The multiple dimensions of cancer pain, whether treated singly or together, all contribute to the pain experience and all require input from different health professionals. The plan of treatment may include several cancer specialists from various health care disciplines, and the patient may be cared for by a number of different specialists. Care givers must plan for effective communication to promote continuity in pain management. Nurses by virtue of their sustained contact with patients and their families in a variety of settings are best prepared to assume a central role in the assessment and management of cancer pain. The focus of assessment and management activities of the nurse is concerned with the patient as a whole person, on the patient's and family's response to pain.

In current clinical practice, nurses assume a great deal of responsibility for helping to manage cancer pain as a symptom. A useful delineation of nursing responsibilities for cancer pain management has been framed within the Johnson Behavioural System Model for nursing practice by (Wilkie, 1990). This model suggests that nurses have two types of responsibilities when providing care. Primary responsibility lies in diagnosing and intervening with people who have actual or potential health problems, and a secondary responsibility exists to collaborate with physicians in the diagnosis and treatment of human illness. Associated with these responsibilities are independent and interdependent functions. Examples of the independent function include the evaluation of the responses of patients and their families to cancer, and pain and the evaluation of analgesic effect, side-effects and response to therapy. A related but interdependent function is the suggestion of alternative therapies where a prescription is required.

## ■ Assessment

Although pain assessment has been covered in Chapter 5, a discussion of the pain assessment tools that are particularly useful in cancer pain management will also be presented here. Assessment is the vital first step toward the satisfactory control of cancer pain (WHO, 1986). There are eight dimensions considered essential to thorough assessment related to the multi-dimensional conceptualization of cancer pain:

1. Location
2. Intensity
3. Factors influencing the occurrence of pain
4. Observed behaviours including vital signs
5. Psychosocial factors
6. Effects of pain
7. Effects of therapy
8. Established patterns of coping (Donovan, 1987).

A systematic assessment of the cancer patient's pain is essential in understanding his or her experience and devising a realistic plan for control. Owing to the multidimensional and individual nature of the pain experience, pain assessment could become a laborious process for the patient as well as the nurse. An ideal tool for nursing assessment would provide information about the eight dimensions described above to guide the selection of appropriate therapy.

Few of the tools currently available meet all of the criteria completely but each has a contribution to make to the process of assessment. Three pain questionnaires are sufficiently short to be considered for routine use with cancer patients. The London Hospital Pain Observation Chart (Raiman, 1986a, b) can be used to monitor and record physical and psychological aspects of pain over a period of time, and incorporates sites and intensities of pain and actions taken, such as nursing care related to analgesia administration and positioning. The Memorial Pain Assessment Card (MPAC) (Fishman et al., 1987), has been reported to be useful in the assessment of clinical pain in medically ill adults. The MPAC is a short, easy to administer, multidimensional tool, consisting of a pain adjective rating scale, a pain intensity visual analogue scale (VAS), a pain relief VAS and mood rating scale. As described in Chapter 5, the McGill Pain Questionnaire (MPQ) (Melzack, 1975) provides information about the sensory, affective and evaluative dimensions of pain. In addition to these parameters, the MPQ elicits information about: the location of pain; the intensity and periodicity of pain; the accompanying symptoms; the effects of sleep, activity, and eating; and the pattern of analgesic use. A short form has been developed by Melzack (1987). See also Chapter 5 for a fuller discussion. The Wisconsin Brief Pain Questionnaire (Daut et al., 1983), now called the Brief Pain Inventory (Cleeland, 1989), was developed primarily for clinical use with patients in pain who were too ill to be subjected to longer or more exhausting assessment techniques. It asks patients to represent the location of their pain on a drawing, and explores other issues concerning duration of pain relief and cause of pain, providing a list of descriptors to help the patient describe the pain quality.

It is useful to know that a number of tools are now available to help us assess our patients' pain, since this facilitates selecting interventions and evaluating therapeutic efficacy. Nurses need to instruct patients in the use of the selected scale for reporting pain, evaluate the patient's ability to understand and use the scale, implement the plan for pain control, and use the scale to monitor the effectiveness of the plan once implemented. The patients' own vocabulary that they choose to describe the pain should be identified and used in any ongoing assessment. A thorough discussion of tools to assess pain appears in Chapter 5, and in Donovan (1987) and Cleeland and Syrjala (1992) with specific relevance to cancer pain. These sources will help the nurse select the best tool for a given situation. The impact of a systematic nursing pain assessment tool and pain flow sheets on pain management has been studied by Evans Faries et al. (1991), and the results of this study support other research and recommendations in the literature that the use of systematic pain records can improve pain management. Any cancer patient with pain should have a baseline assessment conducted in addition to ongoing assessment for the evaluation and revision of treatment plans in order to ensure effective care.

### ■ Planning

During a series of studies to develop tests, and evaluate methods of observation and assessment of pain, Raiman (1986a) demonstrated that one of the main problems was low treatment aims, i.e. pain does not exist, pain does not matter, or pain is acceptable. In developing goals for pain relief, the nurse must involve the patient in order to develop realistic goals. Hanks (1983) advocates the setting of realistic goals and recommends that three stages of pain relief should be aimed at: pain-free at night, pain-free at rest, and pain-free on movement – in that order. However, freedom from pain on movement is difficult to achieve in nerve compression and bone pain.

### ■ Interventions

There are a wide variety of methods for managing cancer-related pain, some of which are presented in Table 12.5. These are by no means exhaustive.

Methods of managing pain can be categorized into three major approaches. Firstly, treatment may be aimed at the underlying pathology (the pathological or organic cause of the pain). Possible treatments include radiotherapy, chemotherapy, endocrine therapy, surgery and biological therapy. These are considered as primary control methods directed towards controlling the disease process itself. The second approach is used to change the individual's perception or sensation of pain (analgesics, anaesthetics and neurosurgical techniques). Finally, the third approach consists of a number of interventions aimed at diminishing the suffering component of pain. Each will be discussed in turn.

*Table 12.5* *Methods of managing cancer-related pain*

| | |
|---|---|
| Radiation | |
| Chemotherapy | |
| Hormonal therapy | } Treat underlying pathology |
| Surgery | |
| | |
| Pharmacological, i.e. non-opioid, opioid, adjuvant | |
| Neurosurgical procedures | |
| Anaesthetic procedures | } Change perception or sensation of pain |
| Acupuncture and acupressure | |
| Counterirritant and cutaneous stimulation | |
| | |
| Hypnosis | |
| Distraction | |
| Relaxation, imagery and meditation | } Reduce suffering from pain |
| Biofeedback | |

## Treatment of underlying pathology

Chemotherapy, radiotherapy and surgery are the main methods used to treat cancer when cure is the intent, but they are also useful when palliation is the goal. Hormonal therapy is a fourth treatment modality often used for the palliative treatment of particular tumours, e.g. breast and prostate tumours (Abrams and Hansen, 1989). Treatment of the cancer itself with these various forms of therapy, minimizes or eliminates the source of pain.

Radiotherapy has long been used to treat painful bone metastases, most often in cancers of the breast, lung and prostate (Ford and Yarnold, 1983). The mechanism by which irradiation achieves pain control is not clear. It is considered probable that local effects on tissue, in particular the release of pain-mediating humoral agents, and the direct effect of radiotherapy on the tumour cells are important in the achievement and maintenance of pain relief. In addition, it may be helpful in relieving pain owing to spinal cord or nerve root compression, brain metastases or primary brain tumour, and hepatic metastases.

Surgery as an approach for treating cancer pain can take a variety of forms. A number of clinical conditions and tumours may benefit from various types of surgery and relief of pain may be expected to occur as an outcome of such procedures, e.g. immobilization of a pathological fracture, simple mastectomy of a fungating breast cancer and formation of a colostomy to relieve intestinal obstruction (Azzarelli and Crispino, 1987).

## Changes in perception and sensation of pain

As can be seen from the list in Table 12.5, the number of interventions in this category is extensive. Pharmacological drug therapy is an essential component of this area of cancer pain relief and is a major responsibility of nurses. There is a wide range of publications addressing the issue of pharmacological management of cancer pain from which further information can be gleaned (e.g. Catalano, 1987; Foley, 1985; Gorman, 1991; Hanks, 1987; Lindley et al., 1990; Twycross and Lack, 1990).

### Pharmacological therapy

The World Health Organisation has created guidelines to assist clinicians to use the wide variety of drugs available for the pharmacological management of cancer pain systematically (WHO, 1986). A systematic therapy plan consists of both antitumour therapy and a stepwise method of symptomatic therapy, known as the 'analgesic ladder'. The analgesic ladder is illustrated in Fig.12.2. Studies testing the effectiveness of the symptomatic component of the WHO guidelines have been conducted internationally, including England (Walker et al., 1988).

It is important to 'keep it simple', therefore the use of an 'analgesic ladder', using a few drugs familiar to the practitioner, is the key to successful pain control. If pain fails to respond to a non-opioid drug, then a weak opioid may be used. If a weak opioid fails then a strong opioid is the next logical step. For mild to moderate pain, regular oral paracetamol or aspirin are appropriate. If these drugs fail to bring relief, they should be replaced by the regular administration of a drug from the next 'rung', a weak opioid, i.e. codeine, dihydrocodeine or dextropropoxyphene. If pain relief is still not achieved with the maximum recommended dose of one of these analgesics, then movement should be upwards to the next 'strong analgesic rung', strong opioid, and regular oral morphine should be commenced. In patients with severe pain, morphine – a strong opioid – is the drug of choice. If the cancer pain is severe, then morphine should be administered from the start. Changing from one weak opioid to another will not achieve better pain control. The decision to start a strong opioid is made by a logical series of decisions, not as a last resort.

Another key concept underlying the use of analgesics in cancer pain management is 'by the clock' whereby analgesics are given on a regular basis. The dose of analgesics should be titrated against the patient's pain, being gradually increased until he or she is comfortable. The next dose is given before the previous one has completely worn off; in this way it is possible to relieve the pain continuously.

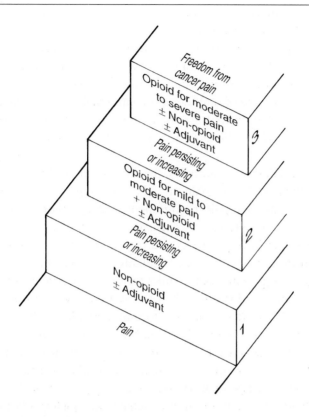

**Figure 12.2** *The WHO three-step analgesic ladder. Reproduced with permission from Cancer Pain Relief and Palliative Care: Report of a WHO Expert Committee. World Health Organisation, Geneva, 1990 (Technical Report Series No. 804) Figure 1.*

*Non-opioid analgesics (non-steroidal anti-inflammatory drugs)*   Non-opioid analgesics have four major pharmacological properties: analgesic, antipyretic, antiplatelet and anti-inflammatory. They have a peripheral site of action and produce an analgesic effect by inhibiting prostaglandin synthesis. Non-steroidal anti-inflammatory drugs (NSAIDs) are most effective in treating mild to moderate pain when an inflammatory component is present. They are of particular value in helping control the pain of metastatic bone cancer, mechanical pain resulting from compression of tendons and muscles and non-obstructive visceral pain (Ventafridda et al., 1980). Some of the commonly used NSAIDS are aspirin, ibuprofen, diclofenac sodium and naproxen.

*Opioid analgesics*   The most common weak opioids are codeine and dextropropoxyphene. Codeine is preferred, but dextropropoxyphene is a useful alternative (WHO, 1986). When the pain is no longer controlled by a weak opioid combined with aspirin or paracetamol (and if necessary an adjuvant), the patient should commence morphine.

Morphine is pre-eminent as an oral analgesic in advanced cancer. It produces its analgesic effect by binding of the opiate receptors at the peripheral and central nervous systems and altering the perception of pain (see Chapters 1 and 6). The use of oral therapy is preferable because the patient's mobility is not restricted. In contrast, the parenteral administration of a drug restricts the patient to either hospital or home, and requires additional people to perform it.

Morphine requirements are individualized by titration of the dose against the intensity of the individual's pain. Initial dose requirement will be dependent on the previous analgesic requirement and age. For more detailed guidance, the reader is referred to *A Guide to Symptom Relief in Advanced Cancer* by Regnard and Davies (1996) and the advice of the Expert Working Group of the European Association of Palliative Care (1996).

When analgesic requirements for mild to moderate pain reach the 'top analgesic rung' many doctors prescribe twice-daily controlled-release morphine (e.g. MST Continus®). The formulation allows the release of morphine over a period of about 12 hours. MST Continus® is unsuitable for the initial treatment of severe pain. Here the flexibility of the use of morphine sulphate tablets or solution given 4 hourly, which allows a rapid increase in the dose to an effective level, is required. Controlled-release morphine also takes too long (i.e. about 4 hours) to achieve satisfactory plasma levels. However, once dosage has been stabilized, it may be possible to revert to 12 hourly MST Continus® therapy.

When oral therapy is impracticable, owing to vomiting, dysphagia, coma or profound weakness, administration via the rectal or parenteral route will be required. Morphine suppositories may be a useful alternative to injections. The suppositories may be directly substituted for ordinary oral morphine: the same dose and time interval may be used. When parenteral medication is required, diamorphine is preferred to morphine; because of its greater solubility, only a small volume of fluid is needed for injection. Continuous intravenous opioids are unnecessary since there is no evidence that, in chronic cancer pain, the intravenous route provides more effective analgesia than regular subcutaneous administration. Extradural or intrathecal opioids may have a place in treating some patients, but these routes are not free of side-effects, including delayed respiratory depression and itching. The method requires practitioners skilled in this technique.

When patients cannot tolerate oral administration, continuous subcutaneous infusion has a valuable role. Subcutaneous diamorphine may be given intermittently at regular intervals but an increasingly popular method is to administer the drug continuously via a subcutaneous butterfly needle from a battery-operated syringe driver, eliminating the need for repeated injections. Some care givers use diamorphine alone in the syringe but the majority administer a mixture of the drug and various anti-emetic and/or anxiolytic agents. Practitioners should seek advice from colleagues informed about this technique (pharmacists, pain teams, the Macmillan nurse and symptom-control teams) and from published information, which is readily available (Latham, 1991; Pritchard and Mallett, 1996). A transdermal system for drug delivery has been developed for fentanyl, which delivers opioid continuously through the skin (Zech et al., 1992). This is emerging as an alternative mode of administration for patients who require long-term parenteral administration, or who cannot take oral therapy.

Side-effects of morphine therapy must be treated systematically. As we saw in Chapter 6, the most common are drowsiness, constipation, nausea and vomiting. Many of the questions often asked by health professionals on the topic of oral morphine have been addressed thoroughly in the booklet *Oral Morphine in Advanced Cancer* by Twycross and Lack (1989). Detailed reviews on opioid analgesics in the management of pain in patients with cancer are readily available, e.g. Hanks (1987). A core care plan, which will inform the individual plan of care for a patient receiving oral morphine sulphate therapy, can be found in Fig. 12.3. Patients should receive explicit information where emphasis should be placed on the need for regular administration of analgesics, in the case of oral morphine solution or tablets, every 4 hours. The first and last doses of the day should be 'anchored' to the patient's waking and bedtime. Ideally, the patient's drug regimen should be written out in full for the patient and family to work from, including the names of drugs, the reason for use, the dose and the number of times per day the drug should be taken. The patient and family should be warned about possible initial side-effects. A useful source of information for patients and their families is Twycross and Lack (1991) *Oral Morphine: Information For Patients, Families and Friends.*

In the majority of patients, morphine sulphate is effective and acceptable; however, occasionally a patient may show an intolerance that necessitates a change to an alternative powerful analgesic. Practitioners who have responsibility for treating cancer patients will need to consider carefully the alternatives available: dextromoramide, phenazocine and oxycodone.

*Adjuvant analgesics* Adjuvant analgesics are a third group of drugs used to treat the patient with cancer pain. These are drugs other than analgesics which indirectly relieve pain. They include corticosteroids, tricyclic antidepressants, anticonvulsants, antibiotics and antispasmodics. They may be effective without concurrent analgesics.

Corticosteroids have a wide application in advanced cancer because they

| **Situation requiring nursing intervention** | **Oral morphine sulphate** |
|---|---|

The administration of oral morphine sulphate solution for chronic pain associated with malignant disease.

*Common potential problems*

Unrelieved pain leading to insomnia, withdrawal from valued activities, depression, anxiety and inability to perform self-care activities, side-effects associated with therapy, for example, nausea, constipation, drowsiness, confusion and urinary retention and fears of addiction and/or tolerance.

*Nursing intention*

1.  Achievement of adequate pain relief.

2.  Ensuring the patient reports alterations in pain levels.

3.  Minimizing side effects and abating concerns about therapy.

*Core care*

1.  Prior to and during therapy a pain assessment detailing site, onset, duration, quality, severity, and aggravating and alleviating factors should be carried out. A selected pain tool to record a baseline and alterations in levels of pain may be a descriptive, numeric or visual analogue in nature, and it should be ensured the patient understands and can use the scale following instruction.

2.  Negotiate with the patient graduated realistic goals of pain relief, for example, pain free for sleeping, pain free at rest and finally pain free on movement within an achievable time frame.

3.  Administer oral morphine sulphate as prescribed at regular intervals (usually every 4 hours). If pain is unrelieved or re-appears before the next dose further additional doses will be required and the medication dosage and/or frequency should be titrated within the prescribed parameters.

4.  Document the degree, onset and duration of pain relief following medication to determine optimal dosage.

5.  Encourage the patient to verbalize alterations in levels of pain and observe for signs of ineffective pain relief, for example, facial expression, guarded movements, inability to concentrate, restlessness and difficulty sleeping.

6.  Instruct concerning the nature of medication, possible side-effects, self-care for such side-effects, necessity to report changes in pain and the need for regular administration. Provide a written explanation in addition to verbal presentation.

7.  Drowsiness and confusion (muddled thoughts, disorientation and hallucinations) are early effects and should diminish over 7 days. Warn the patient about initial drowsiness and encourage to persevere in the knowledge that it will lessen. Orientate to time, place and person and maintain a safe environment. Drowsiness may be a reflection of pain relief when previously exhausted mentally and physically from uncontrolled pain. Report excessive and prolonged drowsiness and confusion to the medical officer.

8.  If nausea and vomiting occur, administer anti-emetics regularly as prescribed and monitor effectiveness. Consider modification of the preparation or route of medication if nausea and vomiting remain unresolved, in conjunction with the medical officer.

9.  To control any constipation the patient may be experiencing, suggest a high-fibre diet, increased fluid intake and regular exercise if possible. In conjunction with the medical officer consider prescription of a regular aperient. Monitor bowel action.

10. Respiratory depression is rarely seen in patients receiving morphine sulphate who have severe pain due to malignant disease, but patients who have a limited respiratory reserve, raised intracranial pressure or chronic obstructive airways disease should be observed carefully, particularly when the level of pain is dramatically reduced as a result of other pain-relieving methods.

11. Explore any fears concerning psychological dependence (addiction) and the development of tolerance. Tolerance is characterized by decreasing efficiency with repeated administration, and it may require an increase in dose to maintain the analgesic effect, but it has been illustrated that, with longer durations of opiod administration, the slower the rate of increasing the dose. Psychological dependence rarely, if ever, occurs in cancer patients receiving opioids for chronic pain.

12. To complement the pharmacological approach to pain relief, explore previous pain-coping methods and non-pharmacological approaches, for example, positioning, heat and cold applications, pressure and massage, relaxation, hypnosis and distraction.

13. Consider physical, psychological, environmental and spiritual dimensions of chronic pain which may need to be addressed prior to achieving adequate pain relief.

14. When the patient's pain is resistant or semi-responsive to oral morphine sulphate, consider seeking advice from pain specialists (nursing, medicine and physiotherapy) and, after consultation with the medical officer, the use of co-analgesics, for example, non-steroidal anti-inflammatory drugs (for bone pain) and corticosteroids (for nerve compression) may be beneficial.

can reduce the oedema and inflammation that surround a tumour and there-fore ease the pressure on surrounding structures. A low dose (2–4 mg dexamethasone daily) can improve the appetite and may induce a sense of well-being, whilst high doses (16–24 mg daily) may dramatically relieve tumour mass expansion, reducing symptoms due to raised intracranial pressure or nerve compression.

Anticonvulsants (e.g. carbamazepine, sodium valproate, phenytoin) may play a valuable adjuvant role in controlling the pain of nerve compression. Carbamazepine is useful in the management of the stabbing component of differentiation pain and the antidepressant amytryptyline can be effective in nerve destruction pain (relieving the dyaesthetic pain of differentiation). Muscle spasm caused by nerve involvement or direct irritation by a tumour may be relieved by diazepam or baclofen. Pain in an anxious patient may improve with the use of psychotropic drugs, such as haloperidol. This drug is also commonly used for the management of an agitated confusional state.

The colicky pain of intestinal obstruction may be alleviated by such agents as loperamide or hyoscine. Domperidone or metaclopramide, by their peripheral action on the stomach and small bowel, may help to allay the discomfort of gastric stasis. Metronidazole and antibiotics may relieve the pain of an inflamed infected ulcerating growth.

### Neurosurgical and anaesthetic techniques

All pain is not equally responsive to analgesics, and neurolytic and neurosurgical blocks may be necessary as a supplementary approach in a few cases. Techniques involving anaesthetics are useful, particularly for well-defined localized pain, and the main indication for these techniques is activity-related pain associated with nerve compression. Nerves can be blocked by using either local anaesthetics (e.g. bupivicaine) or neurolytic solutions (e.g. phenol and alcohol). Some of the sites at which neural blockade is commonly per formed are the coeliac plexus and intercostal region. The use of the autonomic nerve block to the coeliac plexus is used to manage mid-abdominal pain associated with cancer of the pancreas and can be very successful. Although these techniques provide an important respite from pain, the effect does not last indefinitely. Cordotomy and the placement of epidural and intrathecal catheters are the most common neurosurgical procedures for pain relief. A cordotomy involves the interruption of the anterolateral spinothalamic tract in the cervical or thoracic region, and is a technique most useful in managing unilateral pain below the waist. Neurolytic and neurosurgical blocks are carried

*Figure 12.3* (opposite) *Core care plan for a patient receiving oral morphine sulphate therapy. Reproduced with permission from Richardson, A. (1992). The Royal Marsden Hospital Manual of Core Care Plans for Nursing. Scutari Press, London, pp. 139–140.*

out only by experienced doctors, in particular anaesthetists, as they are not without risk, and patients are carefully selected because of the potential motor and sensory losses associated with them. Further information on neurological and neurosurgical approaches to cancer pain can be found in Carson (1987).

### Reducing the suffering component of pain

Since the psychological impact of cancer is often devastating, treatments aimed at stress reduction and emotional support should be an integral part of the management of cancer pain. Interventions included in this approach do not affect the underlying pathology or alter the sensation of pain, but rather help in a variety of ways to reduce the suffering generated. Although these interventions are important in the management of cancer-related pain, these areas have received scant attention in cancer populations. Most of the literature is based on the clinical experience of practitioners. Little research has been conducted to evaluate the effectiveness of these strategies system-atically or to develop guidelines for their use, and studies on the efficacy of these approaches are needed urgently. Synder (1985) is concerned that many of the interventions have not been tested thoroughly in the clinical setting. There are many unanswered questions, such as 'Which of these therapies should be used for which patients', and 'How do we decide who should and who should not try a particular therapy?'

Treatment strategies aimed at reducing the suffering component of pain can best be classified as cognitive, behavioural and cognitive-behavioural techniques. As seen in Chapter 7, cognitive methods are those that attempt directly to modify thought processes in order to attenuate or relieve pain. They can be applied to thoughts, images and attitudes. Examples include distraction and imagery. Behavioural methods are those that modify phys-iological reactions to pain or behavioural manifestations of pain. Examples include relaxation, meditation, music therapy, biofeedback and hypnosis. Sometimes cognitive and behavioural strategies are used simultaneously. Relaxation with guided imagery is one such example. Such treatment strate-gies are most likely to be offered in partnership with other health care professionals who specialize in these techniques, such as the cognitive psychotherapist.

Another group of interventions includes those that provide counter irritant cutaneous stimulation. Examples include heat, cold and massage. Although these approaches technically fall into the major treatment approach of chang-ing the sensation/perception of pain, they are mentioned here because they can also be considered a behavioural intervention. A brief discussion of selected techniques and some of the research evidence that supports their effi-cacy in cancer patients will be presented here. For more detail and clinical examples the reader is referred to Chapter 7 and McCaffery and Beebe (1989).

*Distraction*

Distraction can be helpful in reducing pain, and there are many individual distraction techniques and strategies. Examples include conversation, adherence to routines and rituals, breathing exercises, reading and watching television. Researchers have asked patients to report what they used to help control cancer pain. In-patients and out-patients have revealed that such strategies as application of heat or cold, distraction (which included reading and television), relaxation and position changes helped to reduce pain to some degree (Barbour et al. 1986; Donovan, 1987; Wilkie et al., 1988, 1989).

*Hypnosis*

Hypnosis has long been employed in the treatment of cancer-related pain. Although numerous techniques have been used, Barber and Gitelson (1980) have described six hypnotic strategies particularly for the control of cancer-related pain. These include substitution of another sensation (e.g. pressure) for pain and dissociating part of the body from the patient's awareness. One study found that hypnosis and psychosocial support were more effective in reducing pain intensity than psychosocial support without hypnosis training (Spiegal and Bloom, 1983). A second report (Brechner et al., 1987) indicated that patients who were taught self-hypnosis techniques in conjunction with a systematic pharmacological pain therapy plan received better pain control than patients who used only the pharmacological therapy.

*Relaxation and guided imagery*

Relaxation training helps to produce physiological and mental relaxation. Guided imagery in which an individual visualizes pleasant places or things, is frequently used in conjunction with relaxation. Bayuk (1985) provides anecdotal evidence of the helpfulness of relaxation in a group of bone marrow transplant patients. One study found that taped transcripts that used guided imagery or progressive muscle relaxation were equally effective in reducing pain and distress (Graffam and Johnson, 1987). There is a particular need to investigate the usefulness of these techniques when combined with opioid analgesics. Relaxation and biofeedback techniques have been suggested for use with cancer patients (Copley Cobb, 1984) but only a few studies have utilized relaxation exercises and biofeedback with a specific application to the management of cancer-related pain (Fleming, 1985; Fotopoulos et al., 1983).

The majority of the techniques could easily be used by appropriately trained nurses who practise in a variety of settings. Some of the methods such as application of heat or immobilization are commonly used by nurses in the management of cancer pain. Still other techniques are somewhat familiar, but must be learned and practised before they can be effectively used with patients. These include relaxation, imagery and distraction. Finally, such interventions as hypnosis, biofeedback and cognitive therapy programmes require specialized training and are best left to individuals who have undergone such training.

# ■ EVALUATION

Nurses should examine their goals for pain relief in the cancer patient population, let the patients and families know that relief is possible and how it can be attained, use a variety of approaches or interventions to relieve pain, and evaluate the effectiveness of the approach. Nurses are the health team members who spend the greatest amount of time with the patients; thus, nurses are able to collect the most comprehensive information on the patient's response to the treatment plan. The degree, onset and duration of pain relief after the administration of analgesia are of paramount importance in determining optimal revisions to the treatment plan. Unless the nurse collects the appropriate information and documents the patient's response, the treatment plan cannot be altered appropriately (Lindley et al., 1990). If the patient continues to experience pain despite a care plan that combines a variety of medication and non-invasive measures, a reassessment should be performed. Unrelieved insomnia, anxiety, depression and/or psychosocial issues may need to be addressed before the patient can experience pain relief. Full relief may not be experienced until chemotherapy or radiotherapy have been completed. Alternate administration routes or increased dosages of analgesics may help break the pain cycle. Twycross (1972) has outlined the many reasons for failure to relieve pain, which include incorrect use of analgesia, inadequate communication and emotional support and unnecessary fears about morphine.

Pain management is intimately linked with clinical decision-making and this has been studied by Ferrell et al. (1991). The results from this study identified common clinical decisions related to pain, barriers to providing optimum pain relief and ethical/professional conflicts in pain management. Common clinical decisions made by nurses related to when to give medications and choice of analgesics. Nurses identified verbal (e.g. crying, groaning and whimpering) and non-verbal cues (e.g. hesitant movement, facial grimacing, doubling over) and reliance on information from family/caregivers, other nurses and the medical records as central to their decisions regarding pain assessment. Barriers to effective management included doctor knowledge and cooperation, patient/family knowledge and cooperation, as well as nursing knowledge and time. Nurses identified ethical dilemmas that included over- or undermedication, and conflicts with doctors or patients. Effective decision-making will only be possible when nurses and doctors acknowledge their lack of knowledge in the area of cancer pain. Optimum management also requires collaboration between medicine and nursing, and involvement of the patient and family. Clinical protocols and staff support may have a place here in helping nurses who are faced with complex decisions.

Nurses can influence pain relief through an understanding of the multidimensional aspects of pain. Understanding is the key to good pain management, and it is vital that nurses should receive additional education to achieve this understanding. After all, patients with cancer-related pain can be found on most general wards, not just in specialist centres. The inadequate management of pain continues to be a significant problem for persons with cancer and experts suggest that contributing factors include discrepancies in pain assessment, inadequate administration of opioid therapy and insufficient documentation of the patient's pain experience.

A comprehensive approach to pain control advocated by the WHO (1996) should be adhered to, working with a team which includes doctors, nurses and other health professionals. This is crucial for optimum care. Standards of care have been formulated in relation to pain control by the Royal College of Nursing (1991). The management of cancer pain is a multidisciplinary challenge, requiring the closest of cooperation between health professionals, and demanding an integrated approach of a combination of pharmacological and non-pharmacological techniques.

## ■ REFERENCES

**Abrams, R. & Hansen, R.** (1989) Radiotherapy, chemotherapy and hormonal therapy in the management of cancer pain: putting patient, prognosis, and oncologic opinions in perspective. In: Abram, S. (ed.) *Cancer Pain*. Kluwer, Boston, pp. 49–66.

**Ahles, T., Blanchard, E. & Ruckdeschel, J.** (1983) The multidimensional nature of cancer-related pain. *Pain* **17**, 277–288.

**Azzarelli, A. & Crispino, S.** (1987) Palliative surgery in cancer pain treatment. In: Swerdlow, M. & Ventafridda, V. (eds) *Cancer Pain*. MTP Press, Lancaster, pp. 97–103.

**Barber, J. & Gitelson, J.** (1980) Cancer pain: psychological management using hypnosis. *CA* **30**, 130–136.

**Barbour, L., McGuire, D. & Kirchhoff, K.** (1986) Nonanalgesic methods of pain control used by cancer outpatients. *Oncology Nursing Forum* **13**(6), 56–60.

**Bayuk, L.** (1985) Relaxation techniques. An adjunct therapy for cancer patients. *Seminars in Oncology Nursing* **1**(2), 147–150.

**Bonica, J.** (1979) Cancer pain: the importance of the problem. In: Bonica, J. & Ventafridda, V. (eds) *Advances in Pain Research and Therapy*. Raven Press, New York, pp. 1–11.

**Bonica, J.** (1985) Treatment of cancer pain: current status and future needs. In: Fields, H. (eds) *Advances in Pain Research and Therapy*. Raven Press, New York, pp. 589–616.

**Brechner, T., Reeves, J. & Gianni, J.** (1987) The comparative effectiveness of hypnosis combined with analgesic tailoring versus analgesic tailoring alone in the management of cancer pain. *Pain* **4**(Suppl.), S341.

**Carson, B.** (1987) Neurologic and neurosurgical approaches to cancer pain management. In: McGuire, D. & Yarbro, C. (eds) *Cancer Pain Management*. W.B. Saunders, Philadelphia, pp. 223–244.

**Catalano, R.** (1987) Pharmacologic management in the treatment of cancer pain. In: McGuire, D. & Yarbro, C. (eds) *Cancer Pain Management*. W.B. Saunders, Philadelphia, pp. 151–202.

**Cleeland, A.** (1989) Measurement of pain by subjective report. In: Chapman, C. & Loeser, J. (eds) *Issues In Pain Measurement*. Raven Press, New York.

**Cleeland, C. & Syrjala, K.** (1992) How to assess cancer pain. In: Turk, D. & Melzack, R. (eds) *Handbook Of Pain Assessment*. Guilford Press, New York, pp. 362–387.

**Copley Cobb, S.** (1984) Teaching relaxation techniques to cancer patients. *Cancer Nursing* **7**(2), 157–161.

**Coyle, N. & Foley, K.** (1987) Prevalence and profile of pain syndromes in cancer patients. In: McGuire, D. & Yarbro, C. (eds) *Cancer Pain Management*. W.B. Saunders, Philadelphia, pp. 21–47.

**Dalton, J.** (1989) Nurses' perceptions of their pain assessment skills, pain management practices, and attitudes toward pain. *Oncology Nursing Forum* **16**(2), 225–231.

**Daut, R. & Cleeland, C.** (1982) The prevalence and severity of cancer pain. *Cancer* **50**, 1913–1918.

**Daut, R., Cleeland, C. & Flanery, R.** (1983) Development of the Wisconsin Brief Pain Questionnaire to assess pain in cancer and other diseases. *Pain* **17**, 197–203.

**Donovan, M.** (1987) Clinical assessment of cancer pain. In: McGuire, D. & Yarbro, C. (eds) *Cancer Pain Management*. W.B. Saunders, Philadelphia, pp. 105–132.

**Donovan, M. & Dillon, P.** (1987) Incidence and characteristics of pain in a sample of hospitalised cancer patients. *Cancer Nursing* **10**(2), 85–92.

**Evans Faries, J., Stephens Mills, D., Whitt Goldsmith, K., Phillips, K. & Orr, J.** (1991) Systematic pain records and their impact on pain control: a pilot study. *Cancer Nursing* **14**(6), 306–313.

**Expert Working Group of the European Association for Palliative Care** (1996) Morphine in cancer pain: modes of administration. *British Medical Journal* **312**, 823–826.

**Ferrell, B., Eberts, M., McCaffery, M. & Grant, M.** (1991) Clinical decision making and pain. *Cancer Nursing* **14**(6), 289–297.

**Fishman, B., Pasternak, S., Wallenstein, R., Houde, R., Holland, J. & Foley, K.** (1987) The Memorial Pain Assessment Card: a valid instrument for evaluation of cancer pain. *Cancer* **60**, 1151–1158.

**Fleming, U.** (1985) Relaxation therapy for far-advanced cancer. *The Practitioner* **229**, 471–475.

**Foley, K.** (1979) Pain syndromes in patients with cancer. In: Bonica, J. & Ventafridda, V. (eds) *Advances in Pain Research and Therapy*. Raven Press, New York, pp. 59–75.

**Foley, K.** (1985) The treatment of cancer pain. *New England Journal of Medicine* **313**, 84–95.

**Ford, H. & Yarnold, J.** (1983) Radiation therapy – pain relief and recalcification. In: Stoll, B. & Parbhoo, S. (eds) *Bone Metastasis: Monitoring and Treatment*. Raven Press, New York, pp. 343–354.

**Fotopoulos, S., Cook, M., Graham, C., Cohen, H., Gerkovich, M., Bond, S. & Knapp, T.** (1983) Cancer pain: evaluation of electromyographic and electrodermal feedback. *Progressive Clinical Biological Research* **132D**, 33–53.

**Gorman, D.** (1991) Opioid analgesics in the management of pain in patients with cancer. *Palliative Medicine* **5**, 277–294.

**Graffam, S. & Johnson, A.** (1987) A comparison of two relaxation strategies for the relief of pain and its distress. *Journal of Pain and Symptom Management* **2**, 229–231.

**Greenwald, H., Bonica, J. & Bergner, M.** (1987) The prevalence of pain in four cancers. *Cancer* **60**, 2563–2569.

**Hanks, G.** (1983) Management of symptoms in advanced cancer. *Update* **26**, 1691–1702.

**Hanks, G.** (1987) Opioid analgesics in the management of pain in patients with cancer. *Palliative Medicine* **1**, 1–25.

**Latham, J.** (1991) *Pain Control*. Austen Cornish Publishers in association with the Lisa Sainsbury Foundation, London.

**Lindley, C., Dalton, J. & Fields, S.** (1990) Narcotic analgesics: clinical pharmacology and therapeutics. *Cancer Nursing* **13**(1), 28–38.

**McCaffery, M. & Beebe, A.** (1989) *Pain. Clinical Manual For Nursing Practice*. C.V. Mosby, St. Louis.

**McCaffery, M., Ferrell, B., O'Neil-Page, E. & Lester, M.** (1990) Nurses' knowledge of opioid analgesic drugs and psychological dependence. *Cancer Nursing* **13**(1), 21–27.

**McGuire, D.** (1987) The multidimensional phenomenon of cancer pain. In: McGuire, D. & Yarbro, C. (eds) *Cancer Pain Management*. W.B. Saunders, Philadelphia, pp. 1–20.

**McGuire, D. & Sheidler, V.** (1992) Pain. In: Groenwald, S., Hansen Frogge, M., Goodman, M. & Yarbro, C. (eds) *Manifestations of Cancer and Cancer Treatment. Part V from Cancer Nursing Principles and Practice*, 2nd edn. Jones and Bartlett Publishers, Boston, pp. 385–441.

**Melzack, R.** (1975) The McGill Pain Questionnaire: major properties and scoring methods. *Pain* **1**, 277–299.

**Melzack, R.** (1987) The short-form McGill Pain Questionnaire. *Pain* **30**, 191–197.

**Paice, J., Mahon, S. & Faut-Callahan, M.** (1991) Factors associated with adequate pain control in hospitalised postsurgical patients diagnosed with cancer. *Cancer Nursing* **14**(6), 298–305.

**Potenoy, R.** (1987) Cancer pain: epidemiology and syndromes. *Cancer* **63**, 2298–2307.

**Pritchard, A.** (1988) Management of pain and nursing attitudes. *Cancer Nursing* **11**(3), 203–209.

**Pritchard, P. & Mallet, J.** (1996) *Royal Marsden Hospital Manual of Clinical Nursing Procedures,* 4th edn. Blackwell Science Publications, London.

**Raiman, J.** (1986a) Pain relief: a two-way process. *Nursing Times* **82**(15), 24–28.

**Raiman, J.** (1986b) Towards understanding pain, and planning for relief. *Nursing* **11**, 411–423.

**Rankin, M. & Snider, B.** (1984) Nurses' perceptions of cancer patients' pain. *Cancer Nursing* **7**(2), 149–155.

**Regnard, C. & Davies, A.** (1996) *A Guide to Symptom Relief in Advanced Cancer,* 4th edn. Distributed by Haigh and Hochland Ltd Manchester, International University Booksellers.

**Richardson, A.** (1992) *The Royal Marsden Hospital Manual of Core Care Plans for Cancer Nursing.* Scutari Press, London.

**Royal College of Nursing** (1991) *Standards of Care: Cancer Nursing.* Scutari Press, London.

**Spiegal, D. & Bloom, J.** (1983) Pain in metastatic breast cancer. *Cancer* **52**, 341–345.

**Spross, J., McGuire, D. & Schmitt, R.** (1990) Oncology Nursing Society position paper on cancer pain. Parts I–III. *Oncology Nursing Forum* **17**, 595–603, 751–760, 943–955.

**Synder, M.** (1985) *Independent Nursing Interventions.* John Wiley, New York.

**Twycross, R.** (1972) Principles and practice of pain relief in terminal cancer. *Update* **5**(2), 115–121.

**Twycross, R. & Lack, S.** (1989) *Oral Morphine in Advanced Cancer,* 2nd edn. Beaconsfield Publishers Ltd, Beaconsfield.

**Twycross, R. & Lack, S.** (1990) *Therapeutics In Terminal Cancer,* 2nd edn. Churchill Livingstone, Edinburgh.

**Twycross, R. & Lack, S.** (1991) *Oral Morphine: Information for Patients, Families and Friends,* 2nd edn. Beaconsfield Publishers Ltd, Beaconsfield.

**Ventafridda, V., Fochi, V. & DeConno, D.** (1980) Use of non-steroidal anti-inflammatory drugs in the treatment of pain in cancer. *British Journal of Clinical Pharmacology* **10**, 3435–3465.

**Walker, V., Hoskin, P., Hanks, F. & White, I.** (1988) Evaluation of WHO analgesic guidelines for cancer pain in a hospital-based palliative care unit. *Journal of Pain and Symptom Management* **3**, 145–149.

**Wilkie, D.** (1990) Cancer pain management: state of the art nursing care. *Nursing Clinics of North America* **25**(2), 331–343.

**Wilkie, D., Lovejoy, N., Dodd, M. & Tesler, M.** (1988) Cancer pain control behaviors: description and correlation with pain intensity. *Oncology Nursing Forum* **15**(6), 723–731.

**Wilkie, D., Lovejoy, N., Dodd, M. & Tesler, M.** (1989) Pain control behaviors in patients with cancer. In: Funk, S., Tornquist, E., Champagne, M., Copp, L. & Wiese, R. (eds) *Key Aspects of Comfort: Management of Pain Fatigue, and Nausea.* Springer, New York, pp. 119–126.

**World Health Organization** (1986) *Cancer Pain Relief.* WHO, Geneva.

**World Health Organization** (1990) *Cancer Pain Relief and Palliative Care: A Report of a WHO Expert Committee.* Technical Report Series, No. 804. WHO, Geneva.

**Zech, D., Grond, S., Lynch, J., Dauer, H., Stollenwerk, B. & Lehmann, K.** (1992) Transdermal fentanyl and initial dose finding with patient-controlled analgesia in cancer pain. A pilot study with 20 terminally ill cancer patients. *Pain* **50**, 293–301.

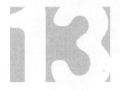

# Chronic non-malignant pain:
# A community-based approach to
# management

Pain is a word applied to many different types of experience and refe. only to the sensation of pain, but also to how it affects us. Chronic noi. malignant pain, the focus of this chapter, is one example of pain where the effects of the pain on the sufferer can assume central importance in determining the extent to which pain adversely impinges on daily life.

This chapter will consider definitions of chronic non-malignant pain, address why treatment in the community is particularly important and focus on the results from a study which taught relaxation as a coping skill to patients in the community with chronic non-malignant pain.

## ■ CHRONIC NON-MALIGNANT PAIN

What exactly is chronic non-malignant pain? McCaffery and Beebe (1989) define it as:

> 'pain that has lasted 6 months or longer, is ongoing on a daily basis, is due to non-life threatening causes, has not responded to currently available treatment methods, and may continue for the reminder of the patient's life' (p. 232).

So when or if the pain might end is not known, and a range of treatment options may have been tried with little success. Such pain often does not have an identifiable physical cause, leading sometimes to sufferers being regarded as malingerers. An example of this sort of pain is chronic low back pain.

Wall (1989) argues such pain is 'not simply a prolongation of acute pain' (p. 15). Sternbach (1989) adds that whilst acute pain may promote survival, chronic pain is usually destructive, physically, psychologically and socially. As Eccleston pointed out in Chapter 3, depression is often associated with chronic pain (Bulmer and Heilbronn, 1982, Kramlinger et al., 1983), as is anxiety. Anger and frustration have also been associated with chronic pain (Wade et al., 1992; Fernandez and Turk, 1995). Sleep disturbance, irritability, fatigue, reduced motor activity and reduced tolerance of pain are all effects of chronic pain (Sternbach, 1989). Having chronic non-malignant pain can lead to changes in roles, relationships and activity levels within the family, as well as at work. This may lead to feelings of loss and isolation (Rose, 1994).

As well as changes in family and work relationships that are important to the sufferer, it may be difficult to sustain open relationships with health professionals. If health professionals try but fail to provide pain relief, it can be frustrating for both sides and all too easy to in some way blame the person in pain for the failure.

Once it has been established that a person has chronic non-malignant pain, the aim of treatment is not necessarily to stop the pain, but, as stated by Williams in Chapter 7, is to help the patient manage or cope with their pain. This is in contrast to telling them there is nothing more that can be done and that they will have to learn to live with it. The most effective treatment for these patients has tended to be demonstrated in multidisciplinary pain clinics where the whole pain experience is considered, and methods of treatment, such as graded exercise and activity, medication reduction, and cognitive and behavioural methods are used (Flor et al., 1992). Pain management needs to be incorporated into everyday life, as pain will need to be dealt with on a day-to-day basis. However, such multidisciplinary treatments can be expensive and are necessarily restricted to a few centres. Accessibility can become a problem. Turk et al. (1993) argued that a treatment that is moderately effective, yet widely accessible is preferable to a more effective treatment that is only accessible by relatively few patients.

One such potentially widely available option appeared to be the use of relaxation for chronic non-malignant pain. People do not always cope well with chronic non-malignant pain, and the effects of this pain can have a wide-ranging and negative impact on their lives. With a move towards community care (Great Britain Parliament, 1990, *National Health Service and Community Care Act*, implemented 1 April 1993) and taking responsibility for one's own health, it may become increasingly important to find a low-cost way of promoting strategies which complement any existing treatment, would be easy to teach and use, and would enable people to exert control over their pain. This could improve their ability to cope with the pain, reducing the impact it has on them, their families and the community.

Chronic non-malignant pain has been described as a highly prevalent, disabling and costly health problem (Loeser et al., 1990). It thus seems crucial to develop, use and assess relaxation as there is the potential to reach many people in the community at present suffering with chronic non-malignant pain, to promote their coping and reduce the impact that pain has on their lives.

The prevalence of chronic non-malignant pain has been demonstrated by Potter (1990). He investigated 1000 consecutive patients presenting to a general practitioner. He found that 11.3% of patients had pain which had lasted more than 3 months. Potter concluded that each general practitioner in his or her practice was likely to have 155 chronic pain patients registered. In Sweden, Brattberg et al. (1989) surveyed a random sample from the general population. They found 40% reported 'obvious pain' lasting for more than 6 months. This suggests that the general practitioner may be seeing only some of those with chronic pain. So treating people with chronic pain is a sizeable problem.

## ■ RELAXATION

### ▮ Background

Relaxation has been described as a 'state of relative freedom from both anxiety and skeletal muscle tension' (McCaffery and Beebe, 1989, p. 188). Linton (1982b) describes relaxation as breaking the vicious circle of pain leading to chronic tension, which itself produces more pain, which in turn causes more tension. Linton (1982a) reviewed behavioural treatments for chronic non-malignant pains other than headache and found relaxation was generally effective. He did caution that the quality of studies was poor, most lacked adequate and appropriate controls, outcome measures and/or follow-ups. Thus any conclusions about effectiveness were necessarily tentative.

Philips (1988), in a study of 24 patients with chronic non-malignant pain, found induction of relaxation over 20 minutes led to significant reductions in the sensory and affective pain experience. No such changes occurred in the 22 control patients who listened to a presentation on chronic pain over a comparable time period. This suggests relaxation is useful in the very short term, but whether or not these effects could be sustained over time was not investigated. Relaxation was also used in 15 patients with chronic back or joint pain by Linton and Gotestam (1984). They found patients randomly allocated to a relaxation group or relaxation plus operantconditioning group did better than a waiting-list control group on measures of pain, medica-tion use, activity and depression. There were, however, few clear differences between the two treatments. Turner and Jensen (1993) emphasized the impor-tance of practising relaxation in the presence of the therapist so as not to vitiate the efficacy of this treatment.

## ▪ Types of relaxation

Progressive muscle relaxation such as that described by Bernstein and Borkovec (1973) has been used with people who have chronic non-malig-nant pain by Turner (1982), Philips (1988), and Turner and Jensen (1993). It seems, however, that progressive muscle relaxation in isolation is not enough. It needs to be applied to everyday activities. Chang-Liang and Denney (1976) found applied relaxation to be more effective in reducing anxiety than relax-ation only and a no treatment control. This is supported by Affleck et al. (1992) who found those who used relaxation more frequently as part of their daily coping repertoire had less daily pain. The research thus suggests that relaxation strategies can work and that a well-designed study could have enormous potential.

The design of the study outlined in this chapter will now be presented. Full details of this study can be found in Seers (1993).

## ▪ OVERVIEW OF METHODS

A randomized controlled trial was chosen as the most appropriate method to evaluate the effects of teaching relaxation skills to people with chronic non-malignant pain both at the time of teaching and in the longer term. Within this design, qualitative data on the experience of pain was also collected.

### ■ Aims of the study were to:

1. Evaluate the effects of relaxation training with chronic non-malignant pain sufferers immediately after training and in the longer term.
2. Provide a simple treatment programme as a realistic clinical option for health professionals.

### ■ Sample

The sample consisted of all consenting patients attending either the pain clinic or named out-patient clinic at the hospitals involved. Patients were selected by their consultant for inclusion in the study if they fulfilled the following criteria:

1. They were aged 18 years or over.
2. They had pain for more than 3 months.
3. A malignant cause of their pain had been excluded.
4. No surgical treatment or change in medical treatment was proposed at present.

Patients with a diagnosis of dementia or psychosis were excluded.

### ■ Design

Patients from two out-patient clinics who agreed to participate in this study took part in a baseline interview and were then randomly allocated to: (1) an experimental group, which was taught relaxation skills; (2) an attention control group, which was visited by the researcher but not taught relaxation skills; and (3) a waiting-list control group, which was taught relaxation skills after a waiting period.

The two taught groups were reassessed at the end of teaching and 1 and 4 months later. The waiting list group were reassessed 5 months after the baseline interview (to equate with the 4-week teaching plus 4-month follow-up time for the taught groups) and then taught relaxation skills.

### ■ Outcomes

Williams (1988) emphasized that as chronic pain is multidimensional, data must be collected on many axes for adequate assessment. Malone and Strube (1988) supported this when they concluded that non-medical treatments for chronic pain reliably affect mood and subjective symptoms, indicating the importance of using a multidimensional framework for assessment. Outcome assessments were completed by a researcher blind to the treatment allocation. As an additional safeguard, patients were sent the standardized instruments to complete prior to all post-teaching assessments. The baseline interview was completed before the patient was randomized into one of the three groups.

The major outcomes assessed in this study were pain, pain distress, quality of life, coping, self-efficacy, depression and anxiety. These outcomes were assessed using the following measures.

## 1. Pain

This was assessed using:

### (a) McGill Pain Questionnaire (MPQ) (Melzack, 1975)

This 78-item questionnaire yields a pain-rating index. Separate scores of sensory, affective, evaluative and miscellaneous words can also be computed.

### (b) Numerical rating scale

A 0–100 numerical pain-rating scale, where 0 represents 'no pain' and 100 'agonizing pain', was found to be the most practical index with chronic pain patients (Jensen et al., 1986). It was used to rate pain and pain distress now, at its least and at its worst.

## 2. Quality of life

### (a) Sickness impact profile (SIP) (Bergner et al. 1981)

This reflects the patient's perception of their illness related to physical and psychosocial dysfunction. It yields category scores as well as an overall score. It has been shown to be a reliable and valid measure of health status. Bergner et al. (1981) demonstrated a test retest reliability of 0.92 and moderate to high validity. In this study, Watt-Watson and Graydon's (1989) shortened form was used to reduce demands on the patients, and instructions were modified to specify pain-related rather than illness-related dysfunction.

### (b) Patterns of employment

Employment status was ascertained.

## 3. Contact with health professionals

The number of visits to the general practitioner, hospital specialists and/or pain clinic because of the pain were recorded.

## 4. Patient distress/coping

### (a) Coping strategies questionnaire (CSQ) (Rosenstiel Keefe, 1983)

This 42-item questionnaire assesses the frequency with which six cognitive strategies and one behavioural strategy are used by people in pain. It also assesses the extent to which they feel able to control and to decrease their pain. It has demonstrated adequate reliability and validity.

### (b) Self-efficacy questionnaire (Nicholas, 1989)

This 10-item scale reflects how confident patients are that they can function in specific areas of daily life despite the pain. Reasonable reliability and validity have been reported.

### (c) Hospital anxiety and depression scale (Zigmond and Snaith, 1983)

This 14-item self-assessment questionnaire assesses anxiety and depression on a four-point response scale. It has demonstrated adequate reliability and validity.

## ■ PROCEDURES

Ethical clearance was granted from both the relevant hospital ethics committees. Patients who fulfilled the inclusion criteria were selected by their consultant and referred to the researcher. Patients were given an explanation of the study in the clinic and were then given an information sheet to read. They were asked whether they would like to take part and, if so, an appointment for the baseline interview was made. They were thus given time to reflect on their initial decision, and were asked to sign a consent form after they had had time to reflect, read the information sheet and ask any questions. Patients were able to choose whether they were taught at the hospital or in their own homes.

### ▪ Baseline interview

This lasted about 1–1½ hours. The open-ended questions were asked first, with the standardized questionnaires forming the final part of the interview. At the end of this interview, patients were randomized into one of the three study groups.

### ▪ Relaxation teaching package

These sessions lasted about half an hour. All teaching sessions were conducted on a one-to-one basis. Patients were also given a short manual containing an explanation of pain, the rationale for relaxation and a summary of the methods used.

The use of four teaching sessions (once a week for 4 weeks) was decided upon after discussion with several psychologists who regularly taught these techniques, and was based upon Borkovec and Sides (1979), who found studies which employed an average of four sessions demonstrated a change in outcomes, whilst those using an average of two sessions did no better than a control group. The content of each session was based upon the work of Bernstein and Borkovec (1973), Goldfried and Davison (1976), Linton (1982b) and Linton and Gotestam (1984).

## ▪ Attention control teaching sessions

This group was initially included to examine the possibility that visits by the researcher may alone result in an improvement in patient outcomes. The importance of a credible placebo control that arouses similar expectations to the treatment group has been emphasized (Richter et al., 1986). To achieve this, patients were told that people with chronic non-malignant pain often felt that not enough attention was paid to their pain problems. We wanted to pay more attention to and learn about these problems and what the patient did, felt or thought about them. Borkovec et al. (1987) used a similar 'non-directive' therapy with people with chronic non-malignant pain. This control condition was based closely on the manual written by Borkovec during their study. Similar attention control designs have been used in other studies (Holroyd and Andrasik, 1978; Richter et al., 1986). The package used by Nicholas et al. (1992) was not utilized as the current study was designed before this was published.

## ▪ Waiting-list control

Patients in this group were not visited or taught before the reassessment of outcomes 5 months after the baseline interview (to match the 1 month teaching and 4 month follow-up of the two visited groups). Thus the effects of current treatment with no additional intervention were assessed.

## ▪ Procedure during the interview

Patients were always asked to be as honest as possible and the confidential nature of the study was reiterated. To avoid unconscious bias, the standardized questionnaires were given at the end of teaching for patients to complete at home and returned in a stamped addressed envelope. At the 1- and 4-month follow-up interviews, the questionnaires were sent to patients a couple of days before the interview for self-completion. This was done despite the blinding of the assessor at follow-up, to cover the possibility of accidental disclosure of treatment group by the patient.

## ▪ Pilot study

This involved nine patients, three in each of the relaxation, attention control and waiting-list control groups. The purpose of the pilot study was to ensure all proposed methods of data collection were feasible and acceptable to patients, and to explore preliminary methods of data analysis.

The timing and content of the interviews appeared to be acceptable to people with chronic non-malignant pain.

## ▪ Main study

A total of 82 patients fulfilled the criteria for inclusion and were referred to the study. Of these, 75 agreed to take part, a response rate of 91.5%.

## ■ RESULTS AND DISCUSSION

### ▪ Data analysis

Non-parametric tests of association and difference were used after seeking statistical advice because of the mainly ordinal nature of data. Univariate analysis were predominately used to determine whether treatment affected outcomes. As argued by Turner and Jensen (1993), this approach was felt appropriate because tests were undertaken to answer specific, predetermined questions.

### ▪ Demographic details

Of the 75 patients in the main study, 27 were randomized to the relaxation group, 28 to the attention control group and 20 to the waiting-list control group. Patients had experienced pain for between 6 months and 47 years (mean 8.4 years). Over 63% ($n = 47$) had pain all the time.

Patients ranged in age from 21 to 86 years (mean 53 years). Females accounted for 76% ($n = 57$) of the sample. Most of the sample (over 93%; $n = 70$) were Caucasian. Over 50% of patients had pain which involved their back.

Patients had seen between 1 and 9 different traditional specialists (mean 4.4). The number of complementary techniques tried out ranged from 0 to 8 (mean 1.6), with 54 (72%) of patients having tried some form of complementary pain relief. The total number of contacts with both traditional and complementary practitioners ranged from 1 to 13 (mean 6.1).

## ■ RELATIONSHIPS BETWEEN PAIN AND THE MAJOR VARIABLES

These relationships were examined amongst the data from the baseline (pre-teaching) interview. Correlations are reported using the Spearman's rho ($r_s$).

Table 13.1 illustrates that the more pain patients reported, the more their psychological well-being was adversely affected and the more disabled they were.

### ▪ Comparing baseline measures with later outcomes

In the short term, those taught relaxation had significantly less pain immediately after all relaxation sessions, both with the researcher present and during homework practice. Pain scores immediately after the teaching of the attention control group showed no such significant differences. Relaxation thus had an immediate and a longer term beneficial effect, with the attention control group demonstrating no such benefits. This supports the work of Philips (1988). However, given the resources necessary to teach relaxation, a longer term and wider-ranging effect seemed desirable. This study found

*Table 13.1* *Relationship between baselines assessment of pain now and the major variables*

|  | $r_s$ | *p* | *n* |
|---|---|---|---|
| Anxiety | 0.23 | <0.05 | 74 |
| Depression | 0.30 | <0.01 | 73 |
| Sickness Impact Profile | 0.36 | <0.01 | 74 |
| Catastrophizing | 0.33 | <0.01 | 73 |
| Self-efficacy | −0.42 | <0.001 | 73 |

such an effect. Those patients taught relaxation showed significant improvements between baseline and post-teaching outcomes (assessed at the end of teaching and 1 month and 4 months later). Pain (using the MPQ total score), anxiety and disability (SIP total scores) were all significantly lower, and sleep was significantly better at all three follow-up occasions. Patients also used fewer catastrophizing strategies to deal with their pain at the first two follow-ups (the final follow-up showing a trend only). Patients also had higher self-efficacy scores at the final (4 month) follow-up.

There were no such differences for either the attention control or waiting-list control groups. Relaxation thus appears to have the potential to have a beneficial effect.

The present study demonstrated effects of relaxation that were more extensive than those reported by Spinhoven and Linssen (1991). They found that pain intensity was the only outcome variable to be reduced at the end of treatment and at 6 months follow-up. However, they did not assess quality of life or anxiety (both of which showed changes in the present study). It is possible that the group teaching they used may have produced different results.

Why did relaxation work? Patients may have thought differently about their pain (even if it was the same), or done things differently (been more active and less upset by their pain). The physiological relaxation itself may have been effective, and/or patients felt more in control of their pain because they could relax. However, perceptions of control on a 0–6 point scale did not show significant differences during the course of the study, giving less weight to the latter explanation.

Relaxation *per se* may not help, but it may change the way people think, feel and act when in pain. It seemed that relaxation worked at least partly by improving sleep. One might expect this to have a generally beneficial effect on patients. It is important to note that ordinary relaxation can be regarded as rather passive and that patients were taught applied relaxation as a coping strategy to deal with their pain. This point was also made be Linton and Gotestam (1984). The field notes provided valuable insights into how relaxation operated and some, but not all, patients viewed relaxation as a way of coping with, rather than curing, their pain.

## ▪ Clinical versus statistical significance

When the percentage change in scores was examined from before to after treatment, it became clear that, for a result to be statistically significant, a change of about 20% from pre-treatment scores was necessary. The question then arises whether this is clinically significant. Turk et al. (1993) suggested a criterion of 50% symptom reduction may be viewed as a bench mark. A 50% improvement could be regarded as overstringent. A more conservative estimate of a 25% improvement shows a reduction in pain (MPQ), catastrophizing (CSQ) and disability (SIP), with anxiety just outside at an average of 24% improvement. Flor et al. (1992) in their meta-analysis found the average reduction in pain intensity using a multidisciplinary pain treatment programme was 37%. The current study showed an average reduction of between 24% and 30%, and thus compares quite favourably with more complex and expensive treatment programmes.

Thus the criteria for a clinical improvement are somewhat more difficult to demonstrate than those that show a statistically significant improvement. Which one chooses to adopt is a matter of much debate. Clearly relaxation strategies did not cure the pain. However, from the sufferer's perspective, it seems likely that even the fairly modest 25% improvement is better than no improvement at all, especially if they have had intractable pain for many years. When comparing this to ratings of how helpful the technique had been, ratings of 7/10 for relaxation suggested that, for patients at least, it was of clinical significance. The importance of considering the patient's perspective was emphasized by the American Pain Society (1991) who described an outcome as 'the result for the patient' (p. 185).

In addition to the quantitative data analysis, qualitative data were utilized, and will be presented next. These results are reported in more detail in Seers and Friedli (1996).

## ▪ PRESENTATION OF THEMES FROM FIELD NOTES

Extensive field notes were written up after each interview. These included comments made by patients, difficulties that had arisen and the researcher's impressions of the interview.

All field notes were read and emerging themes noted on the text. Although a number of themes emerged (see Appendix), examples of patients' comments in just the first of these categories will now be given.

## ▪ Experiences of health care

This was divided into five sections.

### (i) Believing the pain

It was common for patients to feel their pain was not believed:

> *'Nothing shows up. I feel as if I'm telling lies and no proof I'm in pain. It's so embarrassing – you've got to prove yourself.'*

Having their pain acknowledged as real was crucial to many patients.

### (ii) Treating chronic pain as though it were acute

> *'They treat you as if you're supposed to get better, but I haven't.'*

### (iii) Desperation of doctors

#### (a) Hospital doctors

> *'After the op they didn't answer when I said "why have I got pain?" As far as they were concerned, the op was a success. They were not concerned with how it affected me.' . . . 'just shrugged when asked what can be done.'*

#### (b) General practitioners

> *'It comes to a point, they just give you tablets, they get fed up with you. Can't even listen.'*

### (iv) Blame

> *'The original consultant thought he was omnipotent and wouldn't refer me on. He tried to shift the blame onto me. He was very unpleasant. He said "either you've got something or you're a very good actress." He found inflammation and after that he was nicer to me.'*

### (v) Communication difficulties

It seemed there was sometimes a mismatch between the expectations or perspectives of the patient and those of the doctor:

> *'I asked consultant why I had a pain in my leg when it's my back. He said "I've explained that to you time and time again." So I kept my mouth shut. He hadn't told me though.'*

This outline of some of the field notes gave additional insights into what it was like for these patients to experience chronic non-malignant pain.

## ■ LIMITATIONS OF THE STUDY

Some possible limitations of this study are outlined below.

It is possible that the effectiveness of relaxation was the result of the researchers being better at teaching relaxation than at attention control skills. Although there was no significant difference between the two researchers and any of the outcome measures used, this explanation remains a possibility. As Turk et al. (1993) point out, 'no significant improvement' could be due to inadequate treatment implementation. In a similar vein, Borkovec et al. (1984) highlighted the therapist effect – one may prefer a method or be better trained in that method.

It is possible there were not enough teaching sessions. Turner and Jensen (1993) used 2 hours per week for 6 weeks to teach relaxation. The present study used half an hour to an hour per week for 4 weeks. It is not known whether more teaching would have changed the effectiveness of relaxation in any way, although a review of such studies by Borkovec and Sides (1979) concluded that studies using four sessions demonstrated changes in outcomes, whilst those using an average of two sessions did no better than a control group.

The study relies to a large extent on self-report. Turner and Jensen (1993) highlighted how demand characteristics may influence self-report, and this may have operated in this study. However, the inclusion of a control group should have controlled for any such effect.

Attrition of sample size during a longitudinal study like this can be problematic. Other similar studies have reported quite high attrition rates: Turner and Jensen (1993) lost 30% from the relaxation group and 40% from the waiting-list control. As in the present study, their 'drop-outs' did not differ from 'completers' at pre-treatment assessment on demographic or dependent variables. Peters et al. (1992) reported a very high drop-out rate of 52% from the control condition. The drop-out rate in the present study (drop-outs plus exclusions) was 10/75 (13%). If the four patients who were lost to follow-up are included as drop-outs, this total increases to 14/75 or 18.7%. This is lower than attrition rates from other studies. One explanation for this might be that the one-to-one teaching in the current study could have encouraged rapport with the patient and thus increased the likelihood of completing the study. However, as Turk et al. (1993) caution, when patients are not available for follow-up, the follow-up sample can no longer be considered random. This has to be considered when assessing longer term follow-up.

## ■ COMPARING RESULTS WITH MULTIDISCIPLINARY PROGRAMMES

Flor et al. (1992) in their meta-analysis concluded that multidisciplinary programmes demonstrated improvements over and above single treatment modalities. As pain is so complex, it is likely that a combination of techniques will be appropriate. However, when considering costs and access to such programmes, the present study's four ½–1 hour sessions would be substantially cheaper and have wider availability than, for example, a multidisciplinary in-patient pain management programme, which admitted people for 4 weeks as in-patients (Williams et al., 1993). The present study has the added advantage of allowing and indeed encouraging people to apply their strategies in their own environment, rather than having to transfer skills learnt elsewhere. Whilst there may be a small number of patients for whom in-patient treatment is appropriate for a number of reasons, many more could be treated by the more simple relaxation treatment option outlined in this study. It seems likely that relaxation is one of the active ingredients of the multidisciplinary programme.

## ■ RELEVANCE FOR PRACTICE

If patients have several unsuccessful referrals in an attempt to relieve pain, they may be told there is nothing more that can be done. By default, the patient then becomes responsible for their own care, often with very little or no back-up from health care professionals. However, they do not always cope well. If nurses were skilled in teaching relaxation, they would have the potential to facilitate patients' efforts at coping. This is in accord with the 'partnership' approach between nurses and patients, and the role of nurses as offering practical advice and assistance to cope with problems more effectively as advocated in the Department of Health's (1989) *Strategy for Nursing*. It could also ultimately reduce the impact of pain and distress caused by chronic non-malignant pain.

Nurses are in an ideal position to implement such a programme as they fulfil diverse roles and thus have the opportunity to work with people in many settings, whether as a practice nurse, district nurse, health visitor or hospital nurse. Nurses could use a package as described in this study as a realistic clinical option in their day-to-day practice. This study has shown such a package can be effective.

## ■ CONCLUSIONS

Chronic non-malignant pain is detrimental to the patient, their family and the community, yet it is one of the most prevalent and difficult problems that health professionals treat (Keefe, 1982). The extent to which health needs are met has clearly been described as part of quality of care (Buchan et al., 1990). The baseline assessments in this study revealed the high degree of disability these patients experienced, suggesting that their health needs have not been met.

Relaxation was found to be an effective and a realistic treatment option, improving many aspects of the experience of pain; gains that were maintained over time. Such a relaxation package that could be taught to nurses would be a valuable asset for educators, especially with the increasing emphasis on community care and new training relevant to it. Several authors, including Sofaer (1985), Pilowsky (1988), Davis and Seers (1991) and IASP (1991, 1993), have pointed out deficiencies in current education on pain and have included relaxation strategies in proposals for an educational programme or curriculum on pain.

The study demonstrated a selective effect for relaxation over and above any non-specific effects. This simple and cheap method could be promoted, especially for use by clients at home.

## ■ ACKNOWLEDGEMENTS

I would like to thank Karin Friedli, the research assistant who worked with me on the study described within this chapter, for all her hard work and dedication. The Department of Health funded this study through a post-doctoral Nursing Research Fellowship.

## ■ REFERENCES

**Affleck, G., Urrows, S., Tennen, H. & Higgins, P.** (1992) Daily coping with pain from rheumatoid arthritis: patterns and correlates. *Pain* **51**, 221–229.

**American Pain Society** (1991) American Pain Society quality assurance standards for relief of acute pain and cancer pain. In: Bond, M.R., Charlton, J.E. & Woolf, C.J. (eds) *Proceedings of the VIth World Congress on Pain.* Elsevier, Amsterdam, pp. 185–189.

**Bergner, M., Bobbitt, R.A., Carter, W.B. & Gilson, B.S.** (1981) The sickness impact profile: development and final revision of a health status measure. *Medical Care* **19**, 787–805.

**Bernstein, D.A. & Borkovec, T.D.** (1973) *Progressive Relaxation Training. A Manual for the Helping Professions.* Research Press, Champaign.

**Borkovec, T.D. & Sides, J.K.** (1979) Critical procedural variables related to the physiological effects of progressive relaxation: a review. *Behavioural Research and Therapy* **17**, 119–125.

**Borkovec, T.D., Johnson, M.C. & Block, D.L.** (1984) Evaluating experimental designs in relaxation research. In: Woolfolk, R.L. & Lehrer, P.M. (eds) *Principles and Practice of Stress Management.* Guildford Press, New York, pp. 368–403.

**Borkovec, T.D., Mathews, A.M., Chambers, A., Ebrahimi, S., Lytle, R. & Nelson, R.** (1987) The effects of relaxation training with cognitive or nondirective therapy and the role of relaxation-induced anxiety in the treatment of generalized anxiety. *Journal of Consulting and Clinical Psychology* **55**, 883–888.

**Brattberg, G., Thorslund, M. & Wilkman, A.** (1989) The prevalence of pain in a general population. The results of a postal survey in a country of Sweden. *Pain* **37**, 215–222.

**Buchan, H., Gray, M., Hill, A. & Coulter, A.** (1990) Score on quality. *Health Service Journal* **100**, 362–363.

**Bulmer, D. & Heilbronn, M.** (1982) Chronic pain as a variant of depressive disease. The pain prone disorder. *Journal of Nervous and Mental Disease* **170**, 381–406.

**Chang-Liang, R. & Denney, D.R.** (1976) Applied relaxation as training in self control. *Journal of Counseling Psychology* **23** 183–189.

**Davis, P. & Seers, K.** (1991) Teaching nurses about managing pain. *Nursing Standard* **5**, 30–32.

**Department of Health** (1989) *A Strategy for Nursing.* HMSO, London.

**Fernandez, E. & Turk, D.C.** (1995) The scope and significance of anger in the experience of chronic pain. *Pain* **61**, 165–175.

**Flor, H., Fydrich, T. & Turk, D.C.** (1992) Efficacy of multidisciplinary pain treatment centers: a meta-analytic review. *Pain* **49**, 221–230.

**Goldfried, M.R. & Davison, G.C.** (1976) *Clinical Behavior Therapy.* Holt, Rinehart & Winston, New York.

**Great Britain Parliament** (1990) *National Health Service and Community Care Act.* HMSO, London.

**Holroyd, K.A. & Andrasik, F.** (1978) Coping and the self control of chronic tension headache. *Journal of Consulting and Clinical Psychology* **46**, 1036–1045.

**International Association for the Study of Pain** (1986) Pain terms. A current list with definitions and notes on usage. *Pain* **27**, S215–S221.

**International Association for the Study of Pain** (1991) *Core Curriculum for Professional Education in Pain.* IASP, Seattle.

**International Association for the Study of Pain** (1993) *Pain Curriculum for Basic Nursing Education. IASP Newsletter* September/October, 4–6.

**Jensen, M.P., Karoly, P. & Braver, S.** (1986) The measurement of clinical pain intensity: a comparison of six methods. *Pain* **27**, 117–126.

**Keefe, F.J.** (1982) Behavioral assessment and treatment of chronic pain: current status and future directions. *Journal of Consulting and Clinical Psychology* **50**, 896–911.

**Kramlinger, K.G., Swanson, D.W. & Maruta, T.** (1983) Are patients with chronic pain depressed? *American Journal of Psychiatry* **140**, 747–749.

**Linton, S.J.** (1982a) A critical review of behavioral treatments for chronic benign pain other than headache. *British Journal of Clinical Psychology* **21**, 321–337.

**Linton, S.J.** (1982b) Applied relaxation as a method of coping with chronic pain: a therapist's guide. *Scandinavian Journal of Behavior Therapy* **11**, 161–174.

**Linton, S.J. & Gotestam, K.G.** (1984) A controlled study of the effects of applied relaxation and applied relaxation plus operant procedures in the regulation of chronic pain. *British Journal of Clinical Psychology* **23**, 291–299.

**Loeser, J.D., Seres, J.L. & Newman, R.L.** (1990) Interdisciplinary, multimodal management of chronic pain. In: Bonica, J.J. (ed.) *The Management of Pain*, 2nd edn. Lea & Febiger, Philadelphia, pp. 2107–2120.

**Malone, M.D. & Strube, M.J.** (1988) Meta-analysis of non-medical treatments for chronic pain. Review article. *Pain* **34**, 231–244.

**McCaffery, M. & Beebe, A.** (1989) *Pain. Clinical Manual for Nursing Practice.* C.V. Mosby, St Louis.

**Melzack, R.** (1975) The McGill Pain Questionnaire: major properties and scoring methods. *Pain* **1**, 277–299.

**Nicholas, M.K.** (1989) *Self-efficacy and Chronic Pain.* Paper presented to British Psychological Society Conference, St Andrews, March.

**Nicholas, M.K., Wilson, P.H. & Goyen, J.** (1992) Comparison of cognitive-behavioral group treatment and an alternative non-psychological treatment for chronic low back pain. *Pain* **48**, 339–347.

**Peters, J., Large, R.G. & Elkind, G.** (1992) Follow-up results from a randomised controlled trial evaluating in- and outpatient pain management programmes. *Pain* **50**, 41–50.

**Philips, H.C.** (1988) Changing chronic pain experience. *Pain* **32**, 165–172.

**Pilowsky, I.** (1988) An outline curriculum on pain for medical schools. *Pain* **33**, 1–2.

**Potter, R.G.** (1990) The frequency of presentation of pain in general practice. *The Pain Society* **8**, 11–14.

**Richter, I.L., McGrath, P.J., Humphreys, P.J., Goodman, J.T., Firestone, P. & Keene, D.** (1986) Cognitive and relaxation treatment of paediatric migraine. *Pain* **25**, 195–203.

**Rose, K.** (1994) Patient isolation in chronic benign pain. *Nursing Standard* **8**, 25–27.

**Rosenstiel, A.K. & Keefe, F.J.** (1983) The use of coping strategies in chronic low back pain patients: relationship to patient characteristics and current adjustment. *Pain* **17**, 33–44.

**Seers, K.** (1993) *Maintaining People with Chronic Non-malignant Pain in the Community: Teaching Relaxation as a Coping Skill.* Report submitted to Department of Health on completion of a post-doctoral nursing research fellowship.

**Seers, K. & Friedli, K.** (1996) The patients' experiences of their chronic non-malignant pain. *Journal of Advanced Nursing* **24**, 1160–1168.

**Sofaer, B.** (1985) Pain management through nurse education. In: Copp, L.A. (ed.) *Perspectives on Pain. Recent Advances in Nursing* 11. Churchill Livingstone, Edinburgh, pp. 62–74.

**Spinhoven, P. & Linssen, A.C.G.** (1991) Behavioral treatment of chronic low back pain. 1. Relations of coping strategy use to outcome. *Pain* **45**, 29–34.

**Sternbach, R.A.** (1989) Acute versus chronic pain. In: Wall, P.D. & Melzack, R. (eds) *Textbook of Pain*, 2nd edn. Churchill Livingstone, Edinburgh, pp. 242–246.

**Turk, D.C., Rudy, T.E. & Sorkin, B.A.** (1993) Neglected topics in chronic pain treatment outcome studies: determination of success. *Pain* **53**, 3–16.

**Turner, J.A.** (1982) Comparison of group progressive-relaxation training and cognitive-behavioural group therapy for chronic low back pain. *Journal of Consulting and Clinical Psychology* **50**, 757–765.

**Turner, J.A. & Jensen, M.P.** (1993) Efficacy of cognitive therapy for chronic low back pain. *Pain* **52**, 169–177.

**Wade, J.B., Dougherty, L.M., Hart, R.P., Rafii, A. & Price, D.D.** (1992) A canonical correlation analysis of the influence of neuroticism and extraversion on chronic pain, suffering and pain behavior. *Pain* **51**, 67–73.

**Wall, P.D.** (1989) Introduction. In: Wall, P.D. & Melzack, R. (eds) *Textbook of Pain*, 2nd edn. Churchill Livingstone, Edinburgh, pp. 1–18.

**Watt-Watson, J.H. & Graydon, J.E.** (1989) Sickness Impact Profile: a measure of dysfunction with chronic pain patients. *Journal of Pain and Symptom Management* **4**, 152–156.

**Williams, A.C.C., Nicholas, M.K., Richardson, P.H., Pither, C.E., Justins, D.M., Chamerlain, J.H., Harding, V.R., Ralphs, J.A., Jones, S.C., Dieudonne, I., Featherstone, J.D., Hodgson, D.R., Ridout, K.L. & Shannon, E.M.** (1993) Evaluation of a cognitive behavioural programme for rehabilitating patients with chronic pain. *British Journal of General Practice* **43**, 513–518.

**Williams, R.C.** (1988) Toward a set of reliable and valid measures for chronic pain assessment and outcome research. Review article. *Pain* **35**, 239–251.

**Zigmond, A.S. & Snaith, R.P.** (1983) The hospital anxiety and depression scale. *Acta Psychiatrica Scandinavica* **67**, 361–370.

## ■ APPENDIX: THEMES EMERGING FROM ANALYSIS OF FIELD NOTES

1. Experience of health care
   (i) Believing the pain
   (ii) Treating chronic pain as if it were acute
   (iii) Desperation of the doctors
   (iv) Blame
   (v) Communication difficulties
2. Psychological state
3. Physical health state
4. Relationship with family/friends
5. Social activities
6. Employment/finance
7. Comments on relaxation and describing
8. Comments on pain
9. Lack of personal control
10. Comments on being involved in research
11. Problems/frustrations or ethical concerns doing the research

# 14

## Pain in the elderly:
## Management strategies

## ■ BACKGROUND

This chapter is based upon a study conducted by Walker (1989) into pain coping among elderly people in the community who suffer from persistent pain. The design of the study originated from personal observations in practice that, although elderly people are more likely than younger people to suffer from pain and disability, most succeed in coping remarkably well in spite of their problems. As individuals grow older, they have an increasingly long history of coping with different types of life events, situations and problems, including pain, which combine to shape well-defined individual differences in personality, beliefs and behaviour patterns. They develop stable ways of coping with pain and physical limitation, which have varying degrees of success in terms of maintaining quality of life. Each individual has a unique combination of social, financial and spiritual resources, and support networks, which together act as buffers against the negative consequences of pain and disability.

Some of the common pain problems associated with old age are outlined below, followed by a report of a study which was designed to understand how older people cope with pain and its attendant problems. The implications for nursing practice are illustrated by a case example.

## ■ THE PREVALENCE OF CHRONIC PAIN IN THE ELDERLY

The prevalence of chronic pain in the elderly is explained by the high incidence of chronic degenerative conditions, such as arthritis, in the ageing population (Office of Population Censuses and Surveys, 1989; Miller and Oertel, 1992). Many elderly people suffer from multiple chronic conditions, the most common of which involve joint problems caused by osteo- and rheumatoid arthritis (Jacobson et al. 1991). The incidence of cardiovascular disorders and cancers increases with age, and these diseases are the most common causes of death among people in the older age groups. Neurogenic pain, caused by postherpetic and trigeminal neuralgias, diabetic neuropathy and stroke, are also more common in the elderly. Other causes include gastrointestinal disorders (many of which are iatrogenic consequences of medication taken for arthritis), respiratory disorders, peripheral vascular disease and leg ulcers (Walker, 1989).

## ■ PAIN SENSATION AND ADAPTATION IN THE ELDERLY

There appears to be a belief, which is commonly held by health professionals, that pain is a natural consequence of growing old and that pain sensitivity decreases with age. Hence the elderly are thought to feel less pain than younger people (McCaffery and Beebe, 1994). Lichtenberg et al. (1984) found that subjective reports of pain were lower among older arthritis patients than younger ones despite greater levels of pain. However, Harkins (1988a) reviewed laboratory studies, which focused on changes in pain threshold and tolerance with age, and found no evidence of significant changes in pain sensitivity with age. Recent evidence supports the view that elderly people with chronic pain tend to report less pain than younger adults (Mosley et al., 1993) but there is no evidence that this is because they feel less pain. Harkins (1988a,b), and McCaffery and Beebe (1994) have argued that the belief that older people feel less pain has led to a stereotype which is unsafe and fosters undertreatment. This assertion is supported by Oberle et al. (1990), who demonstrated that elderly people received significantly less analgesia for postoperative pain than younger patients, although there were no significant differences in pain intensity between the two groups and no differences in the amount of analgesia prescribed. The only difference was that older people reported less preoperative anxiety than younger people.

Kotler-Cope and Gerber (1993) presented evidence to support the view that elderly people report less pain because they are more tolerant to pain. They found that a sample of older patients with chronic pain demonstrated more adaptive pain-coping beliefs prior to hospital admission than younger patients, although both groups benefited from multidisciplinary treatment for their pain. They concluded that elderly patients probably cope better with chronic pain than do younger pain patients.

There are a number of possible reasons for this. Firstly, elderly people may have developed better strategies for coping with pain. There is some evidence that older people tend to use different strategies, though these are not necessarily defined as better. For example, Keefe and Williams (1990) and Corran et al. (1994) compared pain-coping strategies across the age range and found that older patients more frequently used praying and hoping as a strategy, while diverting attention increased as levels of sensory pain increased. Secondly, pain in older people is more likely to be related to a recognized and accepted organic pathology and is, therefore, perceived by them to be less of an immediate threat to survival. Prohaska et al. (1987) found that symptoms which were attributed to ageing elicited more passive acceptance and less emotional distress. Thirdly, older people have probably had more pain in their lives and have, therefore, developed a greater level of tolerance to pain. Corran et al. (1994) identified that elderly attenders at pain clinics were less anxious than younger ones, although pain scores were similar. Overall, the reasons for differences in coping with pain among older people are not clear. This has led Corran et al. (1994) to identify the need for further research into psychosocial sources of age-related differences in pain experience.

Relatively few elderly people attend pain clinics (Marcer et al., 1989) and, since most of the research into chronic pain is conducted on samples drawn from pain clinics, it is necessary to be cautious in the application of their findings to elderly people with chronic pain in the general population. Many researchers have identified a paucity of research into the impact of pain on the elderly (e.g. Ross et al., 1993; Simon, 1993). One of the few researchers who have focused specifically upon pain in the elderly is Ranjan Roy, who has a background in social work. Roy (1987) identified that pain in this group generally coexists with psychological distress and social dysfunction, and that elderly people with chronic pain experience problems which are as serious as their younger counterparts. More recently, Roy has emphasized the importance of considering social context and social factors in the management of chronic pain (Roy, 1992). The study outlined below addressed some of these issues in relation to chronic or persistent pain in the elderly.

# ■ STRESS: A FRAMEWORK FOR INTERPRETING THE CHRONIC PAIN EXPERIENCE

Pain is a stressor which demands coping action because it represents a potential threat to physical and hence social functioning. In the absence of an established diagnosis, pain is associated with uncertainty. Even when the cause of the pain is understood, its course may be unpredictable or its aversive consequences uncontrollable. Thus chronic pain is associated with both anxiety and depression. Pain may be dealt with by taking personal action (personal control) or by seeking help from others (social support). Either course of action is dependent upon the individual's understanding of the nature of the problem, beliefs about ways of dealing with it, and the resources which are available to help. The chronic pain patient may experience feelings of powerlessness and even anger, if they feel that they lack the information or resources needed to help with their pain.

The framework used for the study reported below was based on the assumption that psychological distress (anxiety, depression and anger) is an indicator of poor or maladaptive coping, while psychological well-being (confidence, contentment) indicates successful or adaptive coping (Walker et al., 1989).

# ■ AIMS AND OBJECTIVES

The aim of the study conducted by Walker (1989) was to investigate how elderly people in the community cope with chronic pain and how nurses can contribute to successful coping. The objectives were to identify:

1. Psychosocial factors which influence the ability of elderly people to cope with persistent pain.
2. Current approaches to the nursing management of pain in the community.
3. Nursing strategies likely to improve the management of pain in the elderly in the community.

# ■ METHODOLOGY (Walker, 1989; Walker et al., 1990)

## ▮ Design

Participants were elderly people who lived in the community and received visits from a member of one of 12 district nursing teams selected randomly from one health authority. The participants self-selected themselves for interview on the basis that they had pain, or were being treated for pain which had persisted for at least 6 weeks. Structured interviews were designed to measure a range of factors which predict psychological distress versus well-being. A semi-structured component was included to gain qualitative insights into the experiences of coping with pain in this group. Additional questionnaire data were collected from staff in order to identify their perceptions of the participants' experiences, together with current practices and sources of knowledge.

## ∎ Instruments

In absence of a single instrument which met the criteria for the study, a 12-item seven-point semantic differential measure of mood state, representing a continuum from psychological well-being to psychological distress, was developed for use as the dependent variable for the study (Walker, 1989). Items were drawn from instruments with established validity and statistical tests revealed good internal and test–retest reliability. Scores ranged from –36 to +36 and were used as a measure of how well each individual was coping at the time of interview (the dependent variable).

The independent variables (those which were predicted to influence coping) included a variety of potential stressors and buffers against stress in the elderly population, which were derived from an extensive literature on the psychology of stress, pain and gerontology, and from nurses' observations (Walker, 1989; Walker et al., 1990). They included 'least' and 'worst' levels of pain intensity, perceived control over pain, information about the painful condition, pain-coping strategies, feeling occupied, occupational strategies, regrets about the past, perceived social support, loneliness, other external stressors including financial, health and 'personal' problems (significant life events), and religious beliefs. All independent variables, including pain intensity, were measured using verbal descriptor scales. Visual analogue and numerical rating scales for pain measurement were found not to be successful during pilot studies, an observation which has since received support from Herr and Mobily (1993) who found that a verbal descriptor scale was the preferred method of pain measurement among elderly patients. It is of importance to note that some participants who were substantially confused were able to rate their pain intensity using the verbal descriptor scale, since Marzinski (1991) reported that pain behaviours are not a good indicator of the presence of pain in this group. The McGill Pain Questionnaire (MPQ; Melzack, 1975) was used as an additional measure of the sensory, affective and evaluative dimensions of pain.

## ∎ Sample

Participants were 190 people aged between 61 and 98 who had experienced pain for between 6 weeks and 66 years. Seventy-six per cent were women. Forty per cent lived with their spouse, 32% lived alone, and the remainder were cared for by relatives or in sheltered accommodation.

The types of painful condition experienced included arthritis, cardiovascular disorders, respiratory disease, gastrointestinal disorders, neurogenic pain, leg ulcers and malignancy. The majority of those interviewed experienced multiple pain problems, of which arthritis was not only the most common, but most frequently identified as the worst pain problem.

## ▪ Procedure and analysis

The interviews lasted for up to 3 hours and all responses were recorded in writing at the time. Nurses and care assistants involved in the care of each participant subsequently completed a questionnaire in which they identified the diagnosis and causes of pain, rated pain intensity, psychological state and identified coping problems. Data from patients were analysed using multiple regression analysis, and non-parametric tests of association and group comparison. Multiple regression is a statistical procedure which identifies the combination of independent variables that offer the best fit in predicting the dependent variable (psychological well-being/distress). Qualitative data were analysed using content analysis. A comparison of data obtained from participants and nurses was analysed using non-parametric tests of association and group comparison. Nurses also identified general issues associated with pain management in the community. Statistical results are reported in full in Walker (1989) and Walker et al. (1990). Qualitative findings are reported in Walker (1994).

## ▪ FINDINGS AND DISCUSSION

### ▪ Predictors of coping with chronic pain (Walker, 1989; Walker et al., 1990)

Scores of psychological well-being were spread across the full range and were slightly skewed in a positive direction, indicating that the majority of participants felt positive at the time of interview. [Interestingly, Helme et al. (1992) found that community-dwelling elderly with pain reported less mood disturbance than a similar younger group.] Almost half of the sample experienced continuous pain and 15% reported that their pain was never less than moderate in intensity. Multiple regression identified five variables which explained psychological well-being/distress. These were pain 'under control', feeling informed about the painful condition, being occupied, regrets about the past and personal problems. The detailed findings are reported and discussed below.

### Pain perceived to be 'under control'

Perceived pain control was associated, either directly or indirectly, with every other variable included in the study, a finding which highlights the truly multifactorial nature of pain. Perceived pain control was, not surprisingly, related to levels of pain intensity. However, it was also associated with health and financial problems, and loneliness. Control over pain appeared to increase with advanced age. In fact, the only three individuals to report that their pain was totally under control were all aged over 80, and each suffered from regular episodes of severe or excruciating pain. There was a close relationship between perceived pain control and scores on the evaluative and affective scales of the MPQ, illustrating the strong association between control over pain and psychological state. The results appear to support the view that perceived pain control is influenced by a range of factors other than pain intensity, and that distress is associated with lack of perceived control over pain, rather than the level of pain intensity.

Those who reported that their pain was under control were more likely to be classified, from self-statements, as having internal locus of control. (People with internal locus of control tend to believe that controlling pain depends upon their own actions, as opposed to those with external locus of control who believe that controlling pain depends upon the actions of others, such as doctors, or is a matter of luck, fate or chance.) This observation finds support in an increasing number of pain studies, including those by Crisson and Keefe (1988) and Härkapää et al. (1991), which demonstrated that external locus of control is associated with higher levels of pain and depression. The more strategies people used to control their pain, the greater the degree of control they perceived their pain to be under. Most participants used one or more of a range of pain strategies including exercise, diet, heat applications, hot water bottles, warm clothing, transcutaneous electrical nerve stimulation (TENS), topical ointments and sprays. Adaptive strategies for coping with pain are likely to vary according to the type of pain experienced. For example, Davis et al. (1990) found that heat applications were reported to be particularly useful for older people with arthritic conditions. For those with arthritis pain only, those who relied solely upon prescribed analgesia were less likely to report adequate pain control than those who used alternative strategies. It could be argued that this was because they suffered from more severe pain, but there was no evidence in the data to support this. Indeed, Williamson and Schulz (1992) found that the number of pain medications taken by elderly people, rather than reported pain intensity, was a significant predictor of depression. The findings appear to support those of Brown and Nicassio (1987) in demonstrating that active pain-coping strategies are more adaptive than passive coping strategies. However, the literature on chronic pain now suggests that the use of passive coping strategies, together with beliefs in external locus of control, may be encouraged by medical approaches to treatment which focus predominantly upon medication (Pither and Nicholas, 1991; Waddell, 1992).

There were many reports of drug-induced painful side-effects, including gastric ulceration among those taking non-steroidal anti-inflammatory drugs (NSAIDs) and constipation among those taking opioid analgesics. As a result, many elderly participants reported that they no longer took analgesics on a regular basis. It was disturbing to identify that, of those currently taking NSAIDs, 28% were unable to identify any beneficial effects. It is common in the pain clinic to recommend an intermittent break from such drugs in order to re-evaluate their therapeutic value, and this advice could well be followed in primary care. It is also common advice in the pain clinic to suggest that analgesics should be reserved for the limited occasions when they are considered really necessary, or targeted to relieve pain during such activities as getting up in the morning or exercising, rather than taken on a regular basis. This runs counter to the management of pain in acute or palliative care settings, but is designed to promote personal control and reduce the effects of increasing tolerance to analgesia among those who wish to lead a fulfilling life in spite of persistent pain.

These findings strongly support the view that nurses have a major role to play in teaching patients and encouraging them to use as many personal strategies for controlling their own pain as possible, regardless of their apparent medical utility. Nurses also need to encourage the strategic, rather than regular, use of analgesics for chronic benign pain, and carefully monitor both the beneficial and the deleterious effects of any drugs which are taken on a regular basis.

### Information about the painful condition

It was evident that elderly people were very concerned to know about the causes and treatment of their condition. A total of 26% were uncertain, or did not know what was wrong with them. In contrast, only 8% of those asked said that they would prefer not to know if something serious was wrong. Comments from the remainder, who did want to know, included 'I could put up with it if I knew what it was'. Some were angry at feeling that they had been 'fobbed off' by their doctor. Several people appeared very distressed by their lack of information. Most of these suspected that they had cancer, usually with good reason, but had not been told what was wrong and did not like to ask. Beisecker (1988) found that, although older patients were less likely than younger ones to ask for information, they were as likely to desire information and to want be involved in decision-making about their treatment.

It was evident from these findings that lack of information is a significant source of psychological distress and poor pain control in elderly people, but that information needs to be tailored to meet individual needs and concerns. The provision of information is an important nursing role which appears to be somewhat neglected in the case of elderly patients with chronic painful disorders.

### Feeling occupied

Those who reported higher levels of disability and other health problems felt less occupied. Bearing in mind that three-quarters of the sample were women, the activities most closely related to feelings of occupation were cooking and cleaning. This highlights the importance of providing aids to independence which will enable elderly people with pain to maintain self-care activities. Other reported ways of keeping occupied included hobbies, such as knitting, sewing, woodwork, reading the papers and watching television. However, a more detailed analysis of the results showed that those who engaged in at least one occupation which required active involvement, such as household chores or craft activities, reported a greater level of occupation and increased psychological well-being. Passive pastimes, such as watching television, reading and listening to the radio, appeared to have little therapeutic value unless transformed into an active occupation by discussing or debating them with other people on a regular basis.

These findings suggest that occupation provides more than just distraction. Walker (1989) noted that men were more reliant on physical activity to keep occupied, but tended not to be involved in household chores, particularly if they were married. As a result, many appeared at a total loss when they could no longer engage in gardening or DIY. Heinemann et al. (1988) found that there was a significant reduction in involvement in craft activities following the onset of visual impairment in the elderly, suggesting that elderly people with pain, together with visual and other impairments, require special attention.

These findings indicate that occupational strategies which provide or encourage active involvement are likely to be very helpful for elderly patients with persistent pain. Therefore, nurses have an important role in educating carers (whether spouses, daughters or professional carers) to encourage elderly people who have pain to do as much for themselves as possible, and in making referrals for aids to independence and for social and occupational advice or help, as appropriate.

### Regrets about the past

Regrets about the past were an important determinant of psychological distress and poor pain control. Regrets focused upon a variety of events, few of which were pain-related, including childhood abuse, unsuccessful marriages, death of a child or parent and unfulfilled ambitions. Those with regrets were less likely to perceive their pain as being 'under control' and reported higher levels of persistent pain. However, it is not clear if pain leads to an increased negative focus on the past or if regrets reduce pain tolerance. Stronger religious beliefs were associated with lower levels of regret and distress. Indeed Koenig et al. (1988), in their study of religion in elderly Americans, found that religious commitment provided an important source of spiritual, occupational and social support, each of which were likely to contribute to well-being.

Those with regrets were more likely to report feeling lonely. Coleman (1986) interviewed elderly people for his own study on self-esteem in later life and found regrets to be an important determinant of dissatisfaction with life. He commented that 'loss of contact can be hard to bear, but far worse is an inability to be content in one's own company' (Coleman, 1986, p. 79). This must be especially relevant for people in pain in view of the association identified between regrets and pain control. Haight (1988) found that structured life review increased life satisfaction and reduced psychological distress in elderly people over a prolonged period of time. Mills and Walker (1994) demonstrated that reminiscence is capable of achieving improvements in morale, even among elderly patients suffering from dementia who have predominantly sad memories. These studies both suggest that individual (as opposed to group) reminiscence or life review may be therapeutic for people who have pain and express regret about the past.

It seems likely that those with higher levels of regret are more likely to feel negative about all aspects of their current situation. Therefore, they are more likely to express bitterness and resentment, and least likely to respond to routine medical treatments for pain. It is clearly not possible to address these problems without time and attention, if at all. However, understanding the impact of past traumas and disappointments may assist nurses and carers to feel sympathetic, rather than antagonistic, towards patients who are often very difficult and fail to respond to advice about pain control or pain treatments.

### Personal problems

These related mainly to bereavement and marital relationship problems. It suggests that this variable is closely related to loss of both emotional and functional support, which explains the association found between personal problems, loneliness and financial problems. Loneliness was most acute in the early days of widowhood, suggesting that social support visits are most necessary during the initial period of bereavement. Not surprisingly, those who lived alone were more likely to report feeling lonely than those who lived with their spouse or close partner. However, it was surprising to find that of those who appeared most depressed (with psychological distress scores of less than –10), twelve lived with their spouse while only four lived alone (compared to an expected ratio of 12:9.6). For those who lived alone, receiving social visitors in the home reduced loneliness, although outings from the home had no such effect. It was interesting to note that the majority of elderly people, even when prompted, deliberately excluded home helps or other professional carers from their list of social visitors.

These findings suggest that close social relationships which provide emotional support are a significant buffer against psychological distress in elderly people who have pain. It is most important for nurses to recognize that the presence of problems, such as bereavement and marital disharmony, are likely to reduce pain tolerance as well as causing psychological distress. Referral for professional support, such as bereavement counselling, may be most useful during the early stages of bereavement in order to provide emotional support during a period of major adjustment. Encouragement to go to a day centre may later provide a source of occupation and involvement, but it may not reduce the sense of loneliness owing to lack of emotional support. Older people may become cautious about forging new close relationships with their peers because of the possibility of experiencing further bereavement losses. Therefore, a supportive attitude on the part of nurses and professional carers is highly valued, as indicated below.

### ∎ Patients' expectations of the nursing contribution to pain management in the elderly (Walker, 1989, 1994; Walker et al., 1990)

Interpersonal interaction formed the largest category of response to questions about what nurses can do to help elderly people in pain and themselves in particular. Having someone to talk things over with was considered most frequently to be beneficial: 'Sister listens and tries to understand', 'I like to talk to her – it's a relief and comforting', 'Someone to trust and give confidence will help', 'You can talk to a nurse but doctors talk to you' (Walker, 1994, p. 225). Giving confidence and encouragement was identified as very important. Indeed, Dexter (1992) found that encouragement actually increased the frequency of therapeutic exercises in a community sample of arthritis patients. Lack of time was the most common cause of complaint about the community nursing staff: 'She is in and gone like a shot. She is not the sort of person you could sit and talk to', '(They) only give injections, they don't hang about'. On the other hand, positive comments indicated that some nurses were able to provide reassurance in the time available. 'I always felt that she was not rushed. She gave me the assurance that she had the time, even though she did not really' (Walker, 1994, p. 225).

Overall, nurses who were particularly valued for their help with pain were those who listened, explained, advised and conducted procedures in a manner which was reassuring, considerate, gentle and cheerful. This helped people to share their problems and feel valued, cheered them up, and increased their confidence in their own ability to cope as well as giving confidence in the care received. It appears that time spent with elderly patients, however short, must be 'quality time', in terms of the interpersonal interaction, in order to be perceived as having therapeutic value. It may not always require direct personal contact, for example, Weinberger et al. (1986) demonstrated that biweekly telephone interviews with elderly osteoarthritis sufferers improved physical ability, psychological well-being and pain.

## ■ Nurses' perceptions of elderly patients' pain experiences (Walker, 1989, 1994; Walker et al., 1990)

The association between nurses' assessments and patients' self-reports of pain intensity was modest. The level of agreement between different members of staff reporting on the same patient was better than that between staff and patients. Nurses tended to overestimate levels of least pain and underestimate worst pain, even when they had regular contact with the patient over a long period. These findings are similar to the evidence reviewed by Carr in Chapter 10 and to those of Zalon (1993), who found that nurses tended to underestimate high levels of postoperative pain and overestimate low ones. Comparisons between district nurses and care assistants revealed no differences in the accuracy of estimates of pain intensity levels. However, in very few instances had a nurse actually assessed pain with the patient. Only one district nurse stated that she regularly used formal pain assessment, while two others used it occasionally. One of the benefits of assessing levels of least and worst pain intensity is that it helps to identify trigger factors, and factors which reduce pain, so that direct interventions can be identified to reduce the number and duration of painful episodes.

It appeared that, in the absence of formal assessment, some patients who had high levels of pain but low levels of distress were wrongly judged not to have any pain at all. Judgements about pain were influenced by staff perceptions of the extent to which patients complained about pain. However, the more patients complained, the more likely staff were to perceive that they were exaggerating their pain. Indeed, nurses commonly attributed pain exaggeration to attention-seeking. These findings indicate that patients with the greatest levels of psychological distress may fail to obtain the support they need if they complain too much.

## ■ CONCLUSIONS AND RECOMMENDATIONS

Overall, the findings from this study (Walker, 1989, 1994; Walker et al., 1990) suggest that elderly people who have few strategies to control pain, are uncertain about the causes and consequences of their painful condition, have little which actively occupies them, have regrets about the past, or have suffered loss of close personal relationships are more likely to experience

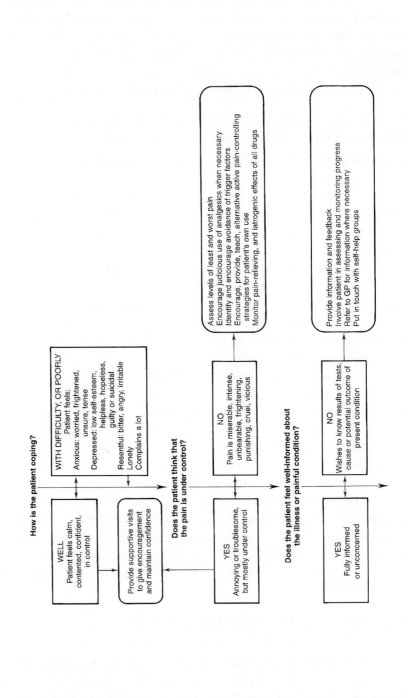

**How is the patient coping?**

WELL
Patient feels calm,
contented, confident,
in control

WITH DIFFICULTY, OR POORLY
Patient feels:
Anxious: worried, frightened,
unsure, tense
Depressed: low self-esteem,
helpless, hopeless,
guilty or suicidal
Resentful: bitter, angry, irritable
Lonely
Complains a lot

Provide supportive visits
to give encouragement
and maintain confidence

**Does the patient think that
the pain is under control?**

YES
Annoying or troublesome,
but mostly under control

NO
Pain is miserable, intense,
unbearable, frightening,
punishing, cruel, vicious

Assess levels of least and worst pain
Encourage judicious use of analgesics when necessary
Identify and encourage avoidance of trigger factors
Encourage, provide, teach, alternative active pain-controlling
strategies for patient's own use
Monitor pain-relieving, and iatrogenic effects of all drugs

**Does the patient feel well-informed about
the illness or painful condition?**

YES
Fully informed
or unconcerned

NO
Wishes to know results of tests,
cause or potential outcome of
present condition

Provide information and feedback
Involve patient in assessing and monitoring progress
Refer to GP for information where necessary
Put in touch with self-help groups

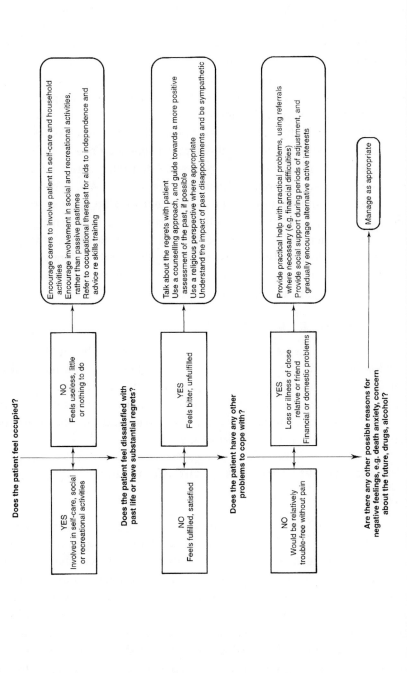

**Does the patient feel occupied?**

YES
Involved in self-care, social or recreational activities

NO
Feels useless, little or nothing to do

Encourage carers to involve patient in self-care and household activities
Encourage involvement in social and recreational activities, rather than passive pastimes
Refer to occupational therapist for aids to independence and advice re skills training

**Does the patient feel dissatisfied with past life or have substantial regrets?**

NO
Feels fulfilled, satisfied

YES
Feels bitter, unfulfilled

Talk about the regrets with patient
Use a counselling approach, and guide towards a more positive assessment of the past, if possible
Use a religious perspective where appropriate
Understand the impact of past disappointments and be sympathetic

**Does the patient have any other problems to cope with?**

NO
Would be relatively trouble-free without pain

YES
Loss or illness of close relative or friend
Financial or domestic problems

Provide practical help with practical problems, using referrals where necessary (e.g. financial difficulties)
Provide social support during periods of adjustment, and gradually encourage alternative active interests

**Are there any other possible reasons for negative feelings, e.g. death anxiety, concern about the future, drugs, alcohol?**

Manage as appropriate

*Figure 14.1* The nursing management of elderly people with persistent pain (Walker et al., 1990).

psychological distress, less likely to tolerate pain and more likely to complain to the nursing staff. What they appear to want from nurses, in addition to the careful conduct of practical procedures and practical medical advice, is empathy, understanding and encouragement, which will help them to cope with pain and the other difficulties or problems they currently face (they do not expect the nurse to solve non-medical problems for them). Unfortunately, many nurses appear not to recognize the significance and therapeutic value of these types of intervention for pain. As a result, they feel helpless when analgesia fails to work and tend to interpret persistent complaints about pain as exaggeration and attention-seeking behaviour. This ensures that elderly people with the greatest psychological needs and poorest control over pain are least likely to gain the support that they need.

The assessment plan, with some recommended interventions, formulated in the light of these research findings, is given in Fig. 14.1. A case example is given below to illustrate how the assessment may be applied. It demonstrates how the majority of interventions for the types of chronic pain most commonly experienced by elderly people are within the remit of the nurse, rather than the doctor. This assessment, together with a detailed medical history and examination, and discussion of appropriate interventions with the patient, took just over one hour.

### ■ CASE EXAMPLE: MRS FROST

Mrs Frost, aged 75, was referred to the pain clinic by her general practitioner for persistent abdominal pain. She described how she had had four major operations for cancer of the bowel over the last 15 years. After the last operation 2 years ago, to remove another growth, the consultant surgeon had found extensive internal adhesions and had told her that she would 'have to live with pain for the rest of my life'.

### ▪ The assessment (this took about 30 minutes)

#### Coping

She was very distressed and reported feeling hopeless, upset and lonely. She said that she wished that she had refused the last operation, since she would be better dead than living like this. She said that she had always been a worrier about everything, and was extremely tense and anxious. She was unable to come off the anxiolytic drug which had been prescribed following the death of her husband 14 years ago and which she had taken continuously ever since (although these drugs are now recognized to increase anxiety and depression in the long term). She had recently seen a psychiatrist for treatment of depression and had received electroconvulsive therapy, which she described as a dreadful experience and worse than useless in its effects on how she was coping. She indicated that if there was nothing we could do for her, she was considering taking her own life.

## Control over pain

She described the pain as unbearable in the mornings when she woke up. After that, it was maintained at a moderate 'nagging, miserable' level through the use of codeine compound analgesics. These gave her constipation and were becoming gradually less effective in controlling the pain. She felt that there was little else that she could do to relieve the pain.

## Information about the pain

Mrs Frost felt that she had been well informed about the cause of the pain. She had been examined at regular intervals and was assured that there was no recurrence of her cancer. She expressed less concern about this possibility than about having to live with the pain.

## Feeling occupied

Mrs Frost lived alone but had led a very active social life until recently, when the pain had become too bad to go out much with her friends. This was one of the main reasons for the referral to the pain clinic at this time. She still played bridge with her friends occasionally, but found it increasingly difficult to concentrate. She had no hobbies at home, paid someone to come in and do her housework, and was increasingly less interested in cooking for herself.

## Regrets

Mrs Frost felt that her life had been full of mixed blessings. Her own mother had died when she was very young. Her stepmother had been very kind to her and she had nursed her for several years before she died, which had been hard. She had no children, which she would have liked, but had a wonderful husband for over 30 years. He died of cancer after a long and painful illness, shortly after her first operation. She had subsequently met and lived with another wonderful man who had died very suddenly 4 years ago. Overall, she felt that she had few regrets about the past as others had been good to her and she had done her best for them.

## Other problems

The main problems faced by Mrs Frost related to her two bereavet
particular, she regularly experienced disturbing flashbacks to the
death, at home, of her last partner. She had always been depende
other people in her life, and now found herself totally alone and
She had been left financially secure and could afford to maintain

lifestyle, but was unable to cope with the emotional pain of her relatively recent losses, and current lack of comfort and support.

**Intervention plan**

As a result of the assessment, the main objectives identified with her were to improve her range of pain-controlling strategies, help her to feel motivated to engage in more active occupations, re-engage in social activities with friends, and help her to come to terms with the traumatic loss of her partner. The medical consultant recommended that she should try to cut down on her use of analgesia during the day in view of the side-effects and increasing tolerance. However, he prescribed a stronger slow-release analgesic to take at night to improve her sleep, enable her to wake up without such unbearable pain, and face the day with more optimism that she could cope. This, it was hoped, would encourage her to arrange to go out with her friends more during the daytime and entertain them to bridge, or a meal, in the evenings. She was given a relaxation tape to listen to at least twice a day to learn to reduce the abdominal muscle tension which might be exacerbating the pain. It was anticipated that this would provide an additional pain-reducing and occupational strategy.

Although she knew the reasons for the pain, the prediction that she would have to live in pain for the rest of her life may have become a self-fulfilling prophecy. She was assured that, since scar tissue tends to soften over time, there was no reason to expect that her pain problem would necessarily become worse, but could actually improve. She was therefore encouraged to take gentle exercise, such as swimming (which she had previously enjoyed), to help her to relax and move more freely. This, it was predicted, would help to ease the pain and provide an additional occupational strategy. She felt that having the opportunity to discuss her problems in the pain clinic had been most helpful. Therefore, in the letter to her general practitioner, it was recommended that she might benefit from counselling to talk through her bereavement losses, come to terms with any other problems, and provide additional emotional support in the short term. In the meantime, she was given the opportunity to telephone or return to the pain clinic, to talk to the nurse, if she felt that she was finding it difficult to cope. It was hoped that this would provide a sense of support which would help to reduce her feelings of loneliness and despair.

It was clearly not possible to address all of Mrs Frost's problems in one visit to the pain clinic. However, it was possible to explore a range of issues which were of direct relevance to her ability to cope with, and live with, pain. It was evident that the previous medical focus on the treatment of her pain had led to the increasing use of analgesia, more side-effects, poorer pain control and more desperation in the longer term. Psychiatric treatment for her depression may actually have increased her complaints about the physical symptoms of pain because of the failure to address coping with pain. The assessment described above explored factors that influenced her distress in order to identify a range of interventions which would improve her confidence in her own ability to cope, and provide support and reassurance for the future. The cost in terms of the nurse's and doctor's time is small when balanced against the alternative of unmet needs, which often leads to increasing visits to the general practitioner and referrals to other agencies.

This nursing assessment is likely to reveal a unique set of individual needs which can be addressed by a package of interventions, tailored to meet individual needs, which are negotiated with, and hence owned by, the patient. The process is empowering for elderly patients and nurses, since it encourages interpersonal interaction and fosters confidence and understanding on both sides. Recent data collected from patients attending pain clinics (Walker and Sofaer, 1995) suggest that, although younger pain patients are more concerned with the future than those who are older, the assessment and interventions identified in Fig. 14.1 are applicable to patients of all ages who have chronic pain. Personal experience of using this assessment with chronic pain patients supports its effectiveness in practice and a detailed evaluation is currently in progress.

## ■ REFERENCES

**Beisecker, A.E.** (1988) Aging and the desire for information and input in medical decisions: patient consumerism in medical encounters. *The Gerontologist* **28**, 330–335.

**Brown, G.K. & Nicassio, P.M.** (1987) Development of a questionnaire for the assessment of active and passive coping strategies in chronic pain patients. *Pain* **31**, 53–64.

**Coleman, P.G.** (1986) *Ageing and Reminiscence Processes*. John Wiley, Chichester.

**Corran, T.M., Gibson, S.J., Farrell, M.J. & Helme, R.D.** (1994) Comparison of chronic pain experience between young and elderly patients. In: Gebhart, G.F., Hammond, D.L. & Jensen, T.S. (eds) *Progress in Pain Research and Management: Proceedings of the 7th World Congress on Pain*. IASP Press, Seattle.

**Crisson, J.E. & Keefe, F.J.** (1988) The relationship of locus of control to pain coping strategies and psychological distress in chronic pain patients. *Pain* **35**, 147–154.

**Davis, G.C., Cortez, C. & Rubin, B.R.** (1990) Pain management in the older adult with rheumatoid arthritis or osteoarthritis. *Arthritis Care and Research* **3**, 127–131.

**Dexter, P.A.** (1992) Joint exercises in elderly persons with symptomatic osteoarthritis of the hip or knee. *Arthritis Care and Research* **5**, 36–41.

**Haight, B.** (1988) The therapeutic role of a structured life review process in homebound elderly subjects. *Journal of Gerontology* **43**, 40–43.

**Härkapää, K., Järvikoski, A., Mellin, G., Hurri, H. & Luomi, J.** (1991) Health locus of control beliefs and psychological distress as predictors for treatment outcomes in low-back patients: results of a 3-month follow-up of a controlled intervention study. *Pain* **46**, 35–41.

**Harkins, S.W.** (1988a) Studies in the study of pain and suffering in relation to age. *International Journal of Technology and Aging* **1**, 146–155.

**Harkins, S.W.** (1988b) Pain in the elderly. In: Dubner, R., Gebhart, G.F. & Bond, M.R. (eds) *Proceedings of the Vth World Congress on Pain*. Elsevier, Amsterdam.

**Heinemann, A.W., Colorez, A., Frank, S. & Taylor, D.** (1988) Leisure activity participation of elderly individuals with low vision. *The Gerontological Society of America* **28**, 181–184.

**Helme, R.D., Corran, T.M. & Gibson, S.J.** (1992) Pain in the elderly. *Proceedings of the Australian Association of Gerontology* **27**, 22–26.

**Herr, K.A. & Mobily, P.R.** (1993) Comparison of selected pain assessment tools for use with the elderly. *Applied Nursing Research* **6**, 39–46.

**Jacobson, B., Smith, A. & Whitehead, M.** (1991) Rev. edn *The Nation's Health: A Strategy for the 1990s*. London: King Edward's Hospital Fund for London.

**Keefe, F.J. & Williams, D.A.** (1990) A comparison of coping strategies in chronic pain patients in different age groups. *Journal of Gerontology: Psychological Sciences* **45**(5), 161–165.

**Koenig, H.G., Kvale, J.N. & Ferrel, C.** (1988) Religion and well-being in later life. *The Gerontologist* **28**, 18–28.

**Kotler-Cope, S. & Gerber, K.E.** (1993) Is age related to response to treatment for chronic pain? *Abstracts of 7th World Congress on Pain*. IASP, Seattle.

**Lichtenberg, P.A., Skehan, M.W. & Swensen, C.H.** (1984) The role of personality, recent life stress and arthritic severity in predicting pain. *Journal of Psychosomatic Research* **28**, 231–236.

**Marcer, D., Murphy, E.J.J., Pounder, D. & Rogers, P.** (1989) The pain relief clinic: how should we define success? *Journal of the Intractable Pain Society* **7**(2), 9–13.

**Marzinski, L.** (1991) The tragedy of dementia: clinically assessing pain in the confused nonverbal elderly. *Journal of Gerontological Nursing* **17**(6), 25–28.

**McCaffery, M. & Beebe, A.** (1994) *Pain: Clinical Manual for Nursing Practice*. C.V. Mosby, London.

**Melzack, R.** (1975) The McGill Pain Questionnaire: major properties and scoring methods. *Pain* **1**, 277–299.

**Miller, J.F. & Oertel, C.B.** (1992) Powerlessness in the elderly: preventing hopelessness. In: Miller, J.F. (ed.) *Coping with Chronic Illness*. F.A. Davis, Philadelphia.

**Mills, M. & Walker, J.M.** (1994) Mood, memory and dementia: a case study. *Journal of Aging Studies* **8**, 17–27.

**Mosley, T.H., McCracken, L.M., Gross, R.T., Penzien, D.B. & Plaud, J.J.** (1993) Age, pain and impairment: results from two clinical samples. *Abstracts of 7th World Congress on Pain*. IASP, Seattle.

**Oberle, K., Paul, P., Wry, J. & Grace, M.** (1990) Pain, anxiety and analgesics: a comparative study of elderly and younger surgical patients. *Canadian Journal on Aging* **9**, 13–22.

**Office of Population Censuses and Surveys** (1989) *General Household Survey, 1987.* HMSO, London.

**Pither, C.E. & Nicholas, M.K.** (1991) The identification of iatrogenic factors in the development of chronic pain syndromes: abnormal treatment behaviour? *Proceedings of the VIth World Congress on Pain.* Elsevier, Amsterdam.

**Prohaska, T.R., Keller, M.L., Leventhal, E.A. & Leventhal, H.** (1987) Impact of symptoms and aging attribution on emotions and coping. *Health Psychology* **6**, 495–514.

**Ross, M.M., Crook, J., Tunks, E. & Mousseau, J.** (1993) Pain, disability and independent living in later life. *Proceedings of International Conference on Community Health Nursing Research.* Edmonton Board of Health, Edmonton.

**Roy, R.** (1987) A psychosocial perspective on chronic pain and depression in the elderly. *Social Work in Health Care* **12**(2), 27–36.

**Roy, R.** (1992) *The Social Context of the Chronic Pain Sufferer.* University of Toronto Press, Toronto.

**Simon, J.M.** (1993) Hardiness, coping styles and quality of life among community elderly with chronic pain. *Proceedings of International Conference on Community Health Nursing Research.* Edmonton Board of Health, Edmonton.

**Waddell, G.** (1992) Biospsychosocial analysis of low back pain. *Bailliere's Clinical Rheumatology* **6**, 523–551.

**Walker, J.M.** (1989) The Management of Elderly Patients with Pain: a Community Nursing Perspective. Unpublished PhD thesis, Bournemouth University.

**Walker, J.M.** (1994) Caring for elderly people with persistent pain in the community: a qualitative perspective on the attitudes of patients and nurses. *Health and Social Care in the Community* **2**, 221–228.

**Walker, J.M. & Sofaer, B.** (1995) *Factors Affecting Psychological Well-being in Chronic Pain Patients.* Presented at Royal College of Nursing Pain Forum Annual Conference, Eastbourne, April.

**Walker, J.M., Akinsanya, J.A., Davis, B.D. & Marcer, D.M.** (1989) The nursing management of pain in the community: a theoretical framework. *Journal of Advanced Nursing* **14**, 240–247.

**Walker, J.M., Akinsanya, J.A., Davis, B.D. & Marcer, D.M.** (1990) The nursing management of elderly patients with pain in the community: study and recommendations. *Journal of Advanced Nursing* **15**, 1154–1161.

**Weinberger, M., Hiner, S.L. & Tierney, W.M.** (1986) Improving functional status in arthritis: the effect of social support. *Social Science and Medicine* **23**, 899–904.

**Williamson, G.M. & Schulz, R.** (1992) Physical illness and symptoms of depression among elderly outpatients. *Psychology and Aging* **7**, 343–351.

**Zalon, M.I.** (1993) Nurses' assessment of postoperative patients' pain. *Pain* **54**, 323–328.

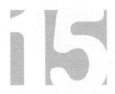

# The influence of nursing expertise on the assessment of pain: A qualitative study

## ■ INTRODUCTION

Clinical expertise is now clearly recognized as a vitally important goal in the development of advanced nursing practice. Major differences have been identified between the knowledge base of novices and experts in clinical practice (Benner, 1984; Tanner et al., 1987; Benner et al., 1992, 1996; McMurray, 1992; Logan and Boss, 1993). However, there is very little research which identifies the impact of expertise on nurses' decision-making as events unfold during patient care. This chapter considers the influence of the nurses' expertise on the assessment of pain in the semi-conscious postoperative patient. The clinical context is the intensive therapy unit (ITU) because it is well known that nurses working in this environment have undergone specialist training, which is likely to impact on their levels of expertise and confidence. Although there are other sources of pain among ITU patients, post-surgical pain is chosen as the focus because it offers a clear and unambiguous situation for evaluating nurses' assessment of pain. This event of practice offers the opportunity to study a particularly difficult area of clinical judgement in nursing. Do nurses with varying levels of expertise assess pain during nursing practice differently?

## ■ THE DEVELOPMENT OF CLINICAL EXPERTISE

Expertise is defined as 'expert skill, knowledge or judgement' (*Concise Oxford Dictionary*, 1990). Recently, several studies which have used retrospective accounts from practice have shed some light on the development of clinical expertise. Benner's (1984) research describes the existence of a five-stage continuum of clinical expertise in nursing based on the Dreyfus and Dreyfus (1980) model of skill acquisition. Her work suggests that nurses progress from novice to expert level along a continuum as they test and refine theoretical and practical knowledge in the context of clinical experiences. Thus she describes expertise in nursing as a synthesis of theoretical and experiential knowledge refined through clinical situations (Benner, 1984). Follow-up studies aimed at explicating this five-stage model found nurses learnt from experiences that provided qualitative differences to their judgement and perception, and thus advanced their practice. The nurses' emotional responses to the experiences and a changing capacity to deal with similar clinical situations more effectively were central to their findings of expertise (Benner et al., 1992, 1996).

A further study of novice and community nurses found a number of factors which figured in the development of clinical expertise. Educational factors, personal factors and experience were the major influences found in the nurses' movement toward expert practice (McMurray, 1992). Logan and Boss (1993) explored the learning patterns of developing nurses in practice. Their findings suggested that nurses needed to acquire technical skills through the synthesis of theoretical and practical knowledge before the mastering of more complex relationship skills could occur.

These studies are helpful to the understanding of the potential differences between nurses of varying levels of expertise and the impact these differences may have on their practice. It is clear the detection of expertise is complex for, while the results of actions are relatively easy to observe, the advanced level of knowledge behind the activity is more difficult to evaluate. Vital to the identification of expertise is the belief that it is possible for practitioners to describe the knowledge that guides their practice (Schon, 1987). There remains much to be learnt of the process of refinement of knowledge through which nurses develop expert judgement in practice.

Pain assessment offers an important area of practice through which the impact of nursing expertise can be considered. Effective clinical assessment of pain is an important requirement of professional nursing practice and this is crucial in the care of the patient returning from major surgery. It is useful at this point to consider findings from a number of studies which provide illumination on nurses' assessment of patients' pain in practice. Chapter 10 has already provided an overview of factors influencing the management of postoperative pain, so the intention here is to select evidence which is particularly useful in setting the scene for the qualitative study which is to follow.

## ■ RESEARCH INTO NURSES' ASSESSMENT OF POSTOPERATIVE PAIN

In reviewing the literature on postoperative pain management, Carr (Chapter 10) found extensive research available to inform nursing practice (see also Kitson, 1994). Literature which focuses upon assessment of pain in semi-conscious patients is particularly helpful. The responses of patients to pain alters under the effect of drugs administered during and following surgery. Thus patients who are still under the paralysing and/or sedating effects of anaesthetic drugs are unable to speak or indicate pain through facial expressions and body movements (McCaffery, 1972). Practical and theoretical knowledge of the physiological responses to pain is considered essential in the care of the acutely dependent semi-conscious patient (Bourbonnais, 1981). Therefore nurses need to be able to recognize physiological changes to pain which include the autonomic nervous system response causing variations in pulse and blood pressure (McCaffery, 1972).

As already shown in Chapter 10, several studies found that nurses are poor assessors of pain and are also unaware of the physiological signs of pain in their patients (Graffam, 1970, 1979, 1981; Jones, 1988). Nurses have also been consistently found to underestimate the intensity of patients' pain (Oberst, 1978; Seers, 1987). Importantly, a number of studies have found that nurses tend to seek non-verbal cues, as well as, or instead of verbal cues of pain (Oberst, 1978; Jacox, 1979; McCaffery, 1983; Saxey, 1986). Clearly, it is vital that nurses do not rely totally upon verbal indicators to identify pain. Seers (1988) summarized several studies which examined the relationship between nurses' characteristics and patients' experience, and the treatment of pain. Nurses' fear of inducing narcotic addiction was found to be a strong influence on the management of patients' pain (Cohen, 1980; White, 1985; Seers, 1987).

Recommendations for education programmes tailored to increase nurses' knowledge of pain assessment and management have long been muted from earlier work (Degner et al., 1982; Sofaer, 1983), especially with regard to improving pharmacological knowledge (Weiss et al., 1983; Hosking, 1985; White, 1985; Saxey, 1986; Royal College of Surgeons, 1990). Interestingly, several studies have found that selected nurse characteristics, such as years in practice and education level, have not been significant in the nurses' inferences of pain in their patients (Oberst, 1978; Dudley and Holm, 1984).

An interesting study explored the decision-making of hospice nurses on pain-control regimens for patients in simulated and retrospective accounts of incidents from their own practice. The researcher found there were significant differences in the nurses' decision-making between simulation and real practice. She warned that findings from simulation may lack validity and recommended that studies which explored facets of nurses' decision-making be conducted in actual practice (Padrick, 1990). More recently, a study sought to examine the practical knowledge of expert intensive care nurses in the management of acute postoperative pain. The researchers found that these nurses recognize an expected pattern of pain for a given surgery, postoperative day and patients' unique response to pain. If the patient's pain was atypical, the nurses sought further data and changed their interventions. Thus expert nurses were found to change their assessment approach according to their judgement of the situation (Guyton-Simmons and Ehrmin, 1994). A further phenomenological study which explored the practice of expert critical-care nurses found that providing comfort through the relief of pain and anxiety were major themes. This research suggests that these nurses are actively searching for signs of pain in their assessment of patients (Walters, 1994).

The findings of these studies suggest that an advanced level of practical and theoretical knowledge is required to identify accurately the significant physiological changes which establish the presence and intensity of pain in a semi-conscious patient. The nurse is faced with a number of alternative causes of physiological changes in a patient following major surgery. Inexperienced nurses may have difficulty in identifying the presence of pain in the semi-conscious postoperative patient. However, there are very few studies of how nurses with varying levels of skills and expertise identify pain in complex clinical situations. Recently, research methods have advanced to offer ways to uncover the hidden knowledge which governs the judgement within nurses' skilful practice. It is now possible to consider the knowledge which governs the nurses' assessment of postoperative pain during patient care.

## ■ THE STUDY

A qualitative study offered the opportunity to consider the influence of nursing expertise on pain assessment in practice. The aim of the study was to identify indicators of clinical expertise amongst nurses working within surgical and intensive care (ITU) units. The focus of the research rested upon the assessment of patients returning from major surgery as a familiar and frequent event in the nurses' practice. Thirty-one qualified nurses working within two cardiothoracic and general surgical ITUs participated in the study. Nurses were sought with a wide range in years of experience and post-basic qualifications, and potentially different levels of clinical expertise. The emic perspective, which focuses upon the views of the participating nurses, was central to the research. The holistic perspective was also taken, in which the context of the phenomena was recognized as a vital component within the study (Morse, 1992).

The nurses were involved in the assessment of semi-conscious patients following major cardiac, lung or abdominal surgery. These events were observed by the researcher as they occurred within the context of the intensive care environment (Field and Morse, 1985). Field notes were taken during observation of the nurse/patient interaction. Reflective interviews followed immediately after these episodes of patient care. The interactive and semi-structured interviews provided verbal accounts of the knowledge and thought processes that guided the nurses' steps of assessment in practice. The focus upon actual everyday episodes of practice provided the base for further discussion of the developmental influences on the nurses' clinical expertise.

An inductive and interactive process of research inquiry supported continuation of analysis of the data as understanding and insight was gained about the phenomena under study (Morse, 1992). A computerized data filing system was used to handle and retrieve the data (Morse, 1991). Inductive data analysis followed the process of unitizing, categorizing and searching for patterns (Lincoln and Guba, 1985). The emerging patterns indicated qualitative differences in the nurses' abilities to assess patients depending on their levels of expertise. These findings revealed valuable insights into the development of skilled assessment of pain in the semi-conscious post-operative patient by ITU nurses.

## ■ FINDINGS

Four major indicators of expertise were identified from the nurses' practice within the study. These dynamic and fluid continuums indicated varying levels of clinical expertise in practice. The indicators had four identifiable levels of skill from the lowest to highest level of practice. The nurses were found at four levels: beginner, competent, proficient and expert across each of the qualitative indicators of expertise. The four indicators ranged from: dependency to autonomous practice; student learner to teacher; task focus to holistic patient assessment; and rigid guidelines to flexible patient care. The differences in the nurses' understanding of the complex issues of pain assessment in the postoperative patient were demonstrated through the indicators of expertise.

# ■ THE BEGINNER NURSES

## ▮ Dependent practitioner

These nurses did not complete a full assessment of the patients on return from theatre. Instead, they followed postoperative charts/care plans, which provided nursing guidelines and the direction of medical staff to plan patient care. The pain management followed the written orders of the doctors in attendance of the patient. The nurses sought the guidance of more experienced staff to complete technical tasks of care successfully. They depended upon senior nurses to assess and make clinical judgements of the patient's condition in practice.

## ▮ Student learner

The inexperienced nurses' knowledge of pain management focused upon the conscious patient following surgery. They were unaware of the possibility of pain in the paralysed and semi-conscious postoperative patient. The nurses were dependent upon more experienced health professionals to teach them how to interpret the salient clinical signs of patients during the initial postoperative period. They also learnt through trial and error experience of caring for patients during similar postoperative situations. Continuing professional education was a powerful influence on the development of the beginners' theoretical knowledge of the assessment of pain.

The impact of increased theoretical knowledge through post-basic pain-management courses was noticeable in the case of one inexperienced ITU nurse. She expressed a heightened awareness of the potential of pain in the paralysed or semi-conscious patient, but lacked sufficient confidence to question set guidelines for pain management.

## ▮ Task-focused patient care

Nurses identified as beginners within the ITU environment were focused on the fulfilment of the technical tasks that provided monitoring and maintenance of the treatments ordered for the patients' care. Observation of the physical systems was discussed but no mention of assessment of pain in the patient was made by these nurses.

## ∎ Rigid guidelines for care

The nurses described following the plan of care as taught by more experienced members of the staff. The tasks were completed with care and attention, and the monitored vital signs of the patients reported to the doctors and/or more senior nurses. The nurses described experiencing intuitive 'gut' feelings of anxiety or confidence regarding the overall condition of the patients. However, they were unable to identify the reasons for their feelings through assessment of the patients. They discussed these feelings with trusted and more experienced staff in their field of practice.

Movement toward the competent level of clinical expertise was found in several nurses' accounts of practice. The nurses moved from a rigid focus on the completion of written directions and technical tasks to a more flexible approach to the assessment of patients' pain and comfort. They described a changing awareness of the patient through previous experiences, the feelings evoked by those experiences and theoretical knowledge of the likely postoperative progression. The impact of increasing knowledge on the nurses' assessment and judgement of pain in the semi-conscious patient was noted by a nurse in the following way:

> 'I remember a patient who came down really awake, with an ET tube in and really distressed, uncomfortable, in pain. I found that was quite a distressing situation for her and for me. When episodes like that happen, you become more aware. And should that happen to me again I would be quite firm – "what do you want to do. Do you want to sedate her or do you want her to wake up." Instances like that do colour your judgement.'

## ∎ Discussion

Beginner nurses did not complete assessments of the postoperative patient. They perceived the need for a triad of support structures to develop these skills within the clinical environment. These nurses required exposure to adequate theoretical knowledge through continuing education to inform their practice. They needed to participate in steadily increasing complex patient situations under the guidance of skilled practitioners to explain the subtle nuances of care. Beginner nurses also needed to acquire analysis skills with which to reflect upon the patient situations. The nurses' analysis of feelings and actions during past unusual and ordinary encounters in care informed their judgements in practice. It was noticeable that reflection on past episodes highlighted knowledge development and progression from the beginner to competent level of expertise. Interestingly, the impact of intuitive feelings on the thinking of beginner nurses has not figured prominently in previous studies of expertise (Benner, 1984; Benner et al., 1992).

# ■ THE COMPETENT NURSES

## ▮ The less dependent practitioner

The competent nurses were more confident in their ability, and less dependent on the direction of others in the assessment and management of patients' pain. The nurses had increased knowledge of physiology, pharmacology and practical skills of caring for postoperative patients. Their knowledge led to a greater awareness and assessment for signs suggestive of the presence of pain. One nurse demonstrated her growing confidence in the following:

> 'I was aware that he had just been paralysed, he hadn't been sedated. I was concerned that he was tachycardic and hypotensive which could have implied that he needed volume. But I was also worried that he was tachycardic because he might have been awake and in pain underneath his paralysis. So it was quite a priority for me to give him some Omnopon just to put that possibility out of my mind.'

Thus these nurses were less dependent on others through increasing ability to link observed physiological signs with judgement of the possibility of pain in the patient.

## ▮ Learner and emerging teacher

The competent nurses described a changing role from learner to emerging teacher, owing to increasing confidence in their skills, knowledge and expertise. The nurses had developed basic theoretical knowledge from continuing education programmes and/or ongoing self-directed learning which informed their ITU practice. However, the nurses continued to seek further information and direction from senior nurses. They sought knowledge of recent changes to practice based on research findings from skilled staff in the field. At the same time the nurses were required to teach less experienced nurses basic guidelines of patient care, which incorporated protocols of pain management. Motivated nurses sought to deepen their theoretical and experiential knowledge by utilizing all opportunities available through continuing education pathways and practice.

## ▮ Shifting from task to consideration of the patient signs

The focus of the competent nurses had shifted slightly from successful completion of the technical tasks to greater consideration of the patient. The nurses had become confident in the technical skills required to complete the tasks involved in practice. They were then able to focus upon their clinical observations and consider the potential of pain as the underlying cause of physiological changes in the patients. The linking of theoretical and practical knowledge was found in a nurse's comment:

> 'It [pain assessment] always comes into play. Like every time I milked his drains today I was wanting to know what his heart rate did. So whether he was awake and whether he was breathing up on the ventilator. I'm assessing for pain the whole time.'

### ▮ Less rigid following of guidelines to patient care

These nurses described a more flexible approach to their care of the patient. The guidelines were still followed but the nurses' practice now incorporated knowledge gleaned from continuing education, their own and others' practice. The nurses also described experiencing intuitive feelings about their patients' condition. They responded to these feelings by monitoring the patients more closely and discussing their concerns with more experienced colleagues. The nurses grew more confident in their 'gut' feelings through reflection on previous experiences in which feelings had preceded deterioration in a patient's condition.

### ▮ Discussion

There was a noticeable increase in the competent nurses' theoretical and experiential knowledge of physiology and pharmacology, the type of surgery and postoperative care. The nurses reported the importance of these fields of knowledge to inform their assessment and judgement of pain in practice. Motivated nurses pursued knowledge from post-basic programmes, reading, study days, other health professionals and from their own experiences in practice. Experiential knowledge was not gained by passive participation in a series of clinical situations over a period of time. Instead the nurses developed experiential knowledge from reflective analysis of situations. The newly learned was synthesized with theoretical knowledge to confirm or discard the underpinnings of previous practice.

## ▪ THE PROFICIENT/EXPERT NURSES

### ▮ Autonomous practitioner

The experienced practitioners followed an increasingly autonomous approach to patient assessment in practice. They drew upon in-depth theoretical and experiential knowledge to guide their assessment and judgement of the presence of pain. These nurses held collaborative relationships with medical and other health professionals, which supported swift responses to the assessed needs of the patients. An example of this form of collaboration is found in the words of a skilled nurse caring for an elderly woman following major cardiac surgery:

*'. . . this particular lady . . . has quite severe osteoarthritis. . . . I asked the doctor . . . what about some Voltarol? I try to follow a plan for her because, after this type of operation, they do have a great deal of pain and when you are trying them off the ventilator you don't want them too sedated. But at the same time you want to try and give them pain relief so they are as pain free as they possibly can be without depressing their respirations or causing hypotension . . . Voltarol I have observed to be extremely good for these people . . . I find they do better, they recover much quicker.'*

## ∎ Teacher

These nurses were constantly responding to requests for advice from less experienced nurses during their practice. They would guide others through complex technical tasks, and teach by demonstration and explanation as they assessed the needs of the patients. The nurses identified many influences on the knowledge that guided their practice. Theoretical knowledge obtained through post-basic courses and updating of relevant changes in their field was pursued by these motivated nurses. Their understanding of current drug therapy, knowledge of surgical procedures and experiential knowledge of caring for patients undergoing similar surgery guided their understanding of postoperative pain.

## ∎ Holistic patient care

The proficient and expert nurses' description of their assessment of the patients were extremely detailed in comparison with nurses at the beginner and competent levels of expertise. They included detailed rationales within the descriptions of the assessment, which gave evidence of in-depth theoretical knowledge of biophysical sciences, especially anatomy, physiology and pharmacology. The nurses' descriptions of assessment for pain were interwoven within the general assessment of the patient. Pain was seen as the greatest priority next to maintenance of life and was assessed continuously during the care of the patients. Accurate assessment and management of pain was described by the nurses as essential for speedy recovery. The importance of freedom from pain to aid respiratory function and patient comfort was seen as vital during recovery from surgery.

These nurses described an awareness of the semi-conscious patient's ability to hear, feel pain and experience feelings of anxiety following major surgery. The expert nurses' ability to identify the presence of pain in the semi-conscious patient was unparalleled. They also demonstrated the ability to interpret early physiological changes and manage care to reduce the likelihood of pain in the most complex patient situations. A skilled nurse described her judgement of a patient's pain thus:

*'Although he appeared to be unconscious ... his blood pressure was rather reactive and I wondered if he was waking up from the anaesthetic but still had a paralysing agent on board. I couldn't visibly tell whether he was conscious or not ... And to cover the fact that the patient might be awake I put the morphine on so he's not in distress under paralysis there.'*

## ▪ Flexible patient care

These nurses were systematic in their assessment but also very flexible, altering their approach to fit the individual patient's situation. The assessment of pain was interwoven throughout the overall description of the assessment in a way not found in the less experienced nurses. Awareness of the potential of pain was evident from the nurses' first moment of contact with the patients. They clearly recognized the possibility that semi-conscious patients may experience pain immediately following surgery. The nurses' assessment of the patient was ongoing and totally flexible, constantly watching for signs indicative of the presence of pain. They considered the clinical signs and the alternative possible causes of changing physiological responses in the postoperative patient. The nurses were very specific in describing the changing physical and psychological cues in the semi-conscious patients and their responses to them. The comprehensiveness of the overall description of pain was the most detailed in this group of all the levels of expertise. An example of one experienced nurse's thoughts on the simultaneous aims of correct technical management and keeping the patient as free as possible from pain follows:

*'I worked in one place which milked the drains all the way down to the bottom and said that clamping them would cause an infection risk. Here they say if you pull them all the way down you are causing a lot of excess pain by pulling on the diaphragm ... Now the research says that perhaps we shouldn't milk them at all. That's the one thing that I've always found that patients remember ... if you milk and clamp or milk down the patient will wake up on that ... so I think when you're milking the drains warn them "I'm just going to pull on these tubes" ... I try to keep them pain free and comfortable before you do these things.'*

The nurses also described their use of intuitive feelings in the identification of the potential needs of the patients. The nurses' 'gut' feelings were perceived to be based on knowledge and past experiences, which had altered their understanding of the potential problems a patient may experience in a clinical situation. The nurses had confidence in their intuitive knowledge and used the feelings as early warning signals of potential problems in the patient. The nurses acted upon these feelings to find the subtle physical or psychological changes in the patients that heralded possible deterioration in their condition.

In-depth theoretical and experiential knowledge provided nurses with strong rationales for early involvement in the patients' care. A nurse noted the importance of reducing pre-operative anxiety, understanding of peri-operative care, early postoperative assessment and collaboration with the health team to manage patients' pain effectively thus:

> 'I think you should go around [to the ward] as the nurse . . . and [the patient] needs to look around ITU so it's an area that they have been before and familiarize themselves with us and talk about what they are scared about . . . Go into the theatre and then you can see why they are in so much pain . . . Then in the early stage after theatre just go around and say "Hi, I'm looking after you". I like to make sure they are pain controlled because the anaes-thetist is there . . . This patient looked comfortable straight away. I looked at the patient's colour, for facial changes and the way he was in the bed . . . I knew he had a high thoracic epidural so I was quite happy that he would come back in this state of complete analgesia . . . I would say pain is on the same level as the A, B, C, with all the readings of the technology.'

## ▪ Discussion

The proficient and expert nurses completed detailed and comprehensive assessments of their patients. Pain was a central focus within these assess-ments and early physiological changes were noted and considered for likely causes. These nurses used in-depth biophysical knowledge and extensive experiential knowledge from the field to interpret the physiological signs and make clinical judgements of the semi-conscious patients' level of pain. These findings support previous evidence of the importance expert ITU nurses place on relieving pain (Walters, 1994). The nurses maintained their current up-to-date knowledge through self-directed continuing professional education and regular involvement in practice. They were highly motivated to access the most recent research-driven changes in their field of ITU practice.

The synthesized theoretical and experiential knowledge gained from reflection on the outcomes of past patient-care episodes was clearly evident within the nurses' assessments of patients' pain. This finding supports the belief that expert nurses are reflective practitioners who utilize theory and past experience to guide skilled practice (Benner, 1993; Guyton-Simmons and Ehrmin, 1994). Intuitive feelings about the patients' condition were felt by many of the nurses within the proficient and expert levels of expertise. The skilled and confident nurses used their feelings as early warning signals to assess the patients for signs of deterioration or improvement. The intuitive knowledge of expert nurses has been well documented (Benner, 1984). Schon (1983) also describes intuitive knowing in action as a major component of expert decision-making.

## ■ CONCLUSION

The findings of this qualitative study are specific to a small group of ITU nurses and, as such, are not generalizable. However, these nurses were identified at varying levels of ability to assess and make judgements of pain in the semi-conscious patients. Experiential and theoretical knowledge plays an important role in the nurses' capacity to identify the likelihood of experiencing pain within the context of their situation. Knowledge gained from post-basic courses, self-directed reading, study days and ward lectures informs nurses' assessment and judgement of the patients' condition. Nurses who are motivated to learn and committed to effective care reflect on their experiences to improve their decisions in future practice.

The variations found in the nurses' ability to assess pain are important. They illuminate our understanding of the role of development of expertise in every aspect of practice (Benner, 1984; Bryckzynski, 1989; Etheredge, 1989; Benner et al., 1992, 1996; McMurray, 1992; Logan and Boss, 1993; Guyton-Simmons and Ehrmin, 1994; Walters, 1994). There is increasing support from these studies to suggest that the development of skilful nursing practice has much to do with effective synthesis of theoretical and experiential knowledge. Nurses need assistance to develop assessment and decision-making skills for practice. They need to understand how to assess, what to assess and how to interpret the clinical signs for effective pain management within the context of the real-life situations. Clearly these skills accompany the growth of knowledge within clinical practice.

The support of skilled practitioners, educational opportunities and effective reflection on experiences were major influences on these nurses' development of expertise in the assessment and management of pain. These findings may have important implications for the content and teaching methods of continuing education programmes. Specialized post-basic courses should provide up-to-date physiological and pharmacological knowledge to inform nurses' clinical practice. These programmes must also be prepared to change and adapt their strategies of teaching to reflect the learning styles and flexible decision-making pathways found in nurses' clinical practice.

## ■ REFERENCES

**Benner, P.** (1984) *From Novice to Expert: Excellence and Power in Clinical Nursing Practice.* Addison-Wesley, Menlo Park, CA.

**Benner, P.** (1993) Transforming RN education: clinical learning and clinical knowledge development. In: Diekelmann, N.L. & Rather, M.L. (eds) *Transforming RN Education.* National League for Nursing Press, New York.

**Benner, P., Tanner, C. & Chesla, C.** (1992) From beginner to expert: gaining a differentiated clinical world in critical nursing. *Advances in Nursing Science* **14**, 13–28.

**Benner, P., Tanner, C. & Chesla, C.** (1996) *Expertise in Nursing Practice, Caring, Clinical Judgement and Ethics.* Springer, New York.

**Bourbonnais, F.** (1981) Pain assessment: development of a tool for the nurse and the patient. *Journal of Advanced Nursing* **6**, 277–282.

**Bryckzynski, K.** (1989) An interpretive study describing the clinical judgement of nurse practitioners. *Scholarly Inquiry for Nursing Practice* **3**, 75–104.

**Cohen, F.L.** (1980) Post-surgical pain relief: patients' status and nurses' medication choices. *Pain* **9**, 265–274.

*Concise Oxford Dictionary of Current English* (1990) Allen, R.E. (ed.) 8th edn. Clarendon Press, Oxford.

**Degner, L.F., Fujii, S. & Levitt, M.** (1982) Implementing a programme to control chronic pain of malignant disease for patients in an extended care facility. *Cancer Nursing* **5**, 263–268.

**Dreyfus, S. & Dreyfus, H.** (1980) *A Five Stage Model of the Mental Activities Involved in Directed Skill Acquisition.* Unpublished report, Air Force Office of Scientific Research (AFSC), University of California, Berkeley.

**Dudley, S.R. & Holm, K.** (1984) Assessment of the pain. Experience in relation to selected nurses' characteristics. *Pain* **18**, 179–186.

**Etheredge, C.** (1989) An Analysis of Expert Critical Care Nurses' Clinical Decision Making. Ed. D. thesis, University of San Francisco.

**Field, P.A. & Morse, J.M.** (1985) *Nursing Research: The Application of Qualitative Approaches.* Chapman and Hall, London.

**Graffam, S.R.** (1970) Nurse response to the patient in distress – development of an instrument. *Nursing Research* **19**, 331–335.

**Graffam, S.R.** (1979) Nurse response to patients in pain; an analysis and an imperative for action. *Nurse Leadership* **2**, 23–25.

**Graffam, S.R.** (1981) Congruence of nurse–patient expectations regarding nursing in pain. *Nursing Leadership* **4**, 12–15.

**Guyton-Simmons, J. & Ehrmin, J.T.** (1994) Problem solving in pain management by expert intensive care nurses. *Critical Care Nurse* October, 37–44.

**Hosking, J.** (1985) Pain relief; knowledge and practice. *Nursing Mirror* **160**(5), Research Suppl. ii–vi.

**Jacox, A.K.** (1979) Assessing pain. *American Journal of Nursing* **79**, 895–900.

**Jones, C.** (1988) Pain assessment. *Surgical Nurse* **1**(16), 5–8.

**Kitson, A.** (1994) Post-operative pain management: a literature review. *Journal of Clinical Nursing* **3**, 7–18.

**Lincoln, Y.S. & Guba E.G.** (1985) *Naturalistic Inquiry.* Sage Publications, Beverley Hills, CA.

**Logan, J. & Boss, M.** (1993) Nurses' learning patterns. *The Canadian Nurse* 18–22.

**McCaffery, M.** (1972) *Nursing Management of the Patient with Pain.* J.B. Lippincott, Toronto.

**McCaffery, M.** (1983) *Nursing Management of the Patient with Pain.* J.B. Lippincott, Philadelphia.

**McMurray, A.** (1992) Expertise in community health nursing. *Journal of Community Health Nursing* **9** (2), 65–75.

**Morse, J.M.** (1991) Pearls, pith and provocation: analyzing unstructured, interactive interviews using the Macintosh computer. *Qualitative Health Research* **1**, 117–122.

**Morse, J.M.** (1992) *Qualitative Nursing Research: A Contemporary Dialogue.* Sage Publications, Newbury Park, CA.

**Oberst, M.T.** (1978) Nurses' inferences of suffering: the effects of nurse–patient similarity and verbalisations of distress. In: Nelson, M.J. (ed.) *Clinical Perspectives in Nursing Research.* Teachers College Press, New York, pp. 38–60.

**Padrick, K.** (1990) Clinical Decision-making in Nursing: A Comparison of Simulations and Practice Situations. Unpublished PhD thesis, Oregon Health Sciences University.

**Royal College of Surgeons of England and The College of Anaesthetists** (1990) *Commission on the Provision of Surgical Services, Report of the Working Party on Pain after Surgery.* Royal College of Surgeons, London.

**Saxey, S.** (1986) The nurse's response to post-operative pain. *Nursing* **3**(10), 377–381.

**Schon, D.** (1983) *The Reflective Practitioner.* Basic Books, New York.

**Schon, D.** (1987) *Educating the Reflective Practitioner.* Jossey-Bass, San Francisco.

**Seers, K.** (1987) Perceptions of pain. *Nursing Times* **83**(48), 37–39.

**Seers, K.** (1988) Factors affecting pain assessment. *Professional Nurses* **3**(6), 201–206.

**Sofaer, B.** (1983) Pain relief: the core of nursing practice. *Nursing Times* **79**(47), 35.

**Tanner, C., Padrick, K., Westfall, U. & Putzier, D.** (1987) Diagnostic reasoning strategies of nurses and nursing students. *Nursing Research* **36**(6), 358–363.

**Walters, A.J.** (1994) An interpretive study of the clinical practice, of critical care nurses. *Contemporary Nurse* **3**(1), 21–25.

**Weiss, O.F., Sriwatanakul, K., Alloza, J.L., Weintraub, M. & Lasagna, L.** (1983) Attitudes of patients, housestaff and nurses toward post-operative analgesic care. *Anaesthesia and Analgesia* **62**, 70–74.

**White, R.** (1985) Policy implications and constraints in the role of the nurse in the management of pain. In: Copp, L.A. (ed.) *Perspectives on Pain.* Churchill Livingstone, Edinburgh.

# Index

Note: pages with illustrations are in **bold** type.